Medical Imaging: Applications of Deep Learning

Medical Imaging: Applications of Deep Learning

Editor: Hubert Henson

FOSTER
ACADEMICS
www.fosteracademics.com

www.fosteracademics.com

FOSTER ACADEMICS

Cataloging-in-Publication Data

Medical imaging : applications of deep learning / edited by Hubert Henson.
p. cm.
Includes bibliographical references and index.
ISBN 978-1-64646-564-4
1. Diagnostic imaging. 2. Imaging systems in medicine. 3. Radiography, Medical.
4. Diagnosis, Radioscopic. I. Henson, Hubert.
RC78.7.D53 H36 2023
616.075 4--dc23

Foster Academics,
118-35 Queens Blvd., Suite 400,
Forest Hills, NY 11375, USA

ISBN 978-1-64646-564-4 (Hardback)

Contents

Preface

I am honored to present to you this unique book which encompasses the most up-to-date data in the field. I was extremely pleased to get this opportunity of editing the work of experts from across the globe. I have also written papers in this field and researched the various aspects revolving around the progress of the discipline. I have tried to unify my knowledge along with that of stalwarts from every corner of the world, to produce a text which not only benefits the readers but also facilitates the growth of the field.

Medical imaging refers to several different technologies that are used to view inside the human body in order to diagnose, monitor or treat medical conditions. Endoscopy, tactile imaging and computerized tomography (CT) scan are some common types of medical imaging procedures. In recent years, deep learning or deep structured imaging has found applications in the field of medical image analysis. Machine learning is a subfield of artificial intelligence (AI) and is used for various purposes such as computer-aided detection/diagnosis, disease prediction, image segmentation, image generation, etc. AI tools are used to accelerate productivity and potentially improve accuracy in the process of medical imaging. This book contains some path-breaking studies in the field of deep learning and medical imaging. The various studies that are constantly contributing towards advancing technologies and evolution of this field are examined in detail. It will serve as a valuable source of reference for medical students, radiologists, and industry researchers engaged in medical imaging research.

Finally, I would like to thank all the contributing authors for their valuable time and contributions. This book would not have been possible without their efforts. I would also like to thank my friends and family for their constant support.

Editor

Neuroimaging Markers for Studying Gulf-War Illness: Single-Subject Level Analytical Method based on Machine Learning

Yi Guan [1,†], Chia-Hsin Cheng [1,†], Weifan Chen [1], Yingqi Zhang [1], Sophia Koo [1], Maxine Krengel [1], Patricia Janulewicz [2], Rosemary Toomey [1], Ehwa Yang [3], Rafeeque Bhadelia [4], Lea Steele [5], Jae-Hun Kim [3], Kimberly Sullivan [2,*] and Bang-Bon Koo [1,*]

1 School of Medicine, Boston University, Boston, MA 02118, USA; guanyi1@bu.edu (Y.G.); chiahsin@bu.edu (C.-H.C.); wfchen@bu.edu (W.C.); yqz2019@bu.edu (Y.Z.); sskoo@bu.edu (S.K.); mhk@bu.edu (M.K.); toomey@bu.edu (R.T.)

2 School of Public Health, Boston University, Boston, MA 02118, USA; paj@bu.edu

3 Department of Radiology, Samsung Medical Center, Sungkyunkwan University School of Medicine, Seoul 06351, Korea; ehwayang@gmail.com (E.Y.); jaehun1115.kim@samsung.com (J.-H.K.)

4 Department of Radiology, Beth Israel Deaconess Medical Center, Harvard Medical School, Boston, MA 02115, USA; rbhadelia@gmail.com

5 Neuropsychiatry Division, Department of Psychiatry and Behavioral Sciences, Baylor College of Medicine, Houston, TX 77030, USA; Lea.Steele@bcm.edu

* Correspondence: tty@bu.edu (K.S.); bbkoo@bu.edu (B.-B.K.)

† Both authors contributed equally to this work.

Abstract: Gulf War illness (GWI) refers to the multitude of chronic health symptoms, spanning from fatigue, musculoskeletal pain, and neurological complaints to respiratory, gastrointestinal, and dermatologic symptoms experienced by about 250,000 GW veterans who served in the 1991 Gulf War (GW). Longitudinal studies showed that the severity of these symptoms often remain unchanged even years after the GW, and these veterans with GWI continue to have poorer general health and increased chronic medical conditions than their non-deployed counterparts. For better management and treatment of this condition, there is an urgent need for developing objective biomarkers that can help with simple and accurate diagnosis of GWI. In this study, we applied multiple neuroimaging techniques, including T1-weighted magnetic resonance imaging (T1W-MRI), diffusion tensor imaging (DTI), and novel neurite density imaging (NDI) to perform both a group-level statistical comparison and a single-subject level machine learning (ML) analysis to identify diagnostic imaging features of GWI. Our results supported NDI as the most sensitive in defining GWI characteristics. In particular, our classifier trained with white matter NDI features achieved an accuracy of 90% and F-score of 0.941 for classifying GWI cases from controls after the cross-validation. These results are consistent with our previous study which suggests that NDI measures are sensitive to the microstructural and macrostructural changes in the brain of veterans with GWI, which can be valuable for designing better diagnosis method and treatment efficacy studies.

Keywords: Gulf War illness; MRI; objective biomarker; machine learning; Kansas case criteria; diffusion; grey matter; neurite density imaging

---

1. Introduction

Gulf War illness (GWI) refers to the variety of chronic symptoms experienced by about 250,000 United States veterans who served in the 1991 Gulf War (GW) [1]. According to the Kansas case criteria, symptoms of GWI fall into six categories: fatigue (fatigue and sleep problems), pain (joint and muscle), neurological (cognitive, mood, headache, and dizziness), respiratory (persistent cough and wheezing), gastrointestinal (diarrhea and nausea), and skin (rashes and other) problems. Exposure to neurotoxicant chemicals (organophosphate pesticides and sarin) during the war and other central nervous system (CNS) damage, such as mild traumatic brain injury (mTBI), are thought to have caused an innate immune over-response in the CNS, resulting in the development of these chronic GWI symptoms [2–7]). In order to meet the Kansas criteria for GWI, veterans must display chronic symptoms in at least three of the six categories, without presenting concurrent psychiatric and medical disorders [8]. However, accurate diagnoses of GWI remained challenging due to the heterogeneous clinical presentation of this condition, as well as the level of subjectivity associated with self-reported symptoms and neurotoxicant exposure history [8–10]. To improve management and treatment of GWI, there is an urgent need for defining sensitive and objective biomarkers of the disorder.

Previous neuroimaging studies demonstrated distinct changes within brains of veterans with GWI, which may underlie physiological symptoms. For example, T1W-MRI studies showed that GW veterans with exposure to the neurotoxicant chemical sarin exhibit reduced gray matter (GM) and white matter (WM) volumes, as well as reductions in hippocampal subfield volumes when compared to non-exposed veterans [11,12]. More recent studies using diffusion tensor imaging (DTI) have shown greater hippocampal mean diffusivity (MD) and increased axial diffusivity (AD) in the WM of sarin and cyclosarin exposed GW veterans, which are correlated to fatigue, pain, or hyperalgesia, and may serve as a potential biomarker for GWI [13–15]. We have previously applied a novel MRI diffusion processing method, neurite density imaging (NDI), on high-order diffusion MRI to demonstrate that the NDI measure scan successfully identify and validate different levels of neurological abnormalities in veterans with GWI from the Boston Gulf War Illness Consortium cohort [16].

ML algorithms have been applied to study a wide range of neurological disorders, including Alzheimer's disease, Parkinson's disease, and traumatic brain injury [17,18]. These studies have reported promising results for identifying diagnostic biomarkers [19,20]. The ML approach have strengths on exploiting features from different domains (i.e., neuropsychological, genetic and neuroimaging) and providing further insights on the potential interactions between different markers for classifying illness [21]. For the current study, we aimed to expand our previous work (on NDI) to cross-compare different types of neuroimaging markers (T1W-MRI, DTI and NDI) to determine whether these measures are useful for single subject-level classification of GWI cases vs. controls. Specifically, we incorporated the machine learning (ML) framework to search out key imaging features valuable for defining GWI. Computerized models were then trained based on the selected features and tested for classifying veterans with GWI.

2. Methods

2.1. Participants

In this study, we included brain imaging data of 119 GW veterans from Boston University Gulf War Illness Consortium (GWIC) (Table 1). GWIC is a multi-site study designed to identify the etiology and potential biomarkers of GWI. The inclusion criterion was deployment to the GW between August 1990 and July 1991. The exclusion criteria included having a diagnosis of chronic medical illnesses that could otherwise account for the symptoms experienced by GW veterans, including autoimmune, CNS, or major psychiatric disorders that could affect the brain and immune functions (e.g., epilepsy, stroke, severe head injury, etc.). Each participant completed an assessment protocol of health surveys, a neuropsychological test battery, brain imaging, and collection of blood and saliva samples [2]. In this study, we utilized brain imaging outcomes to study GWI. All participants provided written informed consent to participate in the study. This study was reviewed and approved by the Boston University institutional review board.

Table 1. Subject Characteristics.

BU Subjects	GW Control	GWI Case
N	21	98
Age (years)	54.06	52.46
Gender (F/M)	3/18	20/78

Gulf War Illness Criteria and Symptom Surveys

GWI case status was defined from the Kansas GWI case definition, which requires multiple or moderate-to-severe chronic symptoms in at least three of six statistically defined symptom domains: fatigue/sleep problems, somatic pain, neurological cognitive/mood symptoms, gastrointestinal symptoms, respiratory symptoms, and skin abnormalities [8]. GWIC participants not meeting Kansas GWI or exclusionary criteria were considered controls. Veterans were excluded from being considered GWI cases, for purposes of the research study, if they reported being diagnosed by a physician with medical or psychiatric conditions that would account for their symptoms or interfere with their ability to report their symptoms. GWIC subjects were administered a general demographic information and medical conditions questionnaire and the Kansas Gulf War and health questionnaire for assessing symptoms [8,10]. Additional validated health symptom surveys were completed by study participants and included the multidimensional fatigue inventory (MFI-20), McGill pain inventory and the Pittsburgh sleep quality index (PSQI) where higher scores suggested worse conditions [22–24].

2.2. *Image Acquisition*

All veterans were scanned on an Achieva 3T whole-body MRI scanner (Philips Healthcare, Best, The Netherlands) at the Center of Biomedical Imaging, Boston University school of Medicine. T1W-MRI were obtained using an MPRAGE sequence developed by the Alzheimer's disease neuroimaging initiative (ADNI) (Repetition time (TR) = 6.8 ms, Echo time (TE) = 3.1 ms, flip angle = 9°, slice thickness = 1.2 mm, 170 slices, Field of view (FOV) = 250 mm, matrix = 256 × 256) (accessible from http://adni.loni.usc.edu/). Diffusion MRI data were obtained using 124 gradient directions utilizing parallel imaging on a 16-channel parallel head coil (70 slices, TR = 13,214 ms, TE = 55 ms, with a matrix size of 128 × 128 yielding a resolution of 2.0 × 2.0 × 2.0 mm^3, no slice gap). Multi-shell diffusion encodings with b-values 1000, 2000 and 3000 s/mm^2 were acquired with a single-shot echo planar imaging (EPI) sequence, and 6 b = 0 s/mm^2 field maps were collected in addition to distortion corrections built into the scanner.

2.3. *Image Processing and Anatomical Defining*

Structural T1W-MRI scans were analyzed with the Freesurfer package (version 6.0) to generate anatomical regions of interest (ROI) for assessing GM morphometric measures, and to provide GM anatomical co-registration references for diffusion images [25]. A total of 78 ROIs defined in the average template space were co-registered to each subject's cortical surface by applying nonlinear co-registration parameters. All results were visually inspected for artifacts or incomplete segmentation. Fractional anisotropy (FA), mean diffusivity (MD), axial diffusivity (AD), and radial diffusivity (RD) maps were created using tract-based spatial statistics (TBSS), part of FSL package that projects all subjects' diffusion tensor imaging (DTI) data onto a mean tract skeleton [26]. A total of 20 major WM tracts were defined using the Johns Hopkins University (JHU) white-matter tractography atlas provided in the FSL package, the same template was also used for special normalization and linear co-registration of diffusion MRIs [27,28].

2.4. *High-Order Diffusion Processing*

Microstructural diffusion measures were reconstructed from multi-shell diffusion MRI images containing 3 b-value encodings using the NDI model [16]. Two parameters, neurite density (ND) index and orientation dispersion (OD) index were extracted from the NDI model. In brief, ND is a fraction of tissue composed of neurites which include axons and dendrites, and OD provides the spatial configuration of the neurite structures based on the composite pattern of intra- and extracellular diffusivity [29]. For WM NDI measures, all subjects' NDI data were registered to a common space based on nonlinear transformation and projected to the WM tract skeleton. Next the major WM tract ROIs were then applied to the skeletonized WM NDI maps to extract ROI-wise NDI measures [26]. For the GM diffusivity assessment, diffusion modeling parameters were determined by voxel wise iterative parameter selection method. We used the maximum likelihood estimation of model fitting error to define the optimal intrinsic free diffusivity parameters [30]. The optimal parameters were used to reconstruct the GM NDI maps and then merged into the 78 GM ROIs to extract ROI-wise NDI measures [30,31].

2.5. T1-Weighted MRI Measures

From the Freesurfer cortical reconstruction process of T1W-MRI, we extracted six measures per subject, including cortical thickness, cortical surface area, cortical volume (cVolume), subcortical GM volume (scVolume), WM volume, curvature (curv). Specifically, cortical thickness, surface area, volume, and curvature are extracted from 62 ROIs based on Desikan–Killiany–Tourville (DKT) atlas, while subcortical ROIs are defined by Freesurfer built-in atlas [31,32].

2.6. Statistical Analysis

From the data processing steps, we generated in total 14 types of imaging measures: 4 NDI, 4 DTI, and 6 T1-weighted morphometric measures. For each type of imaging measure, we conducted statistical comparisons of GWI cases vs. controls using linear regression models adjusting for age and sex, and then corrected for multiple comparison using false discovery rate (FDR) [33]. We reported t-values and FDR-corrected p-values (FDR-p), significant features are defined as FDR-$p < 0.05$.

2.7. Machine Learning Classification

Imaging measures described in the previous sections are used as pre-defined features for training ML classification models. Age- and sex-related confounds were removed from the raw data before training the model. This step is achieved by estimating the effects of age and sex on imaging measures using a linear regression model that is similar to a method applied in an early study [19]. For building the classifier for each imaging measure we adapted a reinforcement learning algorithm with artificial bee colony algorithm for feature selection (BSO: bee swarm optimization), and the K nearest neighbors (KNN) algorithm for classification training and performance evaluation [34,35].

2.7.1. Feature Space Selection and Classifier Training

As mentioned previously, some specific neuroimaging markers (i.e., NDI measures) may be more sensitive for detecting the subtle neurological changes occurring in GWI cases [16]. For training the classifiers, each type of imaging measures (i.e., measurement domains) serves as prior information that will allow us to set up specific feature space for potentially better ML outcomes. Within each feature space, reinforcement learning-based BSO (QBSO) was used to perform iterative search of the subset of features that provides the best classification performance on the training dataset (more details described in QBSO Tuning). Through QBSO, a final subset of features (final solution) was selected to build a final classifier. Final classifiers trained on each feature space were- then tested on the validation dataset (see more details in Ensemble Approach).

QBSO Tuning

This feature selection concept combines the BSO and reinforcement learning (specifically Q-learning) to upgrade simple local search to a more adaptive and efficient search for the final solution [34,35]. Previous study has shown that this hybrid method outperforms other well-known ML algorithms for feature selection [35]. More specifically, the BSO method mimics the foraging behavior of natural bees by performing iterative local search for an optimized solution [36].

From the predefined feature space explained earlier, the initial solution is randomly generated. Then, BSO randomly modifies the initial solution to multiple different secondary solutions, where each will be assigned to a bee (an agent) to perform local search to find local optimum (based on k-fold cross-validation accuracy). In this local search stage, each bee refers to a series of experiments obtained in previous steps to make a decision to do further search in the current search pace, and this local search will continue until no further improvement of accuracy occurs. When the bee reaches this point, each bee's search history is shared to other bees and used for the diversification of searching process.

In the diversification process, the most distant solution will be selected based on the shared information. During this process, the role of reinforcement learning is to allow the agent learn through an interactive environment by trial and error. As the result, the QBSO method will search for a solution (i.e., resulting feature list) that maximizes the reward through multiple iterations. In each iteration, KNN runs on the candidate features (one of the secondary solutions) selected from the bee and tested for 5 iterations of 5-fold cross-validation on the training dataset. We used an average accuracy measure from the 5-fold cross-validation for estimating the reward. Finally, the search process will terminate based on the pre-defined parameters. To set up the optimal parameters, we used a grid-search strategy that is empirically searching the parameters resulting in the highest classification accuracy for the training dataset. The final parameters used in this experiment are listed as follows: flip: 20, max. chance: 9, nBees: 30.

Ensemble Approach

Per each feature space (i.e., one type of imaging measure), QBSO produces a subset of final features that provides the highest average accuracy from the iterative search. QBSO is repeated 5 times in total to generate 5 final solution candidates for a single training dataset. Per each solution, we built 3 different classifiers- KNN, support vector machine, and random forest classifiers. The training dataset was further split into 2 parts (i.e., training and testing) and used to train each classifier. Then the weighted majority voting was used to ensemble those 15 classifiers (i.e., 3 classifiers from each solution) to make a final prediction on the validation dataset. The following weight function was used: $Wi = Pi/(1 - Pi)$, Pi: performance of i-th classifier, $i = [1:15]$.

2.7.2. Comparing Classification with Different Imaging Measures

As mentioned previously, each type of imaging measures was used to set up distinct candidate feature space for training the classifiers. The resulting 14 different classifiers (4 NDI, 4 DTI, and 6 T1W-MRI morphometric measures) were evaluated based on their classification performances. For the benchmark testing, the entire dataset was initially divided into a training dataset and a validation dataset based on a 5-fold partitioning. We took one fold as a validation dataset and used the remaining 4-fold data for performing the QBSO training framework (Section 2.7.1). This process was repeated 5 times as training/validation datasets rotate among the 5 folds (by taking each fold as the validation dataset in each iteration). For the classification performance comparison, we reported performance measures (averaged from 5 iterations after validation) of accuracy, sensitivity, specificity, and F-score. We included F-score as a more representative performance measure for the imbalanced case and control groups [37]. In addition to the average accuracy, we included the standard deviation (SD) of accuracy, as an estimate of variations between iterations, and the highest accuracy value for the top three classifiers.

3. Results

3.1. Group-Level Statistical Comparison and Key Imaging Features

Statistical analysis of NDI measures showed significant differences between GWI cases and controls in both WM tracts and GM ROIs (FDR-$p < 0.05$) (Figure 1). The full result can be found in Table S1. All major WM tracts showed significant decreases in ND and OD for GWI cases compared to controls (Figure 1A). The greatest significant group differences between GWI cases and controls were seen in the bilateral corticospinal tract (CST, t = −3.119 FDR-p = 0.017 (left), t = −3.129, FDR-p = 0.017 (right)) and the bilateral anterior thalamic radiations (ATR, t = −2.891, FDR-p = 0.017 (left), t = −2.808, FDR-p = 0.017 (right)) for WM ND, and in the bilateral cingulum cingulate gyrus bundle (CCG, t = −4.041 FDR-p = 0.002 (left), t = −3.384, FDR-p = 0.007) for WM OD. Both ND and OD showed decreased patterns (FDR-$p < 0.05$) for most GM ROIs as well (Figure 1B). The greatest significant group differences between GWI cases and controls were seen in the left isthmus of cingulate gyrus (t = −3.319, FDR-p = 0.036) and the bilateral thalamus proper (t = −3.168, FDR-p = 0.036 (left), t = −3.015, FDR-p = 0.036) for GM ND, and in the bilateral caudal anterior cingulate gyrus (t = −3.262, FDR-p = 0.016(left), t = −3.182, FDR-p = 0.016 (right)), the bilateral posterior cingulate gyrus (t = −3.832, FDR-p = 0.016 (left), t = −2.461, FDR-p = 0.03 (right)), the bilateral amygdala (t = −3.593, FDR-p = 0.016 (left), t = −3.516, FDR-p = 0.016 (right)) and the bilateral putamen (t = −3.228, FDR-p = 0.016 (left), t = −3.134, FDR-p = 0.016 (right)) for GM OD. The full list of statistically significant imaging features can be found in Table S1.

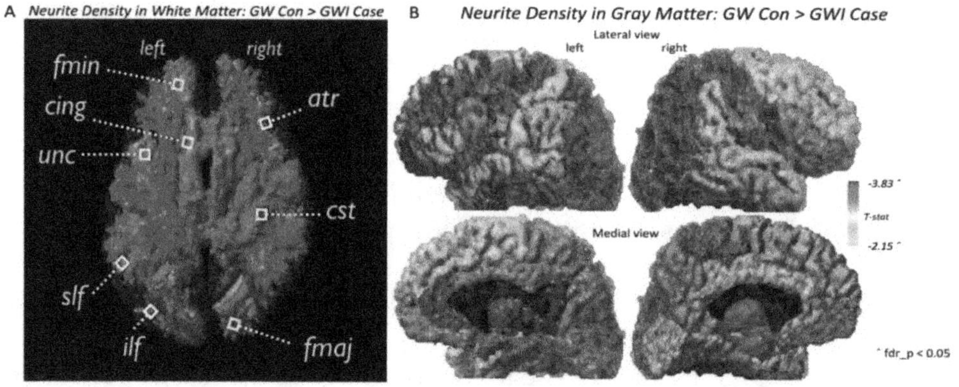

Figure 1. Gulf War illness (GWI) cases vs. Gulf War (GW) control group comparisons of gray matter (GM) and white matter (WM) neurite density imaging (NDI) measures and summary of significant regions. (**A**) 3D tract representation of significant WM ND differences between GWI case and control groups. (**B**) 3D region of interest (ROI) representation of significant GM ND differences between GWI case and control groups. Color bar corresponds to the magnitude of t-value, red indicates greater difference between groups, and vice versa. Fmaj = corpus callosum forceps major, Fmin = corpus callosum forceps minor, atr = anterior thalamic radiations, cst = corticospinal tract, cing = cingulum cingulate gyrus bundle, ilf = inferior longitudinal fasciculus, slf = superior longitudinal fasciculus, unc = uncinate fasciculus.

3.2. Machine Learning Classification Performance

As shown in Figure 2 and Table 2, the best classifier for GWI cases vs. control we had is trained using the WM OD measures, which achieved F-score of 0.941, an accuracy of 90% (SD: 0.063, highest accuracy: 91.7%), sensitivity of 95%, and specificity of 65%. The specific features include the left CST, the corpus callosum forceps minor (fminor), the left inferior fronto-occipital fasciculus (IFOF), the left inferior longitudinal fasciculus (ILF), the left superior longitudinal fasciculus (SLF), and the left superior longitudinal fasciculus temporal (SLFT). All features were statistically significant based on group-level analysis (Figure 1A, Table S1). The second-best classifier is trained using the GM ND measures, which achieved F-score of 0.922, an accuracy of 86.7% (SD: 0.054, highest accuracy:

91.7%), sensitivity of 96%, and specificity of 40%. The specific features used by this GM ND classifier include both cortical and subcortical structures of the limbic system, including the bilateral caudal anterior cingulate gyri (Table 2). The third best classifier was trained using the WM ND measures, which achieved F-score of 0.914, an accuracy of 85% (SD: 0.048, highest accuracy: 91.7%), sensitivity of 96%, and specificity of 30%. For this classifier, the specific features included the bilateral anterior thalamic radiations (ATR), the bilateral IFOF, the bilateral ILF, the left SLF, the right SLFT and the Fminor (Table 2). The full list of imaging features used by the top three classifiers can be found in Table 2 and the full list of classifier performances can be found in Table S2.

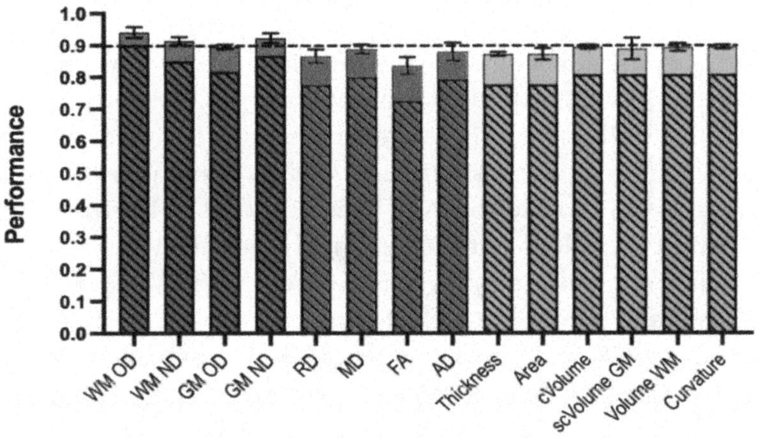

Figure 2. Classification performances of all classifiers. Each bar represents the performance (solid-colored bar: average F-score, shaded area: average accuracy) of each type of classifier trained on one imaging measure, data is presented as mean ± SEM after cross-validation. Grey-colored bars: NDI measure-based classifiers. Blue-colored bars: diffusion tension imaging (DTI) measure-based classifiers. Green-colored bars: T1-weighted structural MRI (T1W-MRI) measure-based classifiers. WM OD = white matter orientation dispersion, WM ND = white matter neurite density, GM OD = grey matter orientation dispersion, GM ND = grey matter neurite density, RD = radial diffusivity, MD = mean diffusivity, FA = fractional anisotropy, AD = axial diffusivity, thickness = cortical thickness, area = cortical surface area, cVolume = cortical volume, scVolume = subcortical GM volume, volume WM = white matter volume.

Table 2. Summary of classification performances and feature characteristics.

Measure	ACC	SEN	SPE	F-Score	Key Features	
WM OD	90%	95%	65%	0.941	L CST ** L IFOF ** L ILF ** L SLF ** L SLFT ** Fminor **	
GM ND	86.7%	96%	40%	0.922	L caudal anterior cingulate * L cuneus L inferior temporal L paracentral * L posterior cingulate * L thalamus proper *	R caudal anterior cingulat R lingual R pars orbitalis R amygdala * R putamen *
WM ND	85%	96%	30%	0.914	L ATR * L IFOF * L ILF * L SLF * Fminor *	R ATR * R IFOF * R ILF * R SLFT *

ACC: accuracy, SEN: sensitivity, SPE: specificity, F-score: F1 score, WM OD: white matter orientation dispersion index, GM ND: gray matter neurite density index, WM ND: white matter neurite density index, L: left hemisphere, R: right hemisphere, CST: corticospinal tract, IFOF: inferior fronto-occipital fasciculus, ILF: inferior longitudinal fasciculus, SLF: superior longitudinal fasciculus, SLFT: superior longitudinal fasciculus temporal, Fminor: corpus callosum forceps minor, ATR: anterior thalamic radiation. *: FDR-$p < 0.05$ in group-level statistical comparison. **: FDR-$p < 0.01$ in group-level statistical comparison.

4. Discussion

In this study, we used various neuroimaging techniques (NDI, DTI, structural T1W-MRI) to identify important features that may help to differentiate between veterans with GWI and control veterans. These features were selected through two different analytical frameworks: (1) group-level statistical analysis, and (2) single subject-level ML classification models. From our group-level, univariate analysis, we identified important imaging features, especially from WM and GM NDI and T1W-MRI regional volumetric measures, which showed high contrasts between veterans with GWI and control veterans. From the multivariate classification results, we could additionally identify unique imaging features that are important for making single-subject level inferences regardless of its relevance to the group differences.

The results from the group-level statistical analysis showed that NDI measures are the most sensitive marker for detecting GWI pathology than other types of neuroimaging measures. For WM NDI measures, all major tracts showed significant decreases for veterans with GWI compared to control veterans (Figure 1A). The greatest significant group differences were seen in the bilateral CST for WM ND and bilateral CCG bundle for WM OD (Table S1). The roles of these tracts in many essential physical and neuropsychological functions have been well described by previous literatures. For instance, earlier studies showed that disruption of the CST WM integrity was associated with motor impairment that occurs in the early stages of many neurological conditions such as Huntington's Disease and Multiple Sclerosis [38,39]. Similarly, disruption of CCG has been associated with impaired executive functioning, pain, memory deficits, and has been a main target for conditions including major depression, schizophrenia, post-traumatic stress disorder (PTSD), and autism spectrum disorder [40]. Changes in these tracts captured by our WM NDI results may also be important to understand specific symptoms such as muscle pain, fatigue, and depression observed in GWI.

From the ML framework, we confirmed that WM OD, GM ND, and WM ND measures were the sources of the top three classifiers (based on average accuracy) (Figure 2, Table 2). The classifier trained using the WM OD measure showed the best performance and consistently reporting six features: the left CST, IFOF, ILF, SLF, SLFT, and the Fminor (Table 2). Due to the completely imbalanced distribution of the data used in this study, performance on classifying controls were more challenging in QBSO and this calls better ideas on handling this issue. For example, synthetic oversampling method such as the synthetic minority oversampling technique (SMOTE) may help addressing this issue [41]. Additionally, in this type of imbalanced sample, assessing the F1-score might serve as a more realistic measure of the classification performance [37]. Although we used average accuracy measure for comparing classifiers, WM OD showed a high F-score (0.941), showing that our proposed ML framework is providing reasonable performance at least in this sample. Compared to the NDI classifiers, the classifiers from DTI measures or T1W-MRI measures all had lower classification performance than NDI measures (Table S2). These results suggest that (1) NDI measures are important imaging markers for defining GWI, and (2) the features defined from ML framework provides distinct information from the group-level statistics on describing GWI. While several features from the group-level statistics may present with overlapping patterns to ML classifiers, there are also unique features reported by ML classifiers but not captured in the group-level analysis framework.

Both our findings on group-level statistics and single subject-level classification model demonstrated the importance of NDI measures for defining GWI. Moreover, considering the other ML methods tested on mild or preclinical stage illness, such as mild cognitive impairment staying with ~78% accuracy levels, the classification performance obtained from NDI QBSO is impressive and brings more attention into the complex diffusion imaging measures for studying preclinical stage or mildly progressive illness [42]. In the current study, we not only identified widespread statistically significant NDI features through group-level analysis, but also demonstrated that WM OD measures trained a better classifier compared to other imaging measures. This is consistent with our previous studies on NDI showing that this technique is sensitive to microstructural and macrostructural brain alterations and useful for detecting neurological abnormalities in GW veterans [16]. Our result also corroborated with our previous findings that showed a higher sensitivity for the novel NDI measures compared to the common DTI measures (e.g., FA, MD, etc.). As we suggested before, this might be due to the higher specificity of NDI for detecting changes in different tissue components [16]. We previously found that there is a strong correlation between alterations in GM ND measure and worse self-reported fatigue and sleep symptoms, and with upregulated levels of proinflammatory cytokines TNFRI and TNFRII [16]. However, based on our current findings, GM ND measures provided slightly lower classification performance than WM OD and ND measures in this study. In addition, while classifier trained on WM OD resulted in nearly identical final solutions across five iterations of validation, GM measures resulted in more variabilities in the selected feature solutions. This might be due to the differences in dimensional size between WM and GM feature space. GM measures have more numbers of features (more complexity in the feature space) to be searched out during the QBSO process than WM measures, and thereby requiring more delicate optimization process especially in this not-a-large dataset problem. Although further investigations based on larger dataset is key to address the issue, this may also indicate that WM OD measures can be better markers for simply classifying veterans with GWI from control veterans, while GM ND can be a sensitive marker to specific symptom domains. Our results also support the diagnostic value of these NDI markers for clinical applications.

Altogether, these results suggest that the microstructural changes measured by NDI may be attributed to GM and WM deficits following chronic neuroinflammation. In line with this finding, other studies have shown that chronic neuroinflammation related to GWI symptoms may be a result of both morphological and functional changes that occurred in glial cells. For instance, a study using a rat model of GWI showed that exposure to the chemical agent, diisopropyl fluorophosphate (DFP: a sarin surrogate), was associated with fewer numbers of both mature and dividing oligodendrocytes in the prefrontal cortex, which in turn interrupted the neuron-glial interactions [43]. DFP injection also induced neuroinflammation and neurodegeneration in multiple brain regions, which is associated with impaired contextual fear learning in these rats [44]. Similarly, mice exposed to DFP demonstrated epigenetic changes to genes related to the immune and neuronal systems and altered proportions of myelinating oligodendrocytes in the frontal cortex, which led to disrupted synaptic connectivity and WM alterations in GWI [45]. A recent in-vivo positron emission tomography study corroborated these findings and reported elevated levels of translocator protein (TSPO), a protein upregulated in activated microglia and astrocytes, in veterans with GWI compared to control veterans [46]. This elevation pattern was observed in many areas including the precuneus, prefrontal, primary motor, and somatosensory cortices [46]. Considering this evidence, our current findings further support the importance of novel NDI measures for detecting microstructural changes in the brain following chronic neuroinflammation in GWI.

Besides NDI measures, some T1W-MRI measures also demonstrated good performances for classifying veterans with GWI vs. control veterans. Among classifiers trained using T1W-MRI measures, the cortical volume, subcortical volume, WM volume, and mean curvature models achieved 80.8% accuracy, and highlighted key features in the frontal and temporal regions (Table S2). The results on the group-level statistical analysis also showed reduced volumes of frontal regions among veterans with GWI (Table S1). GM atrophy has been well studied as a hallmark for various neuropsychological disorders. Previous studies showed that reduced total cortical and regional frontal lobe volumes are associated with poor subjective sleep quality and increased self-reported frequency of hearing chemical alarm among GW veterans [12,47].

For DTI measures, the best performance was demonstrated by the MD classifier with an accuracy of 80% and F-score of 0.887 (Table S2). There is evidence that DTI measures may correlate with GWI symptom severity. An early study on GWI veterans showed that fatigue, pain, and hyperalgesia are associated with increased AD in the right IFOF [15]. Another study showed that changes in frontal-limbic WM connectivity, as indicated by reduced MD and increased FA in the right cingulate bundle, was associated with higher PTSD symptom severity score among a sample of 20 GW veterans [48]. In addition, GW veterans who had been exposed to chemical agents have increased

AD throughout many regions of the brain including the temporal stem, cingulum bundle, IFOF, etc., compared to unexposed veterans [13]. Through our results, we found that while T1W-MRI and DTI measures are less significant based on group-level statistical analysis, a subset of the regional measures may still explain key components of GWI symptoms.

In this study, we showed that neuroimaging markers help to identify GWI Nevertheless, we are expecting that the current approach can be improved in several aspects. One of the limitations of the current work is the imbalanced sample size, where the number of case subjects greatly exceeded the control subjects for building the classification model. This issue is reflected by the higher sensitivity and lower specificity for all the classifiers. To better handle this issue, we are planning to employ an oversampling method on the minority group to balance the samples. In our follow up work, we will also expand our analysis to a larger GW cohort including more control veterans recruited from other sites. Another important future direction is to test if the combination of multiple imaging measures, or combination of imaging and clinical measures (e.g., cognitive scores, inflammatory profiles, etc.) can improve the classification performance. This multivariate approach will be useful for identifying important features from large datasets. In conclusion, our current work provided the first evidence that novel NDI measures are not only useful for defining GWI based on the conventional group-level statistical comparisons, but also constitute key features for building single-subject level ML models for automated diagnostic classification. The features that are highlighted by our analysis suggest neurological changes underlying GWI pathology and support neuroinflammation as a potential target for therapeutic interventions.

Author Contributions: Data analysis and paper writing is done by Y.G. and C.-H.C. W.C. and Y.Z. equally contributed to the ML software development. S.K. helped formal analysis. M.K., P.J., and R.T. worked on data curation. E.Y. and J.-H.K. helped ML optimization. R.B. helped formal analysis and validation. L.S. contributed conceptualization of the research. K.S. contributed conceptualization, funding acquisition, and project administration. B.-B.K. contributed idea development, study design, funding acquisition, leading the technical development, supervision of research works and writing. All authors have read and agreed to the published version of the manuscript.

References

1. White, R.F.; Steele, L.; O'Callaghan, J.P.; Sullivan, K.; Binns, J.H.; Golomb, B.A.; Bloom, F.E.; Bunker, J.A.; Crawford, F.; Graves, J.C.; et al. Recent research on Gulf War illness and other health problems in veterans of the 1991 Gulf War: Effects of toxicant exposures during deployment. *Cortex* **2016**, *74*, 449–475. [CrossRef] [PubMed]
2. Janulewicz, P.; Krengel, M.; Quinn, E.; Heeren, T.; Toomey, R.; Killiany, R.; Zundel, C.; Ajama, J.; O'Callaghan, J.; Steele, L.; et al. The Multiple Hit Hypothesis for Gulf War Illness: Self-Reported Chemical/Biological Weapons Exposure and Mild Traumatic Brain Injury. *Brain Sci.* **2018**, *8*, 198. [CrossRef] [PubMed]
3. Yee, M.K.; Seichepine, D.R.; Janulewicz, P.A.; Sullivan, K.A.; Proctor, S.P.; Krengel, M.H. Self-Reported Traumatic Brain Injury, Health and Rate of Chronic Multisymptom Illness in Veterans from the 1990–1991 Gulf War. *J. Head Trauma Rehabil.* **2016**, *31*, 320–328. [CrossRef] [PubMed]
4. Yee, M.K.; Janulewicz, P.A.; Seichepine, D.R.; Sullivan, K.A.; Proctor, S.P.; Krengel, M.H. Multiple Mild Traumatic Brain Injuries Are Associated with Increased Rates of Health Symptoms and Gulf War Illness in a Cohort of 1990-1991 Gulf War Veterans. *Brain Sci.* **2017**, *7*, 79. [CrossRef]
5. O'Callaghan, J.P.; Kelly, K.A.; Locker, A.R.; Miller, D.B.; Lasley, S.M. Corticosterone primes the neuroinflammatory response to DFP in mice: Potential animal model of Gulf War Illness. *J. Neurochem.* **2015**, *133*, 708–721. [CrossRef]
6. Gade, D.M.; Wenger, J.B. Combat exposure and mental health: The long-term effects among US Vietnam and Gulf War veterans. *Health Econ.* **2011**, *20*, 401–416. [CrossRef]
7. Rathbone, A.T.; Tharmaradinam, S.; Jiang, S.; Rathbone, M.P.; Kumbhare, D.A. A review of the neuro- and systemic inflammatory responses in post concussion symptoms: Introduction of the "post-inflammatory brain syndrome" PIBS. *Brain Behav. Immun.* **2015**, *46*, 1–16. [CrossRef]

8. Steele, L. Prevalence and patterns of Gulf War illness in Kansas veterans: Association of symptoms with characteristics of person, place, and time of military service. *Am. J. Epidemiol.* **2000**, *152*, 992–1002. [CrossRef]
9. Dursa, E.; Barth, S.; Porter, B.; Schneiderman, A. Gulf War Illness in the 1991 Gulf war and Gulf era veteran population: An application of the centers for disease control and prevention and Kansas case definitions to historical data. *J. Mil. Veterans Health* **2018**, *26*, 43–50.
10. Proctor, S.P.; Heeren, T.; White, R.F.; Wolfe, J.; Borgos, M.S.; Davis, J.D.; Pepper, L.; Clapp, R.; Sutker, P.B.; Vasterling, J.J.; et al. Health status of Persian Gulf War veterans: Self-reported symptoms, environmental exposures and the effect of stress. *Int. J. Epidemiol.* **1998**, *27*, 1000–1010. [CrossRef]
11. Chao, L.L.; Abadjian, L.; Hlavin, J.; Meyerhoff, D.J.; Weiner, M.W. Effects of low-level sarin and cyclosarin exposure and Gulf War Illness on brain structure and function: A study at 4T. *Neurotoxicology* **2011**, *32*, 814–822. [CrossRef] [PubMed]
12. Chao, L.L.; Kriger, S.; Buckley, S.; Ng, P.; Mueller, S.G. Effects of low-level sarin and cyclosarin exposure on hippocampal subfields in Gulf War Veterans. *Neurotoxicology* **2014**, *44*, 263–269. [CrossRef] [PubMed]
13. Chao, L.L.; Zhang, Y.; Buckley, S. Effects of low-level sarin and cyclosarin exposure on white matter integrity in Gulf War Veterans. *Neurotoxicology* **2015**, *48*, 239–248. [CrossRef] [PubMed]
14. Chao, L.L.; Zhang, Y. Effects of low-level sarin and cyclosarin exposure on hippocampal microstructure in Gulf War Veterans. *Neurotoxicol. Teratol.* **2018**, *68*, 36–46. [CrossRef]
15. Rayhan, R.U.; Stevens, B.W.; Timbol, C.R.; Adewuyi, O.; Walitt, B.; VanMeter, J.W.; Baraniuk, J.N. Increased Brain White Matter Axial Diffusivity Associated with Fatigue, Pain and Hyperalgesia in Gulf War Illness. *PLoS ONE* **2013**, *8*, e58493. [CrossRef] [PubMed]
16. Cheng, C.H.; Koo, B.B.; Calderazzo, S.; Quinn, E.; Aenll, K.; Steele, L.; Klimas, N.; Krengel, M.; Janulewicz, P.; Toomey, R.; et al. Alterations in high-order diffusion imaging in veterans with Gulf War Illness is associated with chemical weapons exposure and mild traumatic brain injury. *Brain Behav. Immun.* **2020**, *89*, 281–290. [CrossRef]
17. Mateos-Pérez, J.M.; Dadar, M.; Lacalle-Aurioles, M.; Iturria-Medina, Y.; Zeighami, Y.; Evans, A.C. Structural neuroimaging as clinical predictor: A review of machine learning applications. *Neuroimage Clin.* **2018**, *20*, 506–522. [CrossRef]
18. Sakai, K.; Yamada, K. Machine learning studies on major brain diseases: 5-year trends of 2014–2018. *Jpn. J. Radiol.* **2019**, *37*, 34–72. [CrossRef]
19. Moradi, E.; Pepe, A.; Gaser, C.; Huttunen, H.; Tohka, J. Alzheimer's Disease Neuroimaging Initiative. Machine learning framework for early MRI-based Alzheimer's conversion prediction in MCI subjects. *Neuroimage* **2015**, *104*, 398–412. [CrossRef]
20. Provenzano, D.; Washington, S.D.; Rao, Y.J.; Loew, M.; Baraniuk, J. Machine Learning Detects Pattern of Differences in Functional Magnetic Resonance Imaging (fMRI) Data between Chronic Fatigue Syndrome (CFS) and Gulf War Illness (GWI). *Brain Sci.* **2020**, *10*, 456. [CrossRef]
21. Ngiam, K.Y.; Khor, I.W. Big data and machine learning algorithms for health-care delivery. *Lancet Oncol.* **2019**, *20*, e262–e273. [CrossRef]
22. Buysse, D.J.; Reynolds, C.F., 3rd; Monk, T.H.; Berman, S.R.; Kupfer, D.J. The Pittsburgh Sleep Quality Index: A new instrument for psychiatric practice and research. *Psychiatry Res.* **1989**, *28*, 193–213. [CrossRef]
23. Melzack, R. The McGill Pain Questionnaire: Major properties and scoring methods. *Pain* **1975**, *1*, 277–299. [CrossRef]
24. Smets, E.M.; Garssen, B.; Bonke, B.; De Haes, J.C. The Multidimensional Fatigue Inventory (MFI) psychometric qualities of an instrument to assess fatigue. *J. Psychosom. Res.* **1995**, *39*, 315–325. [CrossRef]
25. Fischl, B. FreeSurfer. *Neuroimage* **2012**, *62*, 774–781. [CrossRef]
26. Smith, S.M.; Jenkinson, M.; Johansen-Berg, H.; Rueckert, D.; Nichols, T.E.; Mackay, C.E.; Watkins, K.E.; Ciccarelli, O.; Cader, M.Z.; Matthews, P.M.; et al. Tract-based spatial statistics: Voxelwise analysis of multi-subject diffusion data. *Neuroimage* **2006**, *31*, 1487–1505. [CrossRef]
27. Wakana, S.; Jiang, H.; Nagae-Poetscher, L.M.; van Zijl, P.C.; Mori, S. Fiber tract-based atlas of human white matter anatomy. *Radiology* **2004**, *230*, 77–87. [CrossRef]
28. Mori, S.; Wakana, S.; Van Zijl, P.C.; Nagae-Poetscher, L.M. *MRI Atlas of Human White Matter*; Elsevier: New York, NY, USA, 2005.
29. Zhang, Z.; Schneider, T.; Wheeler-Kingshott, C.; Alexander, D. NODDI: Practical in vivo neurite orientation dispersion and density imaging of the human brain. *Neuroimage* **2012**, *61*, 1000–1016. [CrossRef]

30. Fukutomi, H.; Glasser, M.F.; Zhang, H.; Autio, J.A.; Coalson, T.S.; Okada, T.; Togashi, K.; Van Essen, D.C.; Hayashi, T. Neurite imaging reveals microstructural variations in human cerebral cortical gray matter. *Neuroimage* **2018**, *182*, 488–499. [CrossRef]
31. Desikan, R.S.; Ségonne, F.; Fischl, B.; Quinn, B.T.; Dickerson, B.C.; Blacker, D.; Buckner, R.L.; Dale, A.M.; Maguire, R.P.; Hyman, B.T.; et al. An automated labeling system for subdividing the human cerebral cortex on MRI scans into gyral based regions of interest. *Neuroimage* **2006**, *31*, 968–980. [CrossRef]
32. Fischl, B.; Dale, A.M. Measuring the thickness of the human cerebral cortex from magnetic resonance images. *Proc. Natl. Acad. Sci. USA* **2000**, *97*, 11050–11055. [CrossRef] [PubMed]
33. Noble, W.S. How does multiple testing correction work? *Nat. Biotechnol.* **2009**, *27*, 1135–1137. [CrossRef] [PubMed]
34. Sutton, R.S.; Barto, A.G. *Introduction to Reinforcement Learning*; MIT Press: Cambridge, MA, USA, 1998.
35. Sadeg, S.; Hamdad, L.; Remache, A.R.; Karech, M.N.; Benatchba, K.; Habbas, Z. QBSO-FS: A Reinforcement Learning Based Bee Swarm Optimization Metaheuristic for Feature Selection. In *Advances in Computational Intelligence*; Rojas, I., Joya, G., Catala, A., Eds.; IWANN 2019; Lecture Notes in Computer Science; Springer: Cham, Switzerland, 2019; Volume 11507, pp. 785–796. [CrossRef]
36. Karaboga, D.; Basturk, B. A powerful and efficient algorithm for numerical function optimization: Artificial bee colony (ABC) algorithm. *J. Glob. Optim.* **2007**, *39*, 459–471. [CrossRef]
37. Jeni, L.A.; Cohn, J.F.; De La Torre, F. Facing Imbalanced Data Recommendations for the Use of Performance Metrics. In Proceedings of the 2013 Humaine Association Conference on Affective Computing and Intelligent Interaction, Geneva, Switzerland, 2–5 September 2013; pp. 245–251. [CrossRef]
38. Phillips, O.; Squitieri, F.; Sanchez-Castaneda, C.; Elifani, F.; Griguoli, A.; Maglione, V.; Caltagirone, C.; Sabatini, U.; Di Paola, M. The Corticospinal Tract in Huntington's Disease. *Cereb. Cortex* **2015**, *25*, 2670–2682. [CrossRef] [PubMed]
39. Pawlitzki, M.; Neumann, J.; Kaufmann, J.; Heidel, J.; Stadler, E.; Sweeney-Reed, C.; Sailer, M.; Schreiber, S. Loss of corticospinal tract integrity in early MS disease stages. *Neurol. Neuroimmunol. Neuroinflamm.* **2017**, *4*, e399. [CrossRef] [PubMed]
40. Bubb, E.J.; Metzler-Baddeley, C.; Aggleton, J.P. The cingulum bundle: Anatomy, function, and dysfunction. *Neurosci. Biobehav. Rev.* **2018**, *92*, 104–127. [CrossRef]
41. Fernández, A.; García, S.; Herrera, F.; Chawla, N.V. SMOTE for learning from imbalanced data: Progress and challenges, marking the 15-year anniversary. *J. Artif. Int. Res.* **2018**, *61*, 863–905. [CrossRef]
42. Forouzannezhad, P.; Abbaspour, A.; Li, C.; Fang, C.; Williams, U.; Cabrerizo, M.; Barreto, A.; Andrian, J.; Rishe, N.; Curiel, R.E.; et al. A gaussian-based model for early detection of mild cognitive impairment using multimodal neuroimaging. *J. Neurosci. Methods* **2020**, *333*, 108544. [CrossRef]
43. Belgrad, J.; Dutta, D.J.; Bromley-Coolidge, S.; Kelly, K.A.; Michalovicz, L.T.; Sullivan, K.A.; O'Callaghan, J.P.; Douglas Fields, R. Oligodendrocyte involvement in Gulf War Illness. *Glia* **2019**, *67*, 2107–2124. [CrossRef]
44. Flannery, B.M.; Bruun, D.A.; Rowland, D.J.; Banks, C.N.; Austin, A.T.; Kukis, D.L.; Li, Y.; Ford, B.D.; Tancredi, D.J.; Silverman, J.L.; et al. Persistent neuroinflammation and cognitive impairment in a rat model of acute diisopropylfluorophosphate intoxication. *J. Neuroinflamm.* **2016**, *13*, 267. [CrossRef]
45. Ashbrook, D.G.; Hing, B.; Michalovicz, L.T.; Kelly, K.A.; Miller, J.V.; de Vega, W.C.; Miller, D.B.; Broderick, G.; O'Callaghan, J.P.; McGowan, P.O. Epigenetic impacts of stress priming of the neuroinflammatory response to sarin surrogate in mice: A model of Gulf War illness. *J. Neuroinflamm.* **2018**, *15*, 86. [CrossRef] [PubMed]
46. Alshelh, Z.; Albrecht, D.S.; Bergan, C.; Akeju, O.; Clauw, D.J.; Conboy, L.; Edwards, R.R.; Kim, M.; Lee, Y.C.; Protsenko, E.; et al. In-vivo imaging of neuroinflammation in veterans with Gulf War illness. *Brain Behav. Immun.* **2020**, *87*, 498–507. [CrossRef] [PubMed]
47. Chao, L.L.; Reeb, R.; Esparza, I.L.; Abadjian, L.R. Associations between the self-reported frequency of hearing chemical alarms in theater and regional brain volume in Gulf War Veterans. *Neurotoxicology* **2016**, *53*, 246–256. [CrossRef] [PubMed]
48. Bierer, L.M.; Ivanov, I.; Carpenter, D.M.; Wong, E.W.; Golier, J.A.; Tang, C.Y.; Yehuda, R. White matter abnormalities in Gulf War veterans with posttraumatic stress disorder: A pilot study. *Psychoneuroendocrinology* **2015**, *51*, 567–576. [CrossRef]

2

Objective Diagnosis for Histopathological Images based on Machine Learning Techniques: Classical Approaches and New Trends

Naira Elazab [1], Hassan Soliman [1], Shaker El-Sappagh [2,3], S. M. Riazul Islam [4,*] and Mohammed Elmogy [1]

1 Information Technology Department, Faculty of Computers and Information, Mansoura University, Mansoura 35516, Egypt; naira.elazab@mans.edu.eg (N.E.); hsoliman@mans.edu.eg (H.S.); melmogy@mans.edu.eg (M.E.)
2 Centro Singular de Investigación en Tecnoloxías Intelixentes (CiTIUS), Universidade de Santiago de Compostela, 15705 Santiago de Compostela, Spain; shaker.elsappagh@usc.es
3 Information Systems Department, Faculty of Computers and Artificial Intelligence, Benha University, Benha 13512, Egypt
4 Department of Computer Science and Engineering, Sejong University, Seoul 05006, Korea
* Correspondence: riaz@sejong.ac.kr

Abstract: Histopathology refers to the examination by a pathologist of biopsy samples. Histopathology images are captured by a microscope to locate, examine, and classify many diseases, such as different cancer types. They provide a detailed view of different types of diseases and their tissue status. These images are an essential resource with which to define biological compositions or analyze cell and tissue structures. This imaging modality is very important for diagnostic applications. The analysis of histopathology images is a prolific and relevant research area supporting disease diagnosis. In this paper, the challenges of histopathology image analysis are evaluated. An extensive review of conventional and deep learning techniques which have been applied in histological image analyses is presented. This review summarizes many current datasets and highlights important challenges and constraints with recent deep learning techniques, alongside possible future research avenues. Despite the progress made in this research area so far, it is still a significant area of open research because of the variety of imaging techniques and disease-specific characteristics.

Keywords: medical image analysis; histopathology image analysis; conventional machine learning methods; deep learning methods; computer-assisted diagnosis

1. Introduction

Medical Images are a fundamental section of each patient's digital health file. Such images are produced by individual radiologists who are restricted by speed, professional weaknesses, or a lack of practice. It requires decades and reasonable financial resources to train a radiologist. Additionally, some medical care methods outsource radiology confirmations to less economically developed nations, such as India, via teleradiology. A late or incorrect analysis can cause injury to the patient. Thus, it would be beneficial for medical imaging (MI) analyses to be performed by automatic, precise, and effective machine learning (ML) algorithms. MI analysis is a significant research area for ML, in part because the information is somewhat organized and labeled; i.e., this is probable if the patient was examined in a region with good ML systems [1]. That is significant for two reasons. First, with regards to real patient metrics, MI analysis is a litmus check regarding whether ML techniques would, in actuality, improve individual outcomes and survival. Second, it provides a testbed for human–ML interactions—i.e., how responsive is an individual likely to be to the health changing possibilities being put forward or aided by a nonhuman actor [2]. In recent years, ML has shown significant advances. For a wide variety of applications, including image recognition, medical diagnosis, defect identification and construction health assessments, the potential of this field has also expanded. These new developments in ML are due to many factors, like the creation of self-learning mathematical models that enable computer techniques to execute particular (human-like) tasks based solely on learned patterns, in addition to the increase in the computer power that supports these models' analytical capabilities [3].

There are many imaging types, and their use is becoming more widespread. Types of MI include ultrasound, X-ray, magnetic resonance imaging (MRI), retinal scans, histopathology images (HI), computed tomography (CT), positron emission tomography (PET), and dermoscopy images. Some examples of MIs are shown in Figure 1. Many of these types analyze numerous organs, such as CT and MRI, whereas others are organ-specific, such as retinal and dermoscopy images [4]. The quantity of produced information from each analysis stage differs depending on nature of the MI and the tested organs. HIs are useful for biological studies and to make medical decisions. In addition, they are generally utilized to provide "ground truths" (GTs) for other modalities of MI, such as MRI. A histology slide is a digital record a few megabytes in size, while a magnetic resonance image can be several hundred megabytes. This has a technical effect on how the data is preprocessed and on the architecture design of the algorithm in terms of processor and storage limitations [5].

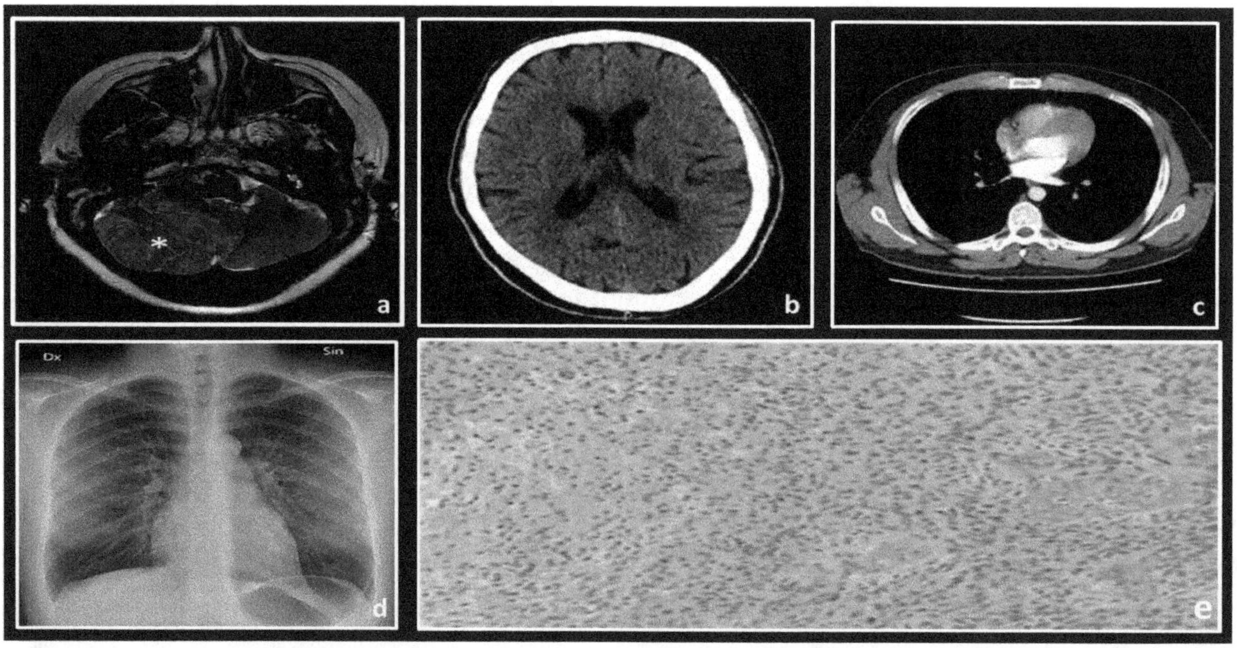

Figure 1. Examples of some medical image types: (**a**) MRI scan of the left side of a brain; (**b**) an axial CT brain scan; (**c**) an axial CT lung scan; (**d**) chest x-ray; (**e**) a histology slide with high-grade glioma.

Pathology analyses are traditionally executed by an individual pathologist observing a dyed specimen on a glass slide with a microscope. Lately, efforts have been made to record the whole slide with a reader and save it as an electronic picture, called a whole slide image (WSI) [6].

Digitizing pathology is just one recent development that produces high levels of visible information designed for automated diagnoses. It enables us to see and understand pathologic cell and muscle samples in good quality images with assistance from personal computer tools. It also brings about the possibility of applying image analysis techniques. Such techniques would assist pathologists and support their explanations, such as hosting and grading. Various classification and segmentation methods for HI have already been discussed in this review. We present and compare conventional techniques and deep learning (DL) methods to choose the most appropriate method for histopathology issues [7].

Natural microscopic architecture data and their features at nuclei, tissue, and different organ levels could be key to illness expansion and infection treatment analysis. Additionally, to examine and diagnose the histological image of biologic microscopic, pathologists have identified the morphological features of tissue that show the current presence of infection, such as cancer [8].

Some characteristics of disease, such as tumor-infiltrating lymphocytes, might be deduced from HI alone. Additionally, HI analysis, which is called the "gold standard" in many disease diagnoses, is nearly included in all kinds of cancer detection and treatment procedures. HI needs specific analysis with respect to organs and a specific task for the visualization of various tissue components under a microscope. With one or more stains, the sections are dyed. These are staining attempts to uncover cellular elements. The contrast is shown by using counterstains [9].

Efficient ML algorithms are presented and used in HI analysis to help pathologists to acquire a quick, stable, and quantified examination result for a more accurate diagnosis. Many different traditional and deep learning methods support the pathologists in accessing more tissues to determine the internal relationship between the visual images and the specific illness. Additionally, since the ML techniques are generally semi- or fully automated, they are effective, encouraging technical feasibility for histopathology examination within the recent big data age [10].

On the other hand, most of the HI analysis stages are based on mathematical basics. Mathematical operations and functions are applied to all analysis stages, starting from the preprocessing to diagnosis stages to provide an intensive analysis for HIs. Figure 2 illustrates the main phases of a common histopathological images pipeline based on conventional ML techniques. First, HIs are supplied to the system as a 2D array for grayscale images or a 3D array for colored images. Then, the preprocessing stage applies some linear algebra operations on the image array to enhance the image quality. This stage helps to distinguish significant structures from others in the processed images. Third, the segmentation stage is applied to differentiate the cells from other background objects by applying some state-of-the-art mathematical algorithms, such as thresholding, level set, watershed transform, and intensity and texture homogeneity transforms. Fourth, the feature extraction stage extracts the most significant features in the segmented images instead of processing each pixel, which reduces the system's computation complexity. Besides, most handcrafted features are based on applying some mathematical techniques to detect the changes in the intensity, color, or texture of the pixels. Common derivative techniques are utilized to detect these changes by applying first or second derivatives to pixel values. Finally, the diagnosis stage is applied to classify or cluster the processed images, depending on the extracted features. The classification and clustering techniques are based on applying some mathematical operations that distinguish the processed images based on the extracted features.

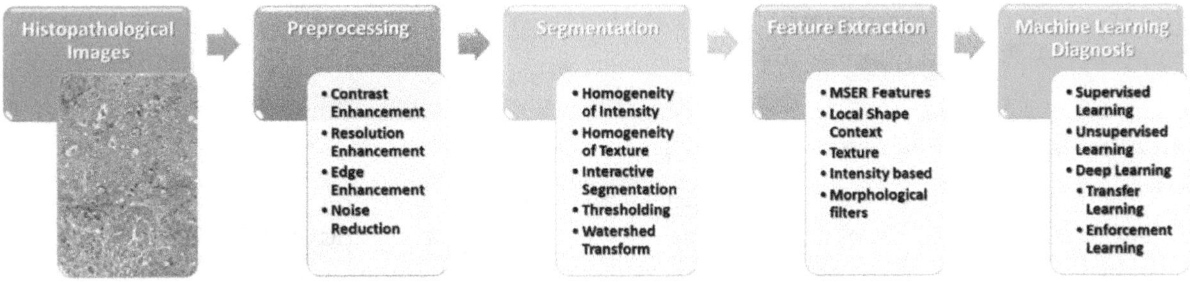

Figure 2. An overview of the HI analysis pipeline.

Numerous segmentation and classification techniques for primitives tissue in HIs were presented in this respect. For selecting the appropriate HIs analysis method, the various ML methods on HIs are reviewed in this study. In this work, the digital HI analysis, applying different ML algorithms and their issues, are described. The paper is presented to describe the necessity of the analysis procedure for segmentation and classification in computer-aided diagnosis (CAD) systems using HI.

The rest of the article is organized into six sections. Section 2 gives a brief overview of the fundamental histopathological analysis. In Section 3, the conventional approaches for HI analysis are described. Section 4 introduces the use of deep learning techniques in HI analysis. The datasets, the discussion, and tasks of HI analysis are elucidated in Sections 5 and 6, respectively. Limitations and future trends in the HI analysis are introduced in Section 7.

2. Histopathological Image Overview

HI has natural and abnormal biological structures, as well as morphological and architectural features defined by pathologists, based on their knowledge. Even given the tissue area, some structures are small, and related patterns typically have high visual appearance variability. In biological systems and anatomy, most visual variability is inherent [11].

Next to obtaining electronic HI via the biopsy test, the guide analysis of images contributes to variability in diagnosis and treatment. To get over this issue, CAD techniques are applied to provide an objective examination of disease. The fundamental steps necessary for applying the CAD examination system appear in Figure 2. This includes electronic image handling methods, such as segmentation, feature extraction, and classification [12].

HI analysis contains the computations executed at various zoom scales (×2, ×4.5, ×10, ×20, and ×40) for multivariate mathematical examination, analysis, and classification. It could be achieved at a lower zoom for tissue stage examination. Demir et al. [13] presented tissue stage and cell stage examination techniques for cancer diagnosis. They examined HI by applying preprocessing, feature extraction, and classification strategies. The new improvement in electronic pathology requirements for the growth of quantitative and automatic digital image examination methods aids pathologists in understanding the number of digitized HIs [14].

2.1. *Types of ML Systems in HI Analysis*

2.1.1. Computer-Aided Diagnosis (CAD)

Many of the searched tasks in electronic HI analysis are CAD systems, which are the pathologists' fundamental functions. The diagnostic method includes the function to map WSI to one of many infection types, indicating a supervised learning function. Considering that the mistakes created by the ML process vary from those created by an individual pathologist [15], the enhancement of classification reliability would be increased by applying the CAD method. CAD could also reduce the instability in understanding and reduce overlooking by analyzing each pixel in WSI. Different related diagnosis functions contain the recognition or segmentation of the region of interest (ROI), such as tumor area in WSI [16,17], rating of immunostaining [18,19], cancer phase [20,21], mitosis recognition [22,23], gland segmentation [24–26], and quantification of general intrusion [27].

2.1.2. Content-based on Image Retrieval (CBIR)

CBIR retrieves pictures related to a query picture. In electronic pathology, CBIR methods help in several scenarios, especially in examining, training, and studying [28–30]. For example, CBIR methods could be utilized for academic applications and novice pathologists to recover appropriate instances of HI of tissues. Additionally, such methods would also be useful to skilled pathologists, especially while detecting uncommon cases. Because CBIR certainly does not need tag data, unsupervised learning could be utilized [31]. Not just precision, but additionally high-speed research of related pictures from several pictures are needed in CBIR. Thus, numerous approaches can reduce picture feature dimensionality—such as primary element examination and small bilinear combination [32]—and quickly estimated the closest neighbor searches [33].

2.1.3. Finding New Clinicopathological Associations

Traditionally, several essential discoveries regarding diseases, such as tumor and contagious conditions, have already been produced by pathologists and analysts. They cautiously and carefully examined pathological specimens. For example, pathologists analyzed the gastric mucosa of individuals with gastritis in [34]. Efforts were made to link the morphological options that come with cancers using their medical behavior. For instance, tumor grading is essential in a patient's diagnosis and in preparing treatment for many kinds of cancer, such as breast and prostate cancer.

There is a noticeable development in the digitization of clinical data, which later improved the genome evaluation technique. Therefore, a wide range of electronic data, such as genome data, electronic pathological images, MRI, and CT scans, are now accessible [35]. By examining the connection between these imaging modalities, new hospital pathological associations, such as the connection involving morphological quality and somatic cancer mutation, are available [36]. CAD techniques could be subdivided into conventional ML and DL methods, illustrated in more detail in the next few sections.

3. Conventional Machine Learning Methods

CAD systems played an essential role and have become an important research topic in HI and diagnostics. Various image processing techniques were applied to examine the disease's diagnosis and prognosis for these HIs. Various image processing and computer vision (CV) techniques have been implemented for gland and nuclei segmentation, cell kind recognition, or classification to extract quantitative measurements of disease characteristics from HIs and automatically assess whether or not a disease exists inside examined samples. It could help to determine the degree of seriousness of the disease, whether present in the sample. Conventional ML methods often contain a few steps to manage HI, as shown in Figure 3. Each step is illustrated in the following sections.

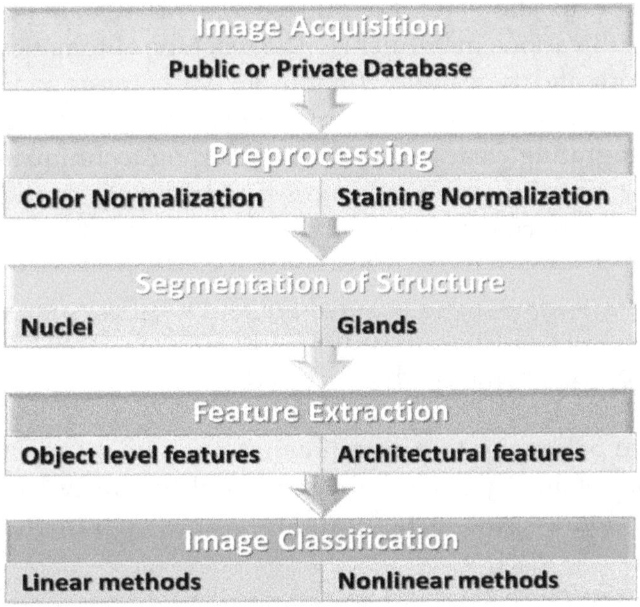

Figure 3. The conventional machine learning methods for HI.

3.1. Preprocessing

Preprocessing could recompense for variations between images, which can vary in color, staining, and other problems, such as noise, which are usually due to the scanning procedure. The gross sections are made with wax to analyze the tissue's architecture and components under the microscope and colored with one or more stains. Pathologists use staining to isolate cellular components for the diagnosis of structural as well as architectural tissue analysis. Hematoxylin–Eosin (H&E) staining is most commonly utilized, and it separates the connective tissue, cytoplasm, and nuclei. Nuclei are stained blue by Hematoxylin, while connective tissue and cytoplasm are stained pink by Eosin. DAB, immune-histochemistry stains, etc. are the other stains. The consistency of the features extracted from the image directly affects classification performance. Thus, it is essential to define the proper conditions under which the image preprocessing techniques will work as the first job. Noise and various illumination fluctuations are detrimental to image processing techniques. If those negative factors are eliminated, it will improve performance. Pre-processing imaging techniques are well adapted to this mission. Pre-processing methods control changes in image brightness and contrast and eliminate noise.

3.1.1. Staining Normalization

HI could have powerful color variations due to various scanners, various staining techniques, and sample age. An efficient color calibration between samples is difficult to accomplish [37]. Hence, color normalization is needed in most of the processing scenarios. Deconvolution-based methods and histogram-based methods are examples of color normalization [38]. Anghel et al. [39] suggested improving stain normalization in low-quality WSIs to increase ML pipeline accuracy. They used an ML pipeline based on convolutional neural networks (CNNs), which classifies pictures to detect prostate cancer, to demonstrate the robustness of this new normalization process. This system makes it possible to pre-process massive datasets and is a crucial requirement for any biomedical imagery learning computer.

3.1.2. Color Normalization

Color normalization is required for bright and fluorescent HI analysis. This process decreases the variations in samples of tissue because of variance in conditions of scanning and staining. There are different techniques for the color normalization of HI, such as the Reinhard approach, descriptor of stain color, and histogram specification [40]. For HI research, MIAQuant [41] was stained by different approaches and obtained with various instruments. The machine automatically extracts and quantifies markers with various colors and types and, for the visual comparison of their positions, aligns the contiguous tissue slices, stained by multiple markers. MIAQuant segments markers efficiently and quantifies them by integrating clear and effective imaging techniques with precise colors from histological images. MIAQuant aligns and measures a picture with contiguous (serialized) parts of the cloth, where the markers are covered with different colors so that the markers can be visually comparable. Its successful findings in biomedicine have inspired us to increase the capacity to communicate different marker positions and, finally, neighboring serialized pieces of tissue. Easy, efficient, and effective processing, pattern detection, and supervised teaching techniques with their improved framework, called MIAQuant-Learn [42], enable you to personalize marker segmentation by all colors.

The quality of HI is the parameter to determine that it can be the most remarkable approach for color normalization. Metrics of quality, such as the structural similarity index metric (SSIM), contains three factors (contrast, luminance, and structural) [43]. These parameters are given in Equations (1)–(3), respectively.

$$\mathrm{N}(\mathrm{x},\ \mathrm{y}) = \frac{2\,\sigma_x\,\sigma_y + c_2}{\sigma_x^2 + \sigma_y^2 + c_2} \tag{1}$$

$$\mathrm{M}\ (\mathrm{x},\ \mathrm{y}) = \frac{2\,\overline{X\,Y} + c_1}{\overline{X}^2 + \overline{Y}^2 + c_1^2} \tag{2}$$

$$\mathrm{R}\ (\mathrm{x},\ \mathrm{y}) = \frac{\sigma_{xy} + c_3}{\sigma_x\sigma_y + c_3} \tag{3}$$

where $\overline{X}$ and $\overline{Y}$ are means of origin and processed image, respectively. σ_x and σ_y are standard deviation, σ_{xy} is the correlation coefficient between the processed and the source image. c_1, c_2, and c_3 are constants that could stabilize SSIM if nearing a zero value. By using Equations (1)–(3), the SSIM is derived from Equation (4). The SSIM value is 0 to 1. The better approach is color normalization, when the value is near to 1.

$$\text{SSIM} = \left(\frac{2\,\overline{X}\,\overline{Y} + c_1}{\overline{X}^2 + \overline{Y}^2 + c_1^2}\right)\left(\frac{2\,\sigma_{xy} + c_2}{\sigma_x^2 + \sigma_y^2 + c_2}\right) \tag{4}$$

3.2. *Recognition and Segmentation of Structures*

One of the main tasks in HI analysis is image segmentation, and it has been applied to solve a wide variety of issues. Image segmentation, in its entirety, similar to clustering, is an unplaced issue as defining a meaningful segment can vary from task to task or even from image to image. For this purpose, the application domain must be aware of the segmentation algorithms, either by taking custom features or algorithmic methods into account or by learning from vast volumes of knowledge [44].

The existence of pathology and the number and the morphological features of detailed textures, such as nuclei and glans, are essential variables to analyze the existence and intensity of pathology—for example, colorectal [45], prostate [46], and breast [47] cancer.

3.2.1. Nuclei and Cells

Nuclei would be the main organelles of a eukaryotic cell, comprising the majority of cell DNA. Nuclei examination often requires recognition, segmentation, and separating overlaps. Recognition of seed factors in nuclei is needed by several segmentation and checking techniques [48]. Several methods had been proposed in the review for nuclei recognition, involving techniques predicted on Euclidean range chart peaks [49], Hough change (recognizing seed factors for circular formed textures, requesting extensive computation) [50], Laplacian of Gaussian filters [51], and radial symmetry [52]. Several methods were shown to represent accurate segmentation. The techniques based on thresholding and morphological procedures are appropriate on a standard background [53]. They may not, however, be powerful in measurement, form, and structure change. Effective shape forms could mix picture attributes with nuclei form types [54]. However, they depend on seed factors. Different techniques were predicated on gradients in polar [55] and graph reductions [56]. Ta et al. [53] suggested an approach, dependent on regularization graphs. The method's specificity was to utilize graphs as image confidential modeling at various grades (areas or pixels) and various component relations, such as grid graph. Dependent on Voronoi's diagrams, they suggested a graph reduction technique for nucleus segmentation of HIs for serious cytologic and breast cancer. A pseudo metric δ: $V \times V \to R$ is illustrated as

$$\delta(u, v) = \min_{\rho \in P_G(u,v)} \sum_{i=1}^{m-1} \sqrt{w(u_i,\, u_i + 1)}\,\left(f(u_i + 1) - f(u_i)\right) \tag{5}$$

where a weight function between two pixels is $w\ (u_i,\ u_i + 1)$, and a set of paths connecting two vertices is PG (u, v). Taking into account the set of K seeds $S = (s_i \subseteq V)$, where $i = 1, 2, \ldots, K$, the energy δ: $V \to R$ presented the metric δ for all the seeds of S, which can be presented as:

$$\delta_s(u) = \min_{s_i \in S} \delta(s_i, u), \qquad \forall_u \in V \tag{6}$$

The zone z of control (known as the Voronoi cell) of the seed $s_i \in S$ is the set of vertices nearer to s_i than any other seeds related to the metric δ. It can be defined, $\forall j = 1, 2, \ldots, K$ and $j \neq i$, as

$$z(s_i) = u \in V : \delta(s_i, u) \leq \delta(s_j,\, u) \tag{7}$$

Then, the energy distribution of the graph is the set of powerful zones $Z(S, \delta) = \{Z(s_i), \forall s_i \in S\}$, for a given set of seeds S and a metric δ.

3.2.2. Glands

It is organs that are shaped by an ingrowth from the epithelial surface. Techniques in thresholding and area growing could recognize nuclei and lumen, which can be applied to initial seed factors for area growing [57]. Segmentation predicated on polar ordinates (the middle of the gland) was performed on the benign and malign gland [48].

Rittscher et al. [58] caught some bright pixels participating in a standard distribution form. Their technique applied three features. The first was the intensity of fluorescent emission. The others were derived from curve descriptors, which could be calculated from eigenvalues of the Hessian matrix. The eigenvalues ($\lambda 1(x, y) \le \lambda 2(x, y)$) of the image $I(x, y)$ encode the curve data of the image. They give helpful cues for shape detection, such as structures of the membrane. However, the eigenvalues are influenced by the brightness of the image [6]. Equations (8) and (9) represent two features, which are autonomous from the image's brightness. These features are known as normalized-curve index and shape index, respectively.

$$\phi(x, y) = \tan^{-1} \frac{\sqrt{(\lambda_1 (x, y)^2 + \lambda_2 (x, y)^2)}}{I(x, y)} \tag{8}$$

$$\theta(x, y) = \tan 2(\lambda_1 (x, y), \lambda_2 (x, y)) \tag{9}$$

This segmentation, based on normalized-curve index and shape index divides an image's pixels into three sets: foreground, indefinite, and background. The indefinite set covers all of the pixels which are not involved in the other two sets. From these sets, the intensity distribution of foreground and background and log-likelihood intensity are derived.

3.3. Feature Extraction

HI was examined by applying several descriptors based on the information of domain experts. Analysis requirements are represented primarily with cytological phrases (i.e., glands, nuclei) and its involvement in the malignant and benign surface. Consequently, many papers dealt with the object stage (applying segmented item attributes) and object connection stage (applying structural attributes). Tumors, such as ductal carcinoma and lobular carcinoma, have an abnormal growth of epithelial cells in these structures. The abnormal growth of tissue, representing a tumor, may result in a large number of nucleus cells or a high number of mitotic cells in a small area. HI captures this function, but it captures other healthy tissues in addition to the nucleus, which can be seen in images of benign tumors. Stroma is a kind of tissue that can be seen in malignant and benign images with the same characteristics. The classification method could be enhanced by choosing more appropriate patches. Histopathological considerations remain paramount in this regard. There are well-known considerations, such as the size of the tumor, the histological shape and subtype, the nature of the sign, circular morphology and degree of differentiation, and the presence of vascular lymph invasion and the involvement of lymph nodes. We have gone from a greater understanding of these causes in recent years, identifying significant factors, such as tumor budding and lymphocytic infiltration. The prognostic importance of resection margins has also been assessed over the last two decades—particularly circumferential margins. Some patients are also notable with histological features associated with various molecular and genetic markers, including KRAS, BRAF, and microsatellite instability. The feature can be divided into literature level artifacts and structural features. Object-level characteristics are characteristics correlated with the nucleus size and shape. Features of the structure describe topological characteristics based on graph theory.

3.3.1. Object-Level Characteristics

Object-level characteristics rely firmly on regarded items (often gland or nuclei) and segmentation methods [6]. These characteristics are appropriate at any resolution. However, generally, they are produced by high-resolution pictures. Object-level characteristics were generally produced to each shade channel and could be collected into shape characteristics, such as region [59]. In the pre-segmentation procedure based on the unregulated medium-shift cluster, Kuse et al. [60] applied a feature extraction method. Thresholds limit the color variation to the image section. After this stage, the kernel is formed, and the contour and area constraints are removed from the overlap. Gray-level co-occurrence Matrix (GLCM) texture functions are finally extracted from a sectioned picture utilizing a classifier specified by support vector machines (SVM). Caicedo et al. [24] merged seven approaches of extraction of features and construct a kernel-based representation of data for each form of function. Inside the SVM classifier, kernels are used to find similarities between data and enforce a content retrieval mechanism.

3.3.2. Structural Characteristics

Structural characteristics are primarily based on graphs. They are comprised of nodes that can be linked by arcs. Lately, characteristics based on the graph were investigated frequently because they are suitable to characterize tumor structure. Three types of brain cancer classification (inflame, health, maligning) were conducted by Demir et al. [13]. They utilized a total weighted graph. Chekkoury et al. [61] made a hybrid between features based on texton and morphologic system to breast cancer. Doyle et al. [62] applied a mix of characteristics for prostate cancer. They show 90% precision in characterizing cancer and benign tissue. To handle the multi-resolution properties of HIs and emulate pathologists' approach to analytics, multi-resolution methods have been proposed. In many resolutions, the Gaussian pyramid method portrayed the pictures. Features for every level have been extracted separately and labeled as image tiles. Color and texture characteristics are typically utilized at low resolutions. The medium-scale architectural arrangement of glands and nuclei at high resolutions may be discriminatory.

3.4. Classification

Techniques for classifying their goal determine the group of recent observations between some classes based on marked training group. Regarding the function, anatomical composition, characteristics, and the preparation of tissue, the classification differs. DiFranco et al. [63] classified the prostate tissue into seven classes: benign hyperplasia, inflammation, Gleason rank 3 and 4, and intraepithelial neoplasia. They acquired 83% accuracy based on sum average, contrast, connected histogram characteristics, and entropy.

Huang et al. [64] proposed a method to enhance hepatocellular carcinoma classifying, which used a subset of feature selection with a support vector machine based on a decision graph for every decision node. Alexandratou et al. [65] presented a literature review for prostate cancer, illustrating good cancer recognition. The overview of conventional HI analysis methods is summarized in Table 1.

Table 1. Overview of HI analysis for different conventional methods.

Study	Organ	Method	Results	Problem with Method
Basavanhallya et al. [66]	Breast	Hierarchical Normalized cut	89% accuracy of segmentation	Discovers false-positive errors because of lumen presence.
Khadi [67]	Meningioma	Classification of texture applying fractal features	92.5% accuracy applying individual texture measurement to meningioma tissue	Misclassification results because of the non-uniformity cell construct.
Demir et al. [68]	Colon	Object graph approach for segmentation	87.59% accuracy of compatible images	Requires variable optimization that reduced results for segmentation
Tosum et al. [69]	Breast	Diagram run-length models to segmentation of the image	The novel descriptor of texture for unsupervised classification had 99.0% accuracy for gland segmentation	Complexity relies on the number of primitives in picture
Chekkoury et al. [61]	Breast	A novel hybrid between features based on texton and morphologic system	86% classification accuracy combining textural features and morphometric	The effects of image compression on classification accuracy
Doyle et al. [62]	Prostate	mix of characteristics	90% accuracy in characterizing cancer and benign tissue	Limited Feature Set
DiFranco et al. [63]	Prostate	classified into seven classes (benign hyperplasia, inflammation, Gleason rank 3,4, and intraepithelial neoplasia)	83% median accuracy based on some characteristics like sum average, contrast	The computation time required for reading and writing data to and from disk, particularly in feature extraction

4. Deep Learning Methods

Recently, DL techniques have often been studied in the effective form of ML methods. Within the last few years, DL techniques outperformed traditional ML methods in varied fields, such as CV, natural language processing (NLP), biomedical fields, and automated analysis for HI [7]. DL methods in the CV are derived from the structure levels for nonlinear transformations on natural input pixels. This structure formed significantly abstract representations, which could be realized in a hierarchical style [70]. A typical instance of a commonly applied structure is the CNN [71].

Multiple criteria can be considered when using the DL techniques to deal with histopathology, since accomplishing the method is partly due to the task-species setting. Among the principal features of HI is that appropriate styles be determined by the magnification stage. The key factors are the size of the patch given to the network, the localization of parts in the image where appropriate histopathology originals can be found, and the homogeneity of staining for WSI [72]. The network structure represents an important position, while many studies keep predefined system structures, as illustrated in Figure 4.

The majority of the DL techniques for localizing, classifying, and segmenting HI are somewhat recent. Deep neural techniques are stated in the new literature of HI analysis, such as [6,13,36]. For example, Irshad et al. [48] were the first mentioned in a review. The critical patterns from an exhaustive analysis of different nuclei identification, segmentation, and classification approaches utilized in HI, specifically in H&E staining protocols, were described and discussed in this review. Ciresan et al. [56] presented one of the first significant efforts to utilize the deep method in mitosis recognition for HI analysis. Arevalo et al. [73] presented a hybrid illustration method to the basal cell of carcinoma areas and utilized a topographic unsupervised technique and a case of characteristic illustrations. They increased the classifier's efficiency by 6% regarding traditional structure-based discrete cosine transform (DCT). Nayak et al. [74] presented an alternative method for the unsupervised Boltzmann technique for understanding image signatures. They classified images of the cancer genome atlas (TCGA) for apparent cell-kidney cancer and glioblastoma variform. The last stage was created utilizing the classifier of multi-class support vector machines (SVM) techniques.

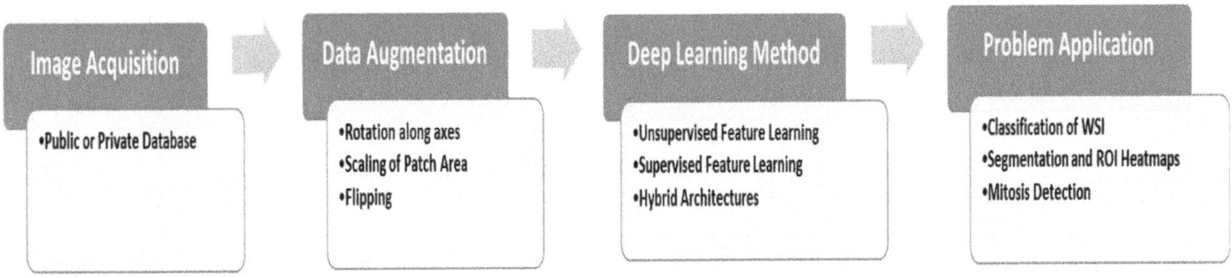

Figure 4. The typical deep learning steps for HI analysis.

Malon et al. [75] proposed a novel mix of features. The authors compiled a feature set of the fundamental nucleus and cytoplasm pixel statistical measurements and combined them with a CNN classifier. Their method increased the efficiency when comparing to the characteristics of handcrafted methods. Xu et al. [76] created an approach that handled marked cases. Numerous examples of the learning platform were presented in this technique, where the colon HI classifier was developed. The researchers presented a thoroughly supervised method and also weakly-marked one. Hou et al. [77] presented a similar strategy by applying numerous cases to understand how to categorize low-grade glioma and glioblastoma images in TCGA. The technique used three phases. First, it understood the masks of discriminative parts utilizing CNN form with few picked discriminative areas. It then created a patch level forecast, applying CNN. Finally, the counting of the class was generated.

Arevalo et al. [78] proposed a stacked form that revealed the most significant features when mixing characteristics from two-layered topographic independent component analysis (TICA) around patches for finding basal cell cancer. They presented an electronic discoloration technique because characteristic detectors are weighed with classification likelihood to spotlight parts, which can be most linked to carcinoma. This technique accomplished 99% of the area under the curve (AUC) for 100,000 patches. Hang et al. [79] were dependent on the understanding book of 1024 characteristics to classify apparent cell cancer and also glioblastoma multiforme. The book was constructed with a stacked unsupervised technique utilized in the spatial chart corresponding platform with the SVM classifier's final step. Some new studies were interested in the classifying of the H&E patch. Han et al. [80] provided a novel deep unsupervised technique for glioblastoma multiforme characterization. They can distinguish two critical phenotypic subtypes at various survival shapes, utilizing the produced unsupervised characteristics. Noel et al. [81] applied a group of 30,000 patches produced from the WSI of the International Conference on Pattern Recognition (ICPR) contest to recognize breast carcinoma, categorizing every pixel utilizing CNN mitosis, stoma, and lymphocytes. They reached 90% accuracy, indicating a better WSI primitive classifier, which could enhance classification performance.

Romo-Bucheli et al. [82] served a CNN form with prospect patches for calculating tubule associateship likelihood to measure tubule nuclei, which was related to high–low chance classes decided by the Oncotype DX test. DL stains' application distinctive from H&E continues to be not adequately researched, such as immunohistochemistry. Chen et al. [83] presented the recognition of immune cells using seven-layer CNN with areas of nature colors from RGB channels, displaying markers of immune cells. They compared the efficiency of their recognition method with pathologists' efficiency, attaining a 99% correlation coefficient. A review of deep-neural models, developed for HI analysis, was presented by Srinidhi et al. [84].

Sumi et al. [85] proposed a deep spatial fusion network that manages the dynamic construction of discriminative characteristics over patches. In the high-resolution histology picture, it also learns to change the bias on patch-wise prediction. To extract characteristics from the cellular level to the tissue level, Patch wise InceptionResNetV2 is used. This approach is used to analyze the spatial interaction between patches. Compared to previous CNN experiments using different architectures, better performance is given by their proposed system. This work needs to be expanded to include other networks that effectively examine more malignant tumor types other than glioblastoma and oligodendroglioma. Maximal tumor resection is especially necessary for larynx surgery, thus maintaining adjacent healthy tissue. Therefore, accurate and swift intraoperative laryngeal histology is vital for optimal surgery results. Zhang et al. [86] hypothesized a DL stimulation of Raman scattering microscopy (SRS) that could automatically and precisely diagnose new, unprocessed surgical specimens with laryngeal squamous cell cancer without fastening, separation or staining. First, they compared 80 pairs of adjacent SRS and regular frozen parts to determine their concordance. They then applied SRS imaging to 45 patients' fresh chirurgical tissues based upon a DL model for automatically producing histologic results. They also applied the main diagnostic features.

Pathology's scientific function is to diagnose diseases to classify differences at cell structures level, such as nucleolus and cytoplasm, tissue (i.e., cell community with complicated structures), and organs that give rise to patient symptoms. It was found that damaged or unresolved cells do not die, and uncontrolled growth is seen by clinical pathology framework and histopathology methods, explaining cancer cells' mass production. Cancer cells also migrate through the blood and lymph systems and cross borders to another body area, reproducing the uncontrolled growth cycle method. This cancer cell phase is called metastatic spreading or metastasis that leaves one area and grows in another part of the body. Breast cancer could be detected by a histopathological methodology. This diagnosis can be made using different ML Models, and DL-based CNN Models. Agarwal et al. [87] showed that CNN models provided significant accurate results in the comparison of ML models, such as U-Net [88], improved precision, and high-performance segmentation. In conjunction with very low-cost consumer graphics processing units, large images can therefore be processed rapidly.

Approaches that rely on Generative Adversarial Networks (GANs) are likely to minimize the need for large volumes of manual notations. Not only have recent innovations enhanced initiatives but so have new technologies. Now, unattended techniques may carry out various tasks for which supervised methods are indispensable. The latest state-of-the-art advances in histopathological images of GANs were summarized in [89]. The overview of the discussed studies is summarized in Table 2.

Table 2. Overview of supervised and unsupervised learning models based on DL techniques.

Study	Organ	Staining	Potential Usage	Method
		Supervised Learning		
Litjens et al. [90]	different tissue	H&E	Prostate and breast carcinoma detection	Convolutional Neural Network based on pixel classifier
Nagpal et al. [91]	Prostate	H&E	Anticipating Gleason indicator	CNN based on sectional Gleason model classifier + k-nearst neighbors (KNN) based on Gleason grade anticipation
Zhao et al. [92]	Breast	H&E	Metastasis Detection + classification	Characteristic pyramid collecting based on the fully convolutional network (FCN) system with the synergistic training technique

Table 2. *Cont.*

Study	Organ	Staining	Potential Usage	Method
Xing et al. [93]	different tissue	H&E, Immunohistochemistry (IHC)	Segmentation of nuclei	CNN + selection based on sparse form Pattern
Gu et al. [94]	Breast	H&E	Tumor detection	U-Net based on multiple resolution model with multiple encoders and a singular decoder system
Tellez et al. [95]	Breast	H&E	Detection of Mitosis	Train of Convolutional Network applying H&E registered to PHH3 slides as a reference
Wei et al. [96]	Lung	H&E	Histological subtypes of lung gland classifier	ResNet-18 on the basis of patch classification
Song et al. [97]	Cervix	Papanicolaou (Pap), H&E	Cells Segmentation	Multiple level CNN system
Agarwalla et al. [98]	Breast	H&E	Segmentation of tumor	CNN and 2D- Long short-term memory (LSTM) to representing training and context collecting
Ding et al. [99]	Colon	H&E	Glands segmentation	Multiple level FCN network with a high-resolution section to avoid the lost in highest pooling layers
Bejnordi et al. [100]	Breast	H&E	Invasive Carcinoma detection	Multiple level CNN which first determines tumor-associated stromal modifications and more categorize into normal/benign versus invasive carcinoma
Seth et al. [101]	Breast	H&E	Ductal carcinoma in-situ (DCIS) segmentation	Compared UNets learned in many resolutions
		Unsupervised Learning		
Xu et al. [102]	Breast	H&E	Segmentation of nuclei	Stacked sparse autoencoders
Bulten and Litjens [103]	Prostate	H&E	Tumor classification	Convolutional adversarial Autoencoders
Hou et al. [104]	Breast	H&E	Segmentation and detection of nuclei	Sparse autoencoder
Sari and Gunduz-Demir [105]	Colon	H&E	Feature extraction and classification	Restricted Boltzmann + clustering
Gadermayr et al. [106]	Kidney	Stain agnostic	Object of interest segmentation in WSIs	CycleGAN + UNet segmentation
Gadermayr et al. [107]	Kidney	Periodic acid–Schiff (PAS), H&E	Glomeruli segmentation	CycleGAN

5. Datasets

The size of the datasets given to researchers for training and testing their methods has dramatically increased in the latest challenges. There is a set of public databases in the electronic pathology subject that include manual annotations for HI, as listed in Tables 3 and 4 [108]. They might help the examination objectively. Slide issue (stain) and image issue (image resolution, zoom level) are similar. However, all these databases are targeted to specific diseases. These databases do not handle several tasks. Additionally, there are many high scale HI datasets, which include WSIs of high resolutions.

TCGA [33] includes around 10,000 images from different types of cancer. Genotype-Tissue Expression (GTE) [109] includes around 20,000 WSIs from different tissues. The Stanford Tissue Microarray Database (TMAD) is available for researchers to access images of microarrays for tissue. It provides images of archiving 349 distinguished probes on 1488 microarray slides of tissue [110]. The CAMELYON dataset is a collection of WSI tissues for the sentinel lymph node. It contains CAMELYON16 and CAMELYON17 challenges that include 399 WSI and 1000 WSI, respectively. The data are currently accessed via registration on the CAMELYON17 website [111]. The Breast Cancer Histopathological Image (BreakHis) contains 9109 macroscopic images for the tissue of the breast tumor obtained from 82 patients in various magnifying factors (40X, 100X, 200X). Up to now, it includes samples of 2480 benign and 5429 malignant WSIs [112].

Table 3. Some common downloadable WSI databases.

Datasets	No Slides	Staining	Diseases
TCGA [33,113]	18,462	H&E	Cancer
GTE [109]	25,380	H&E	Normal
TMAD [110,114]	3726	H&E/IHC	various tissue
TUPAC16 [115]	821 from TCGA	H&E	Breast cancer
Camelyon17 [111]	1000	H&E	Breast cancer (lymph node metastasis)
Köbel et al. [116,117]	80	H&E	Ovarian carcinoma
KIMIA Path24 [118]	24	H&E/IHC	various tissue

Table 4. Some publicly available hand-annotated histopathological images.

Datasets	No of Images	Staining	Organs	Potential Usage
KIMIA960 [119,120]	960	H&E/IHC	Different tissue	Classification
Bio-segmentation [121,122]	58	H&E	Breast	Classification
Bioimaging challenge 2015 [123]	269	H&E	Breast	Classification
GlaS [124]	165	H&E	Colorectal	Gland segmentation
BreakHis [112]	7909	H&E	Breast	Classification
Jakob Nikolas et al. [120,125]	100	IHC	Colorectal	Detection of blood vessel
MITOS-ATYPIA-14 [126]	4240	H&E	Breast	Detection of mitosis, classification
Kumar et al. [119,127]	30	H&E	Different cancer	Segmentation of Nuclear
MITOS [20]	100	H&E	Breast	Detection of mitosis
Janowczyk et al. [128,129]	374	H&E	Lymphoma	classification
Janowczyk et al. [128,129]	85	H&E	Colorectal	Segmentation of gland
Ma et al. [130]	81	IHC	Breast	TIL analysis
Linder et al. [131,132]	1377	IHC	Colorectal	Segmentation of epithelium and stroma

6. Discussion and Histopathological Tasks

Since HI analysis is inherently a cross-disciplinary area, this review has stated that ongoing research is anticipated to have an obvious and tangible impact on automated HI analysis techniques. This paper reviews the recent state of the art CAD techniques for HI. This review also briefly describes the development of histopathology analysis and its problems. Recently, DL outperformed state-of-the-art techniques in various MLs for HI analysis tasks, such as recognition, classification, and segmentation. DL's merit, compared to other forms of learners, is their ability to acquire the performance as well or better than a human's performance. Currently, DL and WSI are revolutionizing the CAD of histopathology, and soon they could help reduce pathologists' workload in most simple tasks. This would allow pathologists to focus on challenging cases and lead to a deeper comprehension of pathologic procedures via ML techniques. More applications of HI analysis using ML techniques have been introduced in this review [108]. Most of the research developed in the field of HI analysis is addressed for some specific tasks.

Tasks for Histopathology Image

Open objective problems targeting issues in HI analysis were presented recently, such as in other medicinal imaging fields. A benefit of trying various methods on an unchanging dataset and in exact issues is the target comparison of advantages and constraints of literature methods. Especially in a sample of pathology, consuming time, and challenging issues of searching WSIs for appropriate tissue basics, such as nuclei and mitosis, could be enhanced. Choosing the most appropriate method to aid and advance the visible model of slides could help pathologists concentrate on significant issues when analyzing the mentioned studies. The difficulty of issues has improved recently. The objectives of problems could be gathered into three major issues, as shown in Figure 5.

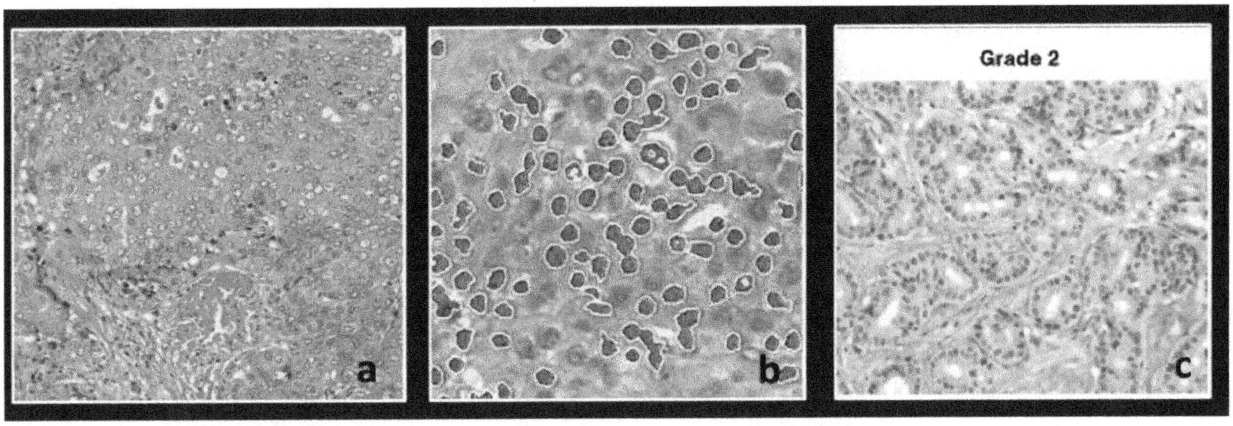

Figure 5. Challenges of HI analysis: (**a**) Mitosis detection, (**b**) Segmentation, and (**c**) Grade classification of a tumor.

- **Recognition of Mitosis**

Recognize mitosis contained in large power domains: There is a powerful relationship with the aggression of carcinoma and faster cell separation in extra mitosis. An essential part of HI tasks is the proper selection of evaluation metrics. A task of mitosis recognition utilizes the F1-score as the best metric to evaluate the participant techniques. The F1-score is calculated using Equation (10).

$$\text{F1-score} = \frac{2\ .precision\ .\ recall}{precision + recall} \tag{10}$$

where Precision = TP/(TP + FP) and Recall = TP/(TP + FN). The threshold of maximum Euclidean distance from centroid for considering the mitotic event, as TP, was estimated to less than 7.5–8 μm.

- **Segmentation of structure**

The segmentation process localized and outlined the border of particular tissue architectures—for example, nuclei of cell or gland. Various kinds of tissue structures have been aimed to structure segmentation in HI. Automatic segmentation system output is typically evaluated by measuring some standard objective parameters, such as the mean boundary distance, the Dice coefficient, and Hausdorff Distance (HD). HD is one of the most insightful and useful metrics, since it measures the greatest segmentation error. For the two datasets, X and Y, the one-sided HD from X to Y is defined as:

$$\text{hd}\ (X;\ Y) = \max_{x \in X} \min_{y \in Y} \|x - y\|2 \quad (11)$$

and similarly, for hd (Y; X):

$$\text{hd}\ (Y;\ X) = \max_{y \in Y} \min_{x \in X} \|x - y\|2 \quad (12)$$

The bidirectional HD between these two sets is then:

$$\text{HD}\ (X;\ Y) = max(hd(X,Y), hd(Y,X)) \quad (13)$$

- **Classification of images**

First, one must find the characteristic set of features for a specific class of tissue, potentially taking into account the primitives of the underlying tissue. In histopathology, various evaluation techniques for ranking the classifications methods have been used. Various evaluation methods for rating the classification methods include

- For nuclear atypia rating, a points-based scheme is used.
- The region under the curve of the receiver operating characteristic (ROC) to classify slides of lymph node comprising metastasis or not.
- Approval with ground truth calculated with Spearman's correlation or quadratic weighted Cohen's kappa to grade cancer.

Equation (14) is used to calculate quadratic weighted Cohen's kappa.

$$K_w = 1 - \frac{\sum_{i,j} w_{i,j}\, p_{i,j}}{\sum_{i,j} w_{i,j}\, e_{i,j}} \quad (14)$$

$$e_{i,j} = p_{i,j} q_{i,j} \quad (15)$$

where $w_{i,j}$ represent weights, $p_{i,j}$ observed probabilities, and $q_{i,j}$ expected probabilities [133]. Though these issues were split into various sets due to their explanation, they could be mixed or regarded as a preliminary phase to another issue. For example, the WSI grading technique of carcinoma could begin by classifying the image as a tumor tissue. Next, the carcinoma was segmented. Finally, grade WSI dependent on the count of mitosis in the ROI of cancer.

7. Limitations and Future Trends

Digital HI recognition is an appropriate issue for ML because pictures themselves include data adequate for diagnosis. Issues in the analysis of digital HI applying ML is mentioned in this review. Because of reasonable efforts produced up to now, these issues being overcome, but there is space for enhancement. Many of these issues are probably resolved when a large amount of well annotated WSIs becomes obtainable. Collecting WSIs from different institutions to note them the exact conditions and creating this information public will be adequate to improve the growth of more advanced electronic HI analysis. Lastly, some possible future issues for the study are recommended, which have not been adequately researched.

- **Novel Objects Discovery**

For instance, unexpected items, irregular organization, uncommon tumor (not contained in the training stage), and aliens' bodies might exist in real diagnostic conditions. However, one can use a discrimination framework containing CNN classes, such as items among the predefined classes [134]. To solve the issue, the recognitions of outlier approaches were applied to HI. However, just a few studies have handled the issue up to now [135]. Recently, some DL-based techniques applied reconstruction error for recognition of outliers in other fields. However, they are not yet used in HI analysis.

- **Interpretable DL Model**

DL is usually disapproved of, since its decision-making process is not clear to individuals and thus frequently explained like a black box. People need to know the process of decision making or the basis of the decision. This might cause new findings in the domain of pathology. Even though this issue has not been fully resolved, some studies have tried to supply solutions, such as combined pathological pictures learning and diagnostic studies incorporated with interesting mechanisms [136]. In other fields, the basis of the decision might be ultimately displayed by visualizing the reaction of the deep network [137] or introducing a useful training picture applying impact functions [138].

- **Intraoperative Diagnosis**

Diagnosis by the pathologist during surgery impacts intraoperative decision making. Therefore, it might be another actual application in HI analysis. Because diagnosis time in an intraoperative examination is limited, a quick classifier while maintaining precision is significant. As a result of time limitation, the quick-freezing part is utilized rather than the formalin-fixed paraffin-embedded part that requires more time to get ready. Thus, for this reason, classification training must be executed, applying freezing part slides. Since the amount of appropriate WSI for analysis is not adequate, and function is more complicated than formalin-fixed paraffin-embedded slides, few studies have analyzed freezing parts [139].

- **Tumor-Infiltrating Immune Cell Analysis**

The microenvironment of carcinoma for immune cells has acquired significant interest recently. Thus, quantitative analysis for the carcinoma permeating of immune cells for slides applying ML methods is going to be among the emerging styles in HI analysis. Functions connected to analysis contain immune cell recognition in the H&E staining picture [140,141] and are recognized as a more specific form of immune cells applying immunohistochemistry [130]. Additionally, the structure of immune cell permeation and immune cell vicinity are supposedly linked to tumor treatment [142], spatial association analysis among immune cells and cells of cancer, and the association among this information and reaction to immunotherapy applying specific techniques, such as methods based on the graph [143], is likewise of good importance.

- **Challenges in HI analysis**

Typical DL architectures need their inputs in a particular structure with specific spatial dimensions. Moreover, these architectures are usually created for RGB pictures, while in digital HI, dealing with pictures in grayscale, HSV color might be desired for a particular system. Transforming pictures between color spaces, resizing pictures to suit GPU's storage, and determining the most effective resolution for applying at tilling are a few of the possible studies required, which will cause various levels of data loss. An acceptable information processing technique seeks to accomplish minimal data loss while using architectures for their maximal capacity. Input images are likely tiled or resized in most applications. It is also essential to balance the appropriate contexts and magnification with memory and computational constraints. Since CNN's can learn from smaller images more easily, images are not larger than the necessary context. A large amount of work was done to integrate low- and high-resolution inputs in different ways and issues to make better decisions [144].

- **Quality of training**

DL's accomplishment depends on the accessibility to high-quality training models to accomplish the required predictive efficiency [145,146]. Some efforts have been built to create extra annotated information by utilizing alternative methods, such as information augmentation [147], picture synthesis [104]. However, it is not even apparent that they are befitting from digital pathology.

- **Clinical translation**

There is a huge rapid development in AI research used in MI, and their possible effect has been shown by systems including the recognition of breast cancer metastasis [148], brain recognition [149], diagnosing diseases in retinal pictures [150], and so on. Regardless of this variety of systems, AI's actual and impactful implementation in medical practice will include many methods still to come.

- **Synthesis rather than marking**

An issue is that mapping of the label to the image domain is often unclear because the label mask can be mapped to many images. The training of the entire Generative Adversarial Network architecture can be difficult. The sizes of the regions-of-interest are given complexity here. Regions can display a diameter of up to several hundred pixels or thousands. This can be a big challenge, as the segmentation networks are implemented patch-wise.

- **Translation of morphology**

The optimal architecture for modified morphology settings does not show. Usually, unclear mappings can be particularly problematic in the event of morphological changes.

8. Conclusions

Different steps to analyze HIs are studied in this review for objective diagnosis automatically. In this survey, a comprehensive overview of different strategies in traditional and DL models has been presented. Different perspectives have tackled the analysis of HI for a wide variety of histology tasks (e.g., segmentation, tumor recognition, tissue classification). We have identified those that have been applied to various types of cancer (e.g., breast, kidney, colon, lung). For CAD in HI, there are primarily three phases: segmentation, feature extraction, and classification. The techniques developed for automatic analysis and evaluation of HIs help the pathologists in objective diagnosis for disease and decreased human error. A reference guide to recent literature methods for analyzing HIs manifests itself in the categorization techniques presented in this survey.

Author Contributions: Conceptualization, N.E. and M.E.; methodology, N.E., H.S., and M.E.; formal analysis, N.E. and M.E.; investigation, N.E., H.S., S.E.-S., S.M.R.I., and M.E.; writing—original draft preparation, N.E., H.S., and M.E.; writing—review and editing, N.E., H.S., S.E.-S., S.M.R.I., and M.E.; supervision, H.S. and M.E.; project administration, M.E. All authors have read and agreed to the published version of the manuscript.

References

1. Litjens, G.; Kooi, T.; Bejnordi, B.E.; Setio, A.A.A.; Ciompi, F.; Ghafoorian, M.; van der Laak, J.A.; van Ginneken, B.; Sanchez, I.C. A survey on deep learning in medical image analysis. *Med. Image Anal.* **2017**, *42*, 60–88. [CrossRef]
2. Ker, J.; Wang, L.; Rao, J.; Lim, T. Deep Learning Applications in Medical Image Analysis. *IEEE Access* **2017**, *6*, 9375–9389. [CrossRef]
3. Perez, H.; Tah, J. Improving the Accuracy of Convolutional Neural Networks by Identifying and Removing Outlier Images in Datasets Using t-SNE. *Mathematics* **2020**, *8*, 662. [CrossRef]

4. Suzuki, K. Overview of deep learning in medical imaging. *Radiol. Phys. Technol.* **2017**, *10*, 257–273. [CrossRef]
5. Pantanowitz, L. Digital images and the future of digital pathology. *J. Pathol. Inform.* **2010**, *1*. [CrossRef]
6. Gurcan, M.N.; Boucheron, L.E.; Can, A.; Madabhushi, A.; Rajpoot, N.M.; Yener, B. Histopathological image analysis: A review. *IEEE Rev. Biomed. Eng.* **2009**, *2*, 147–171. [CrossRef]
7. Greenspan, H.; Ginneken, B.; van Summers, R.M. Guest Editorial Deep Learning in Medical Imaging: Overview and Future Promise of an Exciting New Technique. *IEEE Trans Med. Imaging* **2016**, *35*, 1153–1159. [CrossRef]
8. Rubin, R.; Strayer, D.S.; Rubin, E. *Rubin's Pathology: Clinicopathologic Foundations of Medicine*; Lippincott Williams & Wilkins: Philadelphia, PA, USA, 2008.
9. Hewitson, T.; Darby, I.; Walker, J. Histology Protocols. In *Methods in Molecular Biology*; Humana Press: Totowa, NJ, USA, 2010.
10. Li, C.; Chen, H.; Li, X.; Xu, N.; Hu, Z.; Xue, D.; Qi, S.; Ma, H.; Zhang, L.; Sun, H. A review for cervical histopathology image analysis using machine vision approaches. *Artif. Intell. Rev.* **2020**, *53*, 4821–4862. [CrossRef]
11. He, L.; Long, L.R.; Antani, S.; Thoma, G.R. Histology image analysis for carcinoma detection and grading. *Comput. Methods Programs Biomed.* **2012**, *107*, 538–556. [CrossRef]
12. Ghaznavi, F.; Evans, A.; Madabhushi, A.; Feldman, M. Digital Imaging in Pathology: Whole-Slide Imaging and Beyond. *Annu. Rev. Pathol. Mech. Dis.* **2013**, *8*, 331–359. [CrossRef]
13. Demir, C.; Yener, B. *Automated Cancer Diagnosis Based on Histopathological Images: A Systematic Survey*; Technical Report for Rensselaer Polytechnic Institute: New York, NY, USA, 2005.
14. Belsare, A. Histopathological Image Analysis Using Image Processing Techniques: An Overview. *Signal Image Process. Int. J.* **2012**, *3*, 23–36. [CrossRef]
15. Spanhol, F.A.; Oliveira, L.S.; Petitjean, C.; Heutte, L. Breast cancer histopathological image classification using Convolutional Neural Networks. In Proceedings of the 2016 International Joint Conference on Neural Networks (IJCNN), Vancouver, BC, Canada, 24–29 January 2016; Institute of Electrical and Electronics Engineers (IEEE): Piscataway, NJ, USA, 2016; pp. 2560–2567.
16. Kieffer, B.; Babaie, M.; Kalra, S.; Tizhoosh, H.R. Convolutional neural networks for histopathology image classification: Training vs. using pre-trained networks. Proceeding of the 2017 Seventh International Conference on Image Processing Theory, Tools, and Applications (IPTA), Montreal, QC, Canada, 28 November–1 December 2017; IEEE: Piscataway, NJ, USA, 2017; pp. 1–6.
17. Mungle, T.; Tewary, S.; Das, D.; Arun, I.; Basak, B.; Agarwal, S.; Ahmed, R.; Chatterjee, S.; Chakraborty, C. MRF-ANN: A machine learning approach for automated ER scoring of breast cancer immunohistochemical images. *J. Microsc.* **2017**, *267*, 117–129. [CrossRef]
18. Sheikhzadeh, F.; Ward, R.K.; van Niekerk, D.; Guillaud, M. Automatic labeling of molecular biomarkers of immunohistochemistry images using fully convolutional networks. *PLoS ONE* **2018**, *13*, e0190783. [CrossRef]
19. Wang, D.; Foran, D.J.; Ren, J.; Zhong, H.; Kim, I.Y.; Qi, X. Exploring automatic prostate histopathology image gleason grading via local structure modeling. In Proceedings of the 2015 37th Annual International Conference of the IEEE Engineering in Medicine and Biology Society (EMBC), Milan, Italy, 25–29 August 2015; Institute of Electrical and Electronics Engineers (IEEE): Piscataway, NJ, USA, 2015; Volume 2015, pp. 2649–2652.
20. Roux, L.; Racoceanu, D.; Loménie, N.; Kulikova, M.; Irshad, H.; Klossa, J.; Capron, F.; Genestie, C.; Le Naour, G.; Gurcan, M.N. Mitosis detection in breast cancer histological images An ICPR 2012 contest. *J. Pathol. Inform.* **2013**, *4*, 8. [CrossRef]
21. Shah, M.; Wang, D.; Rubadue, C.; Suster, D.; Beck, A. Deep learning assessment of tumor proliferation in breast cancer histological images. In Proceedings of the 2017 IEEE International Conference on Bioinformatics and Biomedicine (BIBM), Kansas City, MO, USA, 13–16 November 2017; Institute of Electrical and Electronics Engineers (IEEE): Piscataway, NJ, USA, 2017; pp. 600–603.
22. Chen, H.; Qi, X.; Yu, L.; Heng, P.-A. DCAN: Deep Contour-Aware Networks for Accurate Gland Segmentation. In Proceedings of the 2016 IEEE Conference on Computer Vision and Pattern Recognition (CVPR), Las Vegas, NV, USA, 27–30 June 2016; Institute of Electrical and Electronics Engineers (IEEE): Piscataway, NJ, USA, 2016; pp. 2487–2496.

23. Gertych, A.; Ing, N.; Ma, Z.; Fuchs, T.J.; Salman, S.; Mohanty, S.; Bhele, S.; Velásquez-Vacca, A.; Amin, M.B.; Knudsen, B.S. Machine learning approaches to analyze histological images of tissues from radical prostatectomies. *Comput. Med. Imaging Graph.* **2015**, *46*, 197–208. [CrossRef]
24. Caicedo, J.C.; González, F.A.; Romero, E. Content-based histopathology image retrieval using a kernel-based semantic annotation framework. *J. Biomed. Inform.* **2011**, *44*, 519–528. [CrossRef]
25. Caie, P.D.; Turnbull, A.K.; Farrington, S.M.; Oniscu, A.; Harrison, D.J. Quantification of tumour budding, lymphatic vessel density and invasion through image analysis in colorectal cancer. *J. Transl. Med.* **2014**, *12*, 156. [CrossRef]
26. Sirinukunwattana, K.; Pluim, J.P.; Chen, H.; Qi, X.; Heng, P.-A.; Guo, Y.B.; Wang, L.Y.; Matuszewski, B.J.; Bruni, E.; Sanchez, U.; et al. Gland segmentation in colon histology images: The glas challenge contest. *Med. Image Anal.* **2017**, *35*, 489–502. [CrossRef]
27. Qi, X.; Wang, D.; Rodero, I.; Diaz-Montes, J.; Gensure, R.H.; Xing, F.; Zhong, H.; Goodell, L.; Parashar, M.; Foran, D.J.; et al. Content-based histopathology image retrieval using CometCloud. *BMC Bioinform.* **2014**, *15*, 1–17. [CrossRef]
28. Sparks, R.; Madabhushi, A. Out-of-Sample Extrapolation utilizing Semi-Supervised Manifold Learning (OSE-SSL): Content Based Image Retrieval for Histopathology Images. *Sci. Rep.* **2016**, *6*, 27306. [CrossRef]
29. Sridhar, A.; Doyle, S.; Madabhushi, A. Content-based image retrieval of digitized histopathology in boosted spectrally embedded spaces. *J. Pathol. Inform.* **2015**, *6*. [CrossRef]
30. Vanegas, J.A.; Arevalo, J.; González, F.A. Unsupervised feature learning for content-based histopathology image retrieval. In *2014 12th International Workshop on Content-Based Multimedia Indexing (CBMI), Klagenfurt, Austria, 18–20 June 2014*; Institute of Electrical and Electronics Engineers (IEEE): Piscataway, NJ, USA, 2014; pp. 1–6.
31. Zhang, X.; Liu, W.; Dundar, M.; Badve, S.; Zhang, S. Towards Large-Scale Histopathological Image Analysis: Hashing-Based Image Retrieval. *IEEE Trans. Med. Imaging* **2014**, *34*, 496–506. [CrossRef]
32. Flahou, B.; Haesebrouck, F.; Smet, A. Non-Helicobacter pylori Helicobacter Infections in Humans and Animals. In *Helicobacter Pylori Research*; Springer: Tokyo, Japan, 2016; pp. 233–269. [CrossRef]
33. Weinstein, J.N.; Collisson, E.A.; Mills, G.B.; Shaw, K.R.M.; Ozenberger, B.A.; Ellrott, K.; Shmulevich, I.; Sander, C.; Stuart, J.M. The Cancer Genome Atlas Pan-Cancer analysis project. *Nat. Genet.* **2013**, *45*, 1113–1120. [CrossRef]
34. Molin, M.D.; Matthaei, H.; Wu, J.; Blackford, A.; Debeljak, M.; Rezaee, N.; Wolfgang, C.L.; Butturini, G.; Salvia, R.; Bassi, C.; et al. Clinicopathological Correlates of Activating GNAS Mutations in Intraductal Papillary Mucinous Neoplasm (IPMN) of the Pancreas. *Ann. Surg. Oncol.* **2013**, *20*, 3802–3808. [CrossRef]
35. Yoshida, A.; Tsuta, K.; Nakamura, H.; Kohno, T.; Takahashi, F.; Asamura, H.; Sekine, I.; Fukayama, M.; Shibata, T.; Furuta, K.; et al. Comprehensive Histologic Analysis of ALK-Rearranged Lung Carcinomas. *Am. J. Surg. Pathol.* **2011**, *35*, 1226–1234. [CrossRef]
36. Arevalo, J.; Cruz-Roa, A. Histopathology image representation for automatic analysis: A state-of-the-art review. *Rev. Med.* **2014**, *22*, 79–91. [CrossRef]
37. Lyon, H.O.; de Leenheer, A.P.; Horobin, R.W.; Lambert, W.E.; Schulte, E.K.W.; van Liedekerke, B.; Wittekind, D.H. Standardization of reagents and methods used in cytological and histological practice with emphasis on dyes, stains and chromogenic reagents. *J. Mol. Histol.* **1994**, *26*, 533–544. [CrossRef]
38. Khan, A.M.; Rajpoot, N.; Treanor, D.; Magee, D. A Nonlinear Mapping Approach to Stain Normalization in Digital Histopathology Images Using Image-Specific Color Deconvolution. *IEEE Trans. Biomed. Eng.* **2014**, *61*, 1729–1738. [CrossRef]
39. Anghel, A.; Stanisavljevic, M.; Andani, S.; Papandreou, N.; Rüschoff, J.H.; Wild, P.; Gabrani, M.; Pozidis, H. A High-Performance System for Robust Stain Normalization of Whole-Slide Images in Histopathology. *Front. Med.* **2019**, *6*. [CrossRef]
40. Can, A.; Bello, M.; Cline, H.E.; Tao, X.; Ginty, F.; Sood, A.; Gerdes, M.; Montalto, M. Multi-modal imaging of histological tissue sections. In Proceedings of the 2008 5th IEEE International Symposium on Biomedical Imaging: From Nano to Macro, Paris, France, 14–18 May 2008; IEEE: Piscataway, NJ, USA, 2008; pp. 288–291. [CrossRef]
41. Casiraghi, E.; Cossa, M.; Huber, V.; Tozzi, M.; Rivoltini, L.; Villa, A.; Vergani, B. MIAQuant, a novel system for automatic segmentation, measurement, and localization comparison of different biomarkers from serialized histological slices. *Eur. J. Histochem.* **2017**, *61*, 61. [CrossRef]

42. Casiraghi, E.; Huber, V.; Frasca, M.; Cossa, M.; Tozzi, M.; Rivoltini, L.; Leone, B.E.; Villa, A.; Vergani, B. A novel computational method for automatic segmentation, quantification and comparative analysis of immunohistochemically labeled tissue sections. *BMC Bioinform.* **2018**, *19*, 357–397. [CrossRef]
43. Roy, S.; Jain, A.K.; Lal, S.; Kini, J. A study about color normalization methods for histopathology images. *Micron* **2018**, *114*, 42–61. [CrossRef]
44. Mărginean, R.; Andreica, A.; Dioşan, L.; Bálint, Z. Feasibility of Automatic Seed Generation Applied to Cardiac MRI Image Analysis. *Mathematics* **2020**, *8*, 1511. [CrossRef]
45. Gleason, D.F. Histologic grading of prostate cancer: A perspective. *Hum. Pathol.* **1992**, *23*, 273–279. [CrossRef]
46. Kong, J.; Sertel, O.; Shimada, H.; Boyer, K.L.; Saltz, J.H.; Gurcan, M.N. Computer-aided evaluation of neuroblastoma on whole-slide histology images: Classifying grade of neuroblastic differentiation. *Pattern Recognit.* **2009**, *42*, 1080–1092. [CrossRef]
47. Washington, K.; Berlin, J.; Branton, P.; Burgart, L.J.; Carter, D.K.; Fitzgibbons, P.L.; Halling, K.; Frankel, W.; Jessup, J.; Kakar, S.; et al. Protocol for the examination of specimens from patients with primary carcinoma of the colon and rectum. *Arch. Pathol. Lab. Med.* **2009**, *133*, 1539–1551. [CrossRef]
48. Irshad, H.; Veillard, A.; Roux, L.; Racoceanu, D. Methods for Nuclei Detection, Segmentation, and Classification in Digital Histopathology: A Review—Current Status and Future Potential. *IEEE Rev. Biomed. Eng.* **2013**, *7*, 97–114. [CrossRef]
49. Dalle, J.-R.; Li, H.; Huang, C.-H.; Leow, W.K.; Racoceanu, D.; Putti, T. Nuclear pleomorphism scoring by selective cell nuclei detection. In Proceedings of the Workshop on Applications of Computer Vision, Snowbird, UT, USA, 7–8 December 2009.
50. Wahlby, C.; Sintorn, I.-M.; Erlandsson, F.; Borgefors, G.; Bengtsson, E. Combining intensity, edge and shape information for 2D and 3D segmentation of cell nuclei in tissue sections. *J. Microsc.* **2004**, *215*, 67–76. [CrossRef]
51. Jung, C.; Kim, C. Segmenting Clustered Nuclei Using H-minima Transform-Based Marker Extraction and Contour Parameterization. *IEEE Trans. Biomed. Eng.* **2010**, *57*, 2600–2604. [CrossRef]
52. Cosatto, E.; Miller, M.; Graf, H.P.; Meyer, J.S. Grading Nuclear Pleomorphism on Histological Micrographs. In Proceedings of the 2008 19th International Conference on Pattern Recognition, Tampa, FL, USA, 8–11 December 2008; Institute of Electrical and Electronics Engineers (IEEE): Piscataway, NJ, USA, 2008; pp. 1–4.
53. Al-Kofahi, Y.; Lassoued, W.; Lee, W.; Roysam, B. Improved Automatic Detection and Segmentation of Cell Nuclei in Histopathology Images. *IEEE Trans. Biomed. Eng.* **2009**, *57*, 841–852. [CrossRef]
54. Veta, M.; Huisman, A.; Viergever, M.; van Diest, P.J.; Pluim, J. Marker-controlled watershed segmentation of nuclei in H&E stained breast cancer biopsy images. In Proceedings of the IEEE International Symposium on Biomedical Imaging: From Nano to Macro, Chicago, IL, USA, 30 March–2 April 2011; IEEE: Piscataway, NJ, USA, 2011; pp. 618–621. [CrossRef]
55. Aptoula, E.; Courty, N.; Lefèvre, S. Mitosis detection in breast cancer histological images with mathematical morphology. In Proceedings of the 2013 21st Signal Processing and Communications Applications Conference (SIU), Haspolat, Turkey, 24–26 April 2013; Institute of Electrical and Electronics Engineers (IEEE): Piscataway, NJ, USA, 2013; pp. 1–4.
56. Ciresan, D.C.; Giusti, A.; Gambardella, L.M.; Schmidhuber, J. Mitosis Detection in Breast Cancer Histology Images with Deep Neural Networks. In Proceedings of the International Conference on Medical Image Computing and Computer-Assisted Intervention, Nagoya, Japan, 22–26 September 2013; Springer: Berlin/Heidelberg, Germany, 2013; Volume 2, pp. 411–418.
57. Petushi, S.; Garcia, F.U.; Haber, M.M.; Katsinis, C.; Tozeren, A. Large-scale computations on histology images reveal grade-differentiating parameters for breast cancer. *BMC Med Imaging* **2006**, *6*, 14. [CrossRef]
58. Rittscher, J.; Machiraju, R.; Wong, S. *Microscopic Image Analysis for Life Science Applications*; Artech House: Norwood, MA, USA, 2008.
59. Boucheron, L.E. *Object- and Spatial-Level Quantitative Analysis of Multispectral Histopathology Images for Detection and Characterization of Cancer*; University of California at Santa Barbara: Santa Barbara, CA, USA, 2008.
60. Kuse, M.; Sharma, T.; Gupta, S. A Classification Scheme for Lymphocyte Segmentation in H&E Stained Histology Images. In *Static Analysis*; Springer Science and Business Media LLC: Berlin/Heidelberg, Germany, 2010; pp. 235–243.

61. Chekkoury, A.; Khurd, P.; Ni, J.; Bahlmann, C.; Kamen, A.; Patel, A.; Grady, L.; Singh, M.; Groher, M.; Navab, N.; et al. Automated malignancy detection in breast histopathological images. In *Medical Imaging 2012: Computer-Aided Diagnosis*; SPIE: Bellingham, WA, USA, 2012; pp. 332–344.
62. Doyle, S.; Hwang, M.; Shah, K.; Madabhushi, A.; Feldman, M.D.; Tomaszeweski, J.E. Automated Grading of Prostate Cancer Using Architectural and Textural Image Features. In Proceedings of the 2007 4th IEEE International Symposium on Biomedical Imaging: From Nano to Macro, Arlington, VA, USA, 12–15 April 2007; IEEE: Piscataway, NJ, USA, 2007; pp. 1284–1287.
63. Di Franco, M.D.; O'Hurley, G.; Kay, E.W.; Watson, R.W.G.; Cunningham, P. Ensemble-based system for whole-slide prostate cancer probability mapping using color texture features. *Comput. Med. Imaging Graphics* **2011**, *35*, 629–645. [CrossRef]
64. Huang, P.-W.; Lai, Y.H. Effective segmentation and classification for HCC biopsy images. *Pattern Recognit.* **2010**, *43*, 1550–1563. [CrossRef]
65. Alexandratou, E.; Atlamazoglou, V.; Thireou, T.; Agrogiannis, G.; Togas, D.; Kavantzas, N.; Patsouris, E.; Yova, D. Evaluation of machine learning techniques for prostate cancer diagnosis and Gleason grading. *Int. J. Comput. Intell. Bioinform. Syst. Biol.* **2010**, *1*, 297. [CrossRef]
66. Basavanhally, A.; Yu, E.; Xu, J.; Ganesan, S.; Feldman, M.; Tomaszeweski, J.E.; Madabhushi, A. Incorporating domain knowledge for tubule detection in breast histopathology using O'Callaghan neighborhoods. *Inter. Soc. Optics Photonics* **2011**, *7963*, 796310.
67. Al-Kadi, O.S. Texture measures combination for improved meningioma classification of histopathological images. *Pattern Recognit.* **2010**, *43*, 2043–2053. [CrossRef]
68. Demir, C.; Kandemir, M.; Tosun, A.B.; Sokmensuer, C. Automatic segmentation of colon glands using object-graphs. *Med. Image Anal.* **2010**, *14*, 1–12. [CrossRef]
69. Tosun, A.B.; Demir, C. Graph Run-Length Matrices for Histopathological Image Segmentation. *IEEE Transact. Med. Imaging* **2011**, *30*, 721–732. [CrossRef]
70. Krizhevsky, A.; Sutskever, I.; Hinton, G.E. ImageNet classification with deep convolutional neural networks. In Proceedings of the Advances in Neural Information Processing Systems (NIPS), Lake Tahoe, NV, USA, 3–6 December 2012; pp. 1097–1105.
71. Le Cun, Y.; Bottou, L.; Bengio, Y.; Haffner, P. Gradient-based learning applied to document recognition. *Proc. IEEE* **1998**, *86*, 2278–2324. [CrossRef]
72. Lecun, Y.; Bengio, Y.; Hinton, G. Deep learning. *Nature* **2015**, *521*, 436–444. [CrossRef]
73. Arevalo, J.; Cruz-Roa, A.; González, F.A. Hybrid image representation learning model with invariant features for basal cell carcinoma detection. In Proceedings of the IX International Seminar on Medical Information Processing and Analysis, Mexico City, Mexico, 11–14 November2013; SPIE: Bellingham, WA, USA, 2013; Volume 8922, p. 89220M.
74. Nayak, N.; Chang, H.; Borowsky, A.; Spellman, P.T.; Parvin, B. Classification of tumor histopathology via sparse feature learning. In Proceedings of the 2013 IEEE 10th International Symposium on Biomedical Imaging, San Francisco, CA, USA, 7–11 April 2013; IEEE: Piscataway, NJ, USA, 2013; pp. 410–413.
75. Malon, C.D.; Cosatto, E. Classification of mitotic figures with convolutional neural networks and seeded blob features. *J. Pathol. Informat.* **2013**, *4*, 9. [CrossRef]
76. Xu, Y.; Mo, T.; Feng, Q.; Zhong, P.; Lai, M.; Chang, E.I.-C. Deep learning of feature representation with multiple instance learning for medical image analysis. In Proceedings of the 2014 IEEE International Conference on Acoustics, Speech and Signal Processing (ICASSP), Florence, Italy, 4–9 May 2014; Institute of Electrical and Electronics Engineers (IEEE): Piscataway, NJ, USA, 2014; pp. 1626–1630.
77. Hou, L.; Samaras, D.; Kurç, T.M.; Gao, Y.; Davis, J.E.; Saltz, J.H. Efficient Multiple Instance Convolutional Neural Networks for Gigapixel Resolution Image Classification. *arXiv* **2015**, arXiv:abs/1504.07947.
78. Arevalo, J.; Cruz-Roa, A.; Arias, V.; Romero, E.; González, F.A. An unsupervised feature learning framework for basal cell carcinoma image analysis. *Artif. Intell. Med.* **2015**, *64*, 131–145. [CrossRef]
79. Chang, H.; Zhou, Y.; Borowsky, A.; Barner, K.; Spellman, P.; Parvin, B. Stacked Predictive Sparse Decomposition for Classification of Histology Sections. *Int. J. Comput. Vis.* **2014**, *113*, 3–18. [CrossRef] [PubMed]
80. Han, J.; Fontenay, G.V.; Wang, Y.; Mao, J.-H.; Chang, H. Phenotypic characterization of breast invasive carcinoma via transferable tissue morphometric patterns learned from glioblastoma multiforme. Proceeding

of the 2016 IEEE 13th International Symposium on Biomedical Imaging (ISBI), Prague, Czech Republic, 13–16 April 2016; IEEE: Piscataway, NJ, USA, 2016; pp. 1025–1028.

81. Noël, H.; Roux, L.; Lu, S.; Boudier, T. Detection of high-grade atypia nuclei in breast cancer imaging. In *Medical Imaging*; SPIE: Bellingham, WA, USA, 2015; p. 94200R.
82. Romo-Bucheli, D.; Janowczyk, A.; Gilmore, H.; Romero, E.; Madabhushi, A. Automated Tubule Nuclei Quantification and Correlation with Oncotype DX risk categories in ER+ Breast Cancer Whole Slide Images. *Sci. Rep.* **2016**, *6*, 32706. [CrossRef] [PubMed]
83. Chen, T. Deep Learning Based Automatic Immune Cell Detection for Immunohistochemistry Images. In *International Workshop on Machine Learning in Medical Imaging*; Springer: Cham, Switzerlnad, 2014; pp. 17–24.
84. Srinidhi, C.L.; Ciga, O.; Martel, A.L. Deep neural network models for computational histopathology: A survey. *Med Image Anal.* **2020**, 101813. [CrossRef] [PubMed]
85. Sumi, P.S.; Delhibabu, R. Glioblastoma Multiforme Classification On High Resolution Histology Image Using Deep Spatial Fusion Network. In Proceedings of theCEUR Workshop, Como, Italy, 9–11 September 2019.
86. Zhang, L.; Wu, Y.; Zheng, B.; Su, L.; Chen, Y.; Ma, S.; Hu, Q.; Zou, X.; Yao, L.; Yang, Y.; et al. Rapid histology of laryngeal squamous cell carcinoma with deep-learning based stimulated Raman scattering microscopy. *Theranostics* **2019**, *9*, 2541–2554. [CrossRef] [PubMed]
87. Agarwal, A. GPU Based Digital Histopathology and Diagnostic Support System for Breast Cancer Detection: A Comparison of CNN Models and Machine Learning Models. *Nature Rev. Drug Discov.* **2019**, *18*, 463–477.
88. Ronneberger, O.; Fischer, P.; Brox, T. U-Net: Convolutional Networks for Biomedical Image Segmentation. In Proceedings of the International Conference on Medical Image Computing and Computer-Assisted Intervention, Munich, Germany, 5–9 October 2015; pp. 234–241.
89. Tschuchnig, M.E.; Oostingh, G.J.; Gadermayr, M. Generative Adversarial Networks in Digital Pathology: A Survey on Trends and Future Potential. *arXiv* **2020**, arXiv:abs/2004.14936. [CrossRef]
90. Litjens, G.J.S.; Sánchez, C.I.; Timofeeva, N.; Hermsen, M.; Nagtegaal, I.D.; Kovacs, I.; Kaa, C.H.; van de Bult, P.; Ginneken, B.; van Laak, J. Deep learning as a tool for increased accuracy and efficiency of histopathological diagnosis. *Sci. Reports* **2016**, *6*. [CrossRef]
91. Nagpal, K.; Foote, D.; Liu, Y.; Chen, P.-H.C.; Wulczyn, E.; Tan, F.; Olson, N.; Smith, J.L.; Mohtashamian, A.; Wren, J.H.; et al. Publisher Correction: Development and validation of a deep learning algorithm for improving Gleason scoring of prostate cancer. *npj Digit. Med.* **2019**, *2*, 2. [CrossRef] [PubMed]
92. Zhao, Z.; Lin, H.; Chen, H.; Heng, P.-A. PFA-ScanNet: Pyramidal Feature Aggregation with Synergistic Learning for Breast Cancer Metastasis Analysis. *Lecture Notes Comput. Sci.* **2019**, 586–594.
93. Xing, F.; Xie, Y.; Yang, L. An Automatic Learning-Based Framework for Robust Nucleus Segmentation. *IEEE Trans. Med Imaging* **2015**, *35*, 550–566. [CrossRef]
94. Gu, F.; Burlutskiy, N.; Andersson, M.; Wilén, L.K. Multi-resolution Networks for Semantic Segmentation in Whole Slide Images. In *Lecture Notes in Computer Science*; Springer Science and Business Media LLC: Berlin/Heidelberg, Germany, 2018; pp. 11–18.
95. Tellez, D.; Balkenhol, M.; Otte-Holler, I.; van de Loo, R.; Vogels, R.; Bult, P.; Wauters, C.; Vreuls, W.; Mol, S.; Karssemeijer, N.; et al. Whole-Slide Mitosis Detection in H&E Breast Histology Using PHH3 as a Reference to Train Distilled Stain-Invariant Convolutional Networks. *IEEE Trans. Med Imaging* **2018**, *37*, 2126–2136. [CrossRef]
96. Wei, J.W.; Tafe, L.J.; Linnik, Y.A.; Vaickus, L.J.; Tomita, N.; Hassanpour, S. Pathologist-level classification of histologic patterns on resected lung adenocarcinoma slides with deep neural networks. *Sci. Rep.* **2019**, *9*, 1–8. [CrossRef]
97. Song, Y.; Tan, E.-L.; Jiang, X.; Cheng, J.-Z.; Ni, D.; Chen, S.; Lei, B.Y.; Wang, T. Accurate Cervical Cell Segmentation from Overlapping Clumps in Pap Smear Images. *IEEE Transact. Med. Imaging* **2017**, *36*, 288–300. [CrossRef]
98. Agarwalla, A.; Shaban, M.; Rajpoot, N.M. Representation-Aggregation Networks for Segmentation of Multi-Gigapixel Histology Images. *arXiv* **2017**, arXiv:1707-08814.
99. Ding, H.; Pan, Z.; Cen, Q.; Li, Y.; Chen, S. Multi-scale fully convolutional network for gland segmentation using three-class classification. *Neurocomputing* **2020**, *380*, 150–161. [CrossRef]

100. Bejnordi, B.E.; Zuidhof, G.C.A.; Balkenhol, M.; Hermsen, M.; Bult, P.; Ginneken, B.; van Karssemeijer, N.; Litjens, G.J.S.; Laak, J. Context-aware stacked convolutional neural networks for classification of breast carcinomas in whole-slide histopathology images. *J. Med. Imaging* **2017**, *4*, 044504. [CrossRef]
101. Seth, N.; Akbar, S.; Nofech-Mozes, S.; Salama, S.; Martel, A.L. Automated Segmentation of DCIS in Whole Slide Images. In *Case-Based Reasoning Research and Development*; Springer Science and Business Media LLC: Berlin/Heidelberg, Germany, 2019; pp. 67–74.
102. Xu, J.; Xiang, L.; Liu, Q.; Gilmore, H.; Wu, J.; Tang, J.; Madabhushi, A. Stacked Sparse Autoencoder (SSAE) for Nuclei Detection on Breast Cancer Histopathology Images. *IEEE Trans. Med Imaging* **2015**, *35*, 119–130. [CrossRef]
103. Bulten, W.; Litjens, G. Unsupervised Prostate Cancer Detection on H&E using Convolutional Adversarial Autoencoders. *arXiv* **2018**, arXiv:1804.07098.
104. Hou, L.; Agarwal, A.; Samaras, D.; Kurc, T.M.; Gupta, R.R.; Saltz, J.H. Robust Histopathology Image Analysis: To Label or to Synthesize? In Proceedings of the 2019 IEEE/CVF Conference on Computer Vision and Pattern Recognition (CVPR), Long Beach, CA, USA, 16–20 June 2019; Institute of Electrical and Electronics Engineers (IEEE): Piscataway, NJ, USA, 2019; pp. 8525–8534.
105. Sari, C.T.; Gunduz-Demir, C. Unsupervised Feature Extraction via Deep Learning for Histopathological Classification of Colon Tissue Images. *IEEE Transact. Med. Imaging* **2019**, *38*, 1139–1149. [CrossRef] [PubMed]
106. Gadermayr, M.; Gupta, L.; Appel, V.; Boor, P.; Klinkhammer, B.M.; Merhof, D. Generative Adversarial Networks for Facilitating Stain-Independent Supervised and Unsupervised Segmentation: A Study on Kidney Histology. *IEEE Trans. Med Imaging* **2019**, *38*, 2293–2302. [CrossRef] [PubMed]
107. Gadermayr, M.; Gupta, L.; Klinkhammer, B.M.; Boor, P.; Merhof, D. Unsupervisedly Training GANs for Segmenting Digital Pathology with Automatically Generated Annotations. *arXiv* **2018**, arXiv:1805.10059.
108. Komura, D.; Ishikawa, S. Machine Learning Methods for Histopathological Image Analysis. *Comput. Struct. Biotechnol. J.* **2018**, *16*, 34–42. [CrossRef]
109. Search Home—Biospecimen Research Database. Available online: https://brd.nci.nih.gov/brd/image-search/searchhome (accessed on 1 October 2020).
110. TMAD Main Menu. Available online: https://tma.im/cgi-bin/home.pl (accessed on 1 October 2020).
111. Home—CAMELYON17—Grand Challenge. Available online: https://camelyon17.grand-challenge.org/ (accessed on 1 October 2020).
112. Breast Cancer Histopathological Database (BreakHis)—Laboratório Visão Robótica e Imagem. Available online: https://web.inf.ufpr.br/vri/databases/breast-cancer-histopathological-database-breakhis/ (accessed on 1 October 2020).
113. Search GDC. Available online: https://portal.gdc.cancer.gov/legacy-archive/search/f (accessed on 1 October 2020).
114. Marinelli, R.J.; Montgomery, K.; Liu, C.L.; Shah, N.H.; Prapong, W.; Nitzberg, M.; Zachariah, Z.K.; Sherlock, G.; Natkunam, Y.; West, R.B.; et al. The Stanford Tissue Microarray Database. *Nucleic Acids Res.* **2007**, *36*, D871–D877. [CrossRef]
115. Dataset Tumor Proliferation Assessment Challenge 2016. Available online: http://tupac.tue-image.nl/node/3 (accessed on 1 October 2020).
116. Bentaieb, A.; Li-Chang, H.; Huntsman, D.; Hamarneh, G. A structured latent model for ovarian carcinoma subtyping from histopathology slides. *Med Image Anal.* **2017**, *39*, 194–205. [CrossRef]
117. Ovarian Carcinomas Histopathology Dataset. Available online: http://ensc-mica-www02.ensc.sfu.ca/download/ (accessed on 1 October 2020).
118. Babaie, M.; Kalra, S.; Sriram, A.; Mitcheltree, C.; Zhu, S.; Khatami, A.; Rahnamayan, S.; Tizhoosh, H.R. Classification and Retrieval of Digital Pathology Scans: A New Dataset. In Proceedings of the 2017 IEEE Conference on Computer Vision and Pattern Recognition Workshops (CVPRW), Honolulu, HI, USA, 21–16 July 2017; Institute of Electrical and Electronics Engineers (IEEE): Piscataway, NJ, USA, 2017; pp. 760–768.
119. Kumar, N.; Verma, R.; Sharma, S.; Bhargava, S.; Vahadane, A.; Sethi, A. A Dataset and a Technique for Generalized Nuclear Segmentation for Computational Pathology. *IEEE Trans. Med Imaging* **2017**, *36*, 1550–1560. [CrossRef]
120. Pathology Images: KIMIA Path960—Kimia Lab. Available online: https://kimialab.uwaterloo.ca/kimia/index.php/pathology-images-kimia-path960/ (accessed on 1 October 2020).

121. Gelasca, E.D.; Byun, J.; Obara, B.; Manjunath, B.S. Evaluation and benchmark for biological image segmentation. In Proceedings of the 2008 15th IEEE International Conference on Image Processing, San Diego, CA, USA, 12–15 October 2008; Institute of Electrical and Electronics Engineers (IEEE): Pisctaway, NJ, USA, 2008; pp. 1816–1819.
122. Bio-Segmentation Center for Bio-Image Informatics UC Santa Barbara. Available online: https://bioimage.ucsb.edu/research/bio-segmentation (accessed on 1 October 2020).
123. Bioimaging Challenge 2015 Breast Histology Dataset—Datasets CKAN. Available online: https://rdm.inesctec.pt/dataset/nis-2017-003 (accessed on 1 October 2020).
124. BIALab@Warwick: GlaS Challenge Contest. Available online: https://warwick.ac.uk/fac/sci/dcs/research/tia/glascontest/ (accessed on 1 October 2020).
125. Kather, J.N.; Marx, A.; Reyes-Aldasoro, C.C.; Schad, L.R.; Zoellner, F.G.; Weis, C.-A. Continuous representation of tumor microvessel density and detection of angiogenic hotspots in histological whole-slide images. *Oncotarget* **2015**, *6*, 19163–19176. [CrossRef]
126. Dataset—MITOS-ATYPIA-14—Grand Challenge. Available online: https://mitos-atypia-14.grand-challenge.org/dataset/ (accessed on 1 October 2020).
127. Nucleisegmentation. Available online: https://nucleisegmentationbenchmark.weebly.com/ (accessed on 1 October 2020).
128. Janowczyk, A.; Madabhushi, A. Deep learning for digital pathology image analysis: A comprehensive tutorial with selected use cases. *J. Pathol. Informat.* **2016**, *7*. [CrossRef]
129. Andrew Janowczyk—Tidbits from Along the Way. Available online: http://www.andrewjanowczyk.com/ (accessed on 1 October 2020).
130. Ma, Z.; Shiao, S.L.; Yoshida, E.J.; Swartwood, S.; Huang, F.; Doche, M.E.; Chung, A.P.; Knudsen, B.S.; Gertych, A. Data integration from pathology slides for quantitative imaging of multiple cell types within the tumor immune cell infiltrate. *Diagn. Pathol.* **2017**, *12*. [CrossRef] [PubMed]
131. Linder, N.; Konsti, J.; Turkki, R.; Rahtu, E.; Lundin, M.; Nordling, S.; Haglund, C.; Ahonen, T.; Pietikäinen, M.; Lundin, J. Identification of tumor epithelium and stroma in tissue microarrays using texture analysis. *Diagn. Pathol.* **2012**, *7*, 22. [CrossRef] [PubMed]
132. Egfr Colon Stroma Classification. Available online: http://fimm.webmicroscope.net/supplements/epistroma (accessed on 1 October 2020).
133. Jimenez-del-Toro, O.; Otálora, S.; Andersson, M.; Eurén, K.; Hedlund, M.; Rousson, M.; Müller, H.; Atzori, M. *Chapter 10—Analysis of Histopathology Images: From Traditional Machine Learning to Deep Learning*; Academic Press: Cambridge, MA, USA, 2017; pp. 281–314.
134. Zhang, Y.; Zhang, B.; Coenen, F.; Xiao, J.; Lu, W. One-class kernel subspace ensemble for medical image classification. *EURASIP J. Adv. Signal Process.* **2014**, *2014*, 17. [CrossRef]
135. Xia, Y.; Cao, X.; Wen, F.; Hua, G.; Sun, J. Learning Discriminative Reconstructions for Unsupervised Outlier Removal. In Proceedings of the 2015 IEEE International Conference on Computer Vision (ICCV), Las Condes, Chile, 11–15 December 2015; Institute of Electrical and Electronics Engineers (IEEE): Piscataway, NJ, USA, 2015; pp. 1511–1519.
136. Samek, W.; Binder, A.; Montavon, G.; Lapuschkin, S.; Muller, K.-R. Evaluating the Visualization of What a Deep Neural Network Has Learned. *IEEE Trans. Neural Networks Learn. Syst.* **2016**, *28*, 2660–2673. [CrossRef] [PubMed]
137. Zintgraf, L.M.; Cohen, T.S.; Adel, T.; Welling, M. Visualizing Deep Neural Network Decisions: Prediction Difference Analysis. *arXiv* **2017**, arXiv:1702.04595.
138. Koh, P.W.; Liang, P. Understanding Black-box Predictions via Influence Functions. *arXiv* **2017**, arXiv:abs/1703.04730.
139. Abas, F.S.; Gokozan, H.; Goksel, B.; Otero, J.J. *Intraoperative Neuropathology of Glioma Recurrence: Cell Detection and Classification*; SPIE: Bellingham, WA, USA, 2016; p. 979109. [CrossRef]
140. Chen, J.; Srinivas, C. Automatic Lymphocyte Detection in H&E Images with Deep Neural Networks. *arXiv* **2016**, arXiv:abs/1612.03217.
141. Turkki, R.; Linder, N.; Kovanen, P.E.; Pellinen, T.; Lundin, J. Antibody-supervised deep learning for quantification of tumor-infiltrating immune cells in hematoxylin and eosin stained breast cancer samples. *J. Pathol. Informat.* **2016**, *7*, 38. [CrossRef]

142. Feng, Z.; Bethmann, D.; Kappler, M.; Ballesteros-Merino, C.; Eckert, A.; Bell, R.B.; Cheng, A.; Bui, T.; Leidner, R.; Urba, W.J.; et al. Multiparametric immune profiling in HPV—Oral squamous cell cancer. *JCI Insight* **2017**, *2*, e93652. [CrossRef]
143. Basavanhally, A.N.; Ganesan, S.; Agner, S.; Monaco, J.P.; Feldman, M.D.; Tomaszewski, J.E.; Bhanot, G.; Madabhushi, A. Computerized Image-Based Detection and Grading of Lymphocytic Infiltration in HER2+ Breast Cancer Histopathology. *IEEE Trans. Biomed. Eng.* **2009**, *57*, 642–653. [CrossRef]
144. Li, J.; Li, W.; Gertych, A.; Knudsen, B.S.; Speier, W.; Arnold, C. An attention-based multi-resolution model for prostate whole slide imageclassification and localization. *arXiv* **2019**, arXiv:1905.13208.
145. Bera, K.; Schalper, K.A.; Rimm, D.L.; Velcheti, V.; Madabhushi, A. Artificial intelligence in digital pathology new tools for diagnosis and precision oncology. *Nat. Rev. Clin. Oncol.* **2019**, *16*, 703–715. [CrossRef] [PubMed]
146. Niazi, M.K.K.; Parwani, A.V.; Gurcan, M.N. Digital pathology and artificial intelligence. *Lancet Oncol.* **2019**, *20*, 253–261. [CrossRef]
147. Tellez, D.; Litjens, G.J.S.; Bándi, P.; Bulten, W.; Bokhorst, J.-M.; Ciompi, F.; Laak, J. Quantifying the effects of data augmentation and stain color normalization in convolutional neural networks for computational pathology. *Med. Image Anal.* **2019**, *58*, 101544. [CrossRef] [PubMed]
148. Steiner, D.F.; Macdonald, R.; Liu, Y.; Truszkowski, P.; Hipp, J.D.; Gammage, C.; Thng, F.; Peng, L.; Stumpe, M.C. Impact of Deep Learning Assistance on the Histopathologic Review of Lymph Nodes for Metastatic Breast Cancer. *Am. J. Surg. Pathol.* **2018**, *42*, 1636–1646. [CrossRef]
149. Kamnitsas, K.; Ferrante, E.; Parisot, S.; Ledig, C.; Nori, A.V.; Criminisi, A.; Rueckert, D.; Glocker, B. *DeepMedic for Brain Tumor Segmentation*; Springer: Berlin/Heidelberg, Germany, 2016.
150. Voets, M.; Møllersen, K.; Bongo, L.A. Replication study: Development and validation of deep learning algorithm for detection of diabetic retinopathy in retinal fundus photographs. *arXiv* **2018**, arXiv:abs/1803.04337.

3

Machine Learning for the Classification of Alzheimer's Disease and its Prodromal Stage using Brain Diffusion Tensor Imaging Data

Lucia Billeci [1,*], Asia Badolato [2], Lorenzo Bachi [1] and Alessandro Tonacci [1]

1 Institute of Clinical Physiology-National Research Council of Italy (IFC-CNR), Via Moruzzi, 1, 56124 Pisa, Italy; bachi@ifc.cnr.it (L.B.); atonacci@ifc.cnr.it (A.T.)

2 School of Engineering, University of Pisa, Largo Lucio Lazzarino, 1, 56122 Pisa, Italy; asiabadolato@yahoo.it

* Correspondence: lucia.billeci@ifc.cnr.it

Abstract: Alzheimer's disease is notoriously the most common cause of dementia in the elderly, affecting an increasing number of people. Although widespread, its causes and progression modalities are complex and still not fully understood. Through neuroimaging techniques, such as diffusion Magnetic Resonance (MR), more sophisticated and specific studies of the disease can be performed, offering a valuable tool for both its diagnosis and early detection. However, processing large quantities of medical images is not an easy task, and researchers have turned their attention towards machine learning, a set of computer algorithms that automatically adapt their output towards the intended goal. In this paper, a systematic review of recent machine learning applications on diffusion tensor imaging studies of Alzheimer's disease is presented, highlighting the fundamental aspects of each work and reporting their performance score. A few examined studies also include mild cognitive impairment in the classification problem, while others combine diffusion data with other sources, like structural magnetic resonance imaging (MRI) (multimodal analysis). The findings of the retrieved works suggest a promising role for machine learning in evaluating effective classification features, like fractional anisotropy, and in possibly performing on different image modalities with higher accuracy.

Keywords: Alzheimer's disease; mild cognitive impairment; diffusion tensor imaging; magnetic resonance imaging; machine learning; support vector machine

---

1. Introduction

Alzheimer's disease (AD), or Alzheimer's, is a neurodegenerative disorder representing the most common cause of dementia in the elderly population of developed countries. Currently, the number of people affected by Alzheimer is about fifty million, and this number is expected to triple by 2050, due to population aging [1]. Alzheimer's disease is characterized by a progressive and irreversible neurologic deterioration, leading to the decline of cognitive functions and eventually to patient death [2]. Mild cognitive impairment (MCI) is an intermediate pathological condition where patients show heterogeneous symptoms. MCI can represent the prodromal stage of AD, but can also turn to other types of dementia [3]. AD diagnosis is very complex because of different symptoms that patients might show, both at the cognitive and behavioral level. Furthermore, the disease progression modalities are as subjective as the therapeutic responses. Within this framework, the most challenging goal is to develop innovative diagnostic tools to help detecting the disease from its early stages, including MCI. In this context, computer aided diagnosis (CAD) systems are desirable, in order to improve the prediction accuracy, complementing the neuropsychological assessments performed by expert clinicians.

Progresses in neuroimaging techniques have been pivotal to the analysis of structural and functional cerebral modifications connected to Alzheimer's [4]. However, integrating large quantities of data on a large scale is becoming increasingly difficult; therefore, there is a high interest in innovative machine learning (ML) methods that allow for classifying considerable amounts of data following specific algorithms. ML refers to a set of mathematical models that can learn by self-adjusting their output through experience and make predictions or decisions based on new data [5]. Since AD is a complex disease showing heterogenous structural and functional changes at brain level, these techniques can lead to a deeper understanding of new aspects of AD progression. As a matter of fact, ML approaches are particularly sensitive to distributed disease-specific changes observed in many human structural and functional imaging studies. They are designed to identify patterns in data that differentiate between several classes [5]. ML classification offers powerful prediction methods for the disease state of an individual. For example, the support vector machine (SVM) classifier has been used to find a hyperplane for high dimensional training features and to categorize test subjects that were part of a specific clinical group [6].

So far, many studies in the existing literature have analyzed the potential of ML methods applied to the field of neurodegenerative disorders, such as Alzheimer's disease. For this purpose, the use of data derived from magnetic resonance imaging (MRI) [7,8] or positron emission tomography (PET) has been widely investigated [9,10]. However, the diffusion tensor imaging (DTI) technique has drawn researchers' attention for the last fifteen years.

DTI is a non-invasive technology able to provide information on white matter's integrity, which is connected to neuropathological mechanisms. DTI analyzes water diffusion at the microstructural level of the brain, determining the abnormal diffusion pattern in different neurological/neuropsychiatric conditions, including AD [11–13]. By tracking the highly anisotropic diffusion of water along axons, the integrity and trajectory of the major white matter (WM) fiber bundles in the brain can be evaluated through DTI [14]. Diffusion in WM is highly anisotropic being less restricted along the axon, whereas in gray matter (GM), it is usually less anisotropic and in the cerebrospinal fluid (CSF) it is unrestricted in all directions (isotropic) [15]. Based on this assumption, the diffusion process has been modeled by an ellipsoid in which the length of the three principal axes reflects the diffusion tendency along each direction ($\lambda 1$, $\lambda 2$, $\lambda 3$; see Figure 1) [15]. DTI is the only neuroimaging technique that can characterize WM fiber paths and is sensitive to microscopic WM injury in these bundles. It can therefore identify signs of impairment in anatomical connectivity that are not detectable with standard anatomical MRI [14].

Two of the most used features to characterize WM integrity are fractional anisotropy (FA) and mean diffusivity (MD). FA provides useful information about fiber density, axonal diameter, and myelination in WM, and a decrease in its value suggests a loss of fiber tract integrity, thus, WM damage [15]. MD measures the average diffusivity in the non-colinear directions of free diffusion and an increase in its value indicates a loss of anisotropy, thus, representing an increase in free water diffusion [15]. More recently, other features are reported in the literature including axial diffusivity (DA), the rate of water diffusion along the longitudinal axis, and radial diffusivity (DR), or the rate of water diffusion along the perpendicular axes [16,17]. Importantly, several DTI analysis methods can be used, including voxel-wise analysis, region-of-interest (ROI) analysis, tract-based spatial statistics (TBSS; [18]), and tractography. More recently, networks analysis has drawn a great deal of interest [19]. The characterization of global architecture or topological property of anatomical connectivity patterns in the human brain can provide additional insights into structural disruption related to brain disorders [19].

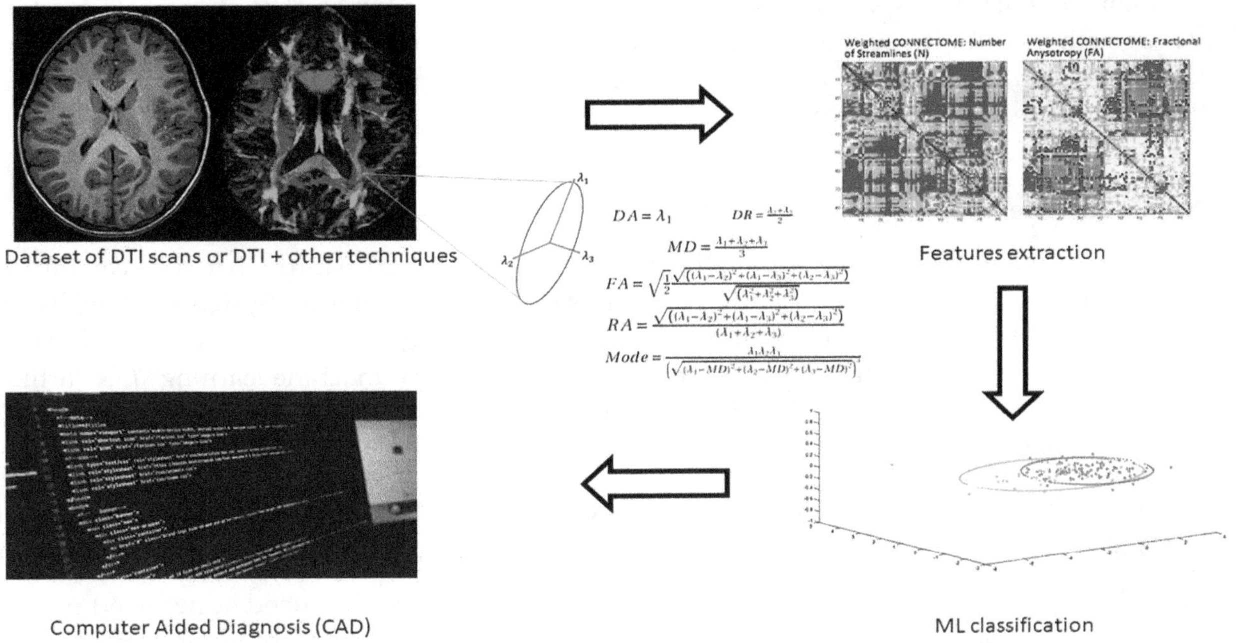

Figure 1. General procedure consisting in four steps: taking a dataset of diffusion tensor imaging (DTI) or multimodal images, features extraction from the dataset, machine learning classification based on most significant features, automated diagnosis obtained by classifying individual scans in a specific clinical class. DA: axial diffusivity; DR: radial diffusivity; MD: mean diffusivity; FA: fractional anisotropy; RA: relative anisotropy.

AD is characterized by a loss of brain barriers that determine a restriction of water motion, thus, compromising the integrity of WM and leading to abnormal diffusivity patterns, and resulting in a measurable difference in the diffusion of water molecules [20]. It has been suggested that such changes precede macroscopic atrophy [21] and, while they are not visible on conventional structural MRI sequences, they can be detected by DTI. Moreover, the literature suggests that WM integrity alterations detected by DTI could be complementary to volumetric alterations [22].

Several studies have applied DTI technique for the characterization of WM integrity in AD (for a review see [23]). In particular, DTI-based studies have shown that AD patients exhibit aberrant FA and MD values in the white matter of specific cerebral regions [24]. Furthermore, other studies have found similar, yet less severe, changes of these values in MCI patients [25]. In particular, voxel-based studies showed that AD and MCI subjects have reduced fractional anisotropy (FA) in multiple posterior WM regions [26] and increased mean diffusivity (MD) in the posterior occipital–parietal cortex and right parietal supramarginal gyrus [27]. ROI-based studies demonstrated higher MD and/or lower FA in the hippocampus [28–30] and posterior cingulate [31,32]. Notably, the results of a previous study showed that measures of diffusivity extracted from the hippocampus are better predictors of MCI conversion to AD than its volume [32]. Altogether, these results suggest that the biomarkers obtained from the DTI technique can be used for AD classification through advanced classification methods [33].

For these reasons, combining DTI data with ML classification algorithms looks promising in detecting specific AD and MCI biomarkers. In this paper, we present the resulting findings of several studies in a systematic review regarding models of CAD that integrate DTI data (or the combination of DTI with other MRI techniques) and ML methods to classify healthy controls and patients affected by AD or MCI.

The main goal of this review is to examine the benefits and the issues of applying DTI combined with ML algorithms in the detection of AD/MCI and to suggest future lines of research. To the author's knowledge, this is the only review in the existing literature focusing on studies that perform DTI-based classification to detect AD and its early stage.

2. Materials and Methods

A systematic literature review covering the period from the year 2010 through to the year 2019 was conducted in PubMed according to the PRISMA (Preferred Reporting Items for Systematic Reviews and Meta-Analyses) guidelines [34]. Articles published before 2010 were not taken into account, due to the limited knowledge of DTI at their disposal. The search strategy was ("machine learning" OR "artificial intelligence" OR "classification") AND "diffusion tensor imaging" AND ("alzheimer's disease" OR alzheimer's OR alzheimer).

To reduce a risk of bias, two authors (L.Bi. and A.B.) independently screened paper abstracts and titles and analyzed the full papers that met the inclusion criteria, as suggested by the PRISMA guidelines.

Overall, the search was limited to articles pertaining to studies that used supervised machine learning methods on data derived from DTI or from other neuroimaging techniques combined with DTI. Moreover, we included only studies that classified AD patients compared to healthy controls, or that also included a sample of MCI subjects. We decided to exclude articles that did not include a sample of AD but only included MCI patients and controls, since this review is mainly focused on the automatic diagnosis of AD, and since we wanted to evaluate the benefits and the issues of using DTI combined with ML methods, according to the literature so far, in a sample which is more uniquely characterized and more homogeneous compared with MCI group. This search led to 51 articles, 36 of which were selected. Among these, 15 articles were excluded: three of them were not focused on AD or MCI disorders, nine did not consider any AD sample and one systematic review and two studies did not involve DTI-based classification. From the remaining 21 articles, a consistent set of information was extracted: the neuroimaging techniques involved, the number of pathologic patients and healthy controls, the list of features, the classification algorithm(s) and the results (accuracy—ACC, sensitivity—SEN, specificity—SPE). When multiple classifiers were tested, only the performance of the one that achieved the best result are reported in Tables 1 and 2. In Figure 1, the general procedure for data analysis and classification applied in the selected articles is represented.

In Appendix A, a comprehensive list of the acronyms and abbreviations used throughout the paper can be found, while Appendix B contains a brief description of the ML approaches mentioned in this paper.

Table 1. Studies that use machine learning to classify only Alzheimer's disease (AD) patients (bold classification methods indicate the preferred ones based on highest performances).

Article	Neuroimaging Technique	Subjects	Measures	Classifier	Classification Results				
					Feature Set/Method		ACC%	SEN%	SPE%
DTI analysis									
Graña et al., 2011 [35]	DTI	20 AD, 25 HC	FA, MD	SVM	**FA**		**100.0**	**100.0**	**100.0**
					MD		~99.0	~97.9	~98.1
Patil et al., 2013 [36]	DTI	34 AD, 58 HC	FA	AdaBoost	**FA (10 features)**		**84.5**	**80.2**	**85.2**
					FA (all features)		75.3	71.0	76.7
Patil and Ramakrishnan, 2014 [37]	DTI	37 AD, 50 HC	FA, MD, DR, DA	SVM, decision stumps, simple logistic	**FA (SVM)**	**MMSE**	**94.2**	**94.4**	**93.0**
						No MMSE	81.6	81.8	81.4
					MD (SVM)	MMSE	89.7	88.9	90.1
						No MMSE	87.4	88.2	86.7
					DR (SVM)	MMSE	91.9	96.8	89.0
						No MMSE	83.9	89.6	81.0
					DA (SVM)	MMSE	93.4	95.1	93.2
						No MMSE	81.6	86.2	79.3
Schouten et al., 2017 [38]	DTI	77 AD, 173 HC	FA, MD, DA, DR	Logistic elastic net regression	FA-TBSS		82.6	83.8	82.1
					MD-TBSS		80.8	84.4	79.2
					DA-TBSS		81.8	84.9	80.4
					DR-TBSS		84.8	79.1	87.3
					FA-ICA		**85.1**	**86.8**	**84.4**
					MD-ICA		84.3	84.2	84.3
					DA-ICA		83.4	89.7	80.6
					DR-ICA		84.0	83.2	84.4
					Connectivity graph		85.0	80.3	87.1
					Degree		75.8	79.9	74.0
					Strength		79.6	79.9	80.9
					Clustering		75.6	76.6	79.5
					Betw.centrality		64.6	66.9	66.8
					Path length		69.6	59.5	72.7
					Transitivity		64.9	62.5	77.2
					Sparse Group Lasso		80.8	37.3	77.4

Table 1. *Cont.*

Article	Neuroimaging Technique	Subjects	Measures	Classifier	Classification Results: Feature Set/Method	ACC%	SEN%	SPE%
Multimodal analysis								
Mesrob et al., 2012 [39]	DTI, sMRI	15 AD, 16 HC	Diff: FA, MD sMRI: GMC	Non-linear SVM	**MD/GMC (15 multivariate)**	**99.6**	**99.2**	**99.9**
					MD/GMC (15 univariate)	72.1	53.6	90.6
					MD/GMC (73 ROIs)	72.4	62.4	82.4
					MD (73 ROIs)	65.2	60.8	69.5
					FA/MD (73 ROIs)	68.6	73.4	63.8
					GMC (73 ROIs)	76.5	78.7	74.3
Dyrba et al., 2013 [40]	DTI, sMRI	137 AD, 143 HC	Diff: FA, MD sMRI: GMD, WMD	Multivariate SVM NB	**GMD (SVM)**	**89.3**	**87.4**	**91.2**
					FA (SVM)	80.3	78.8	81.9
					MD (SVM)	83.3	79.6	86.9
					WMD (SVM)	82.7	77.9	87.4
Li et al., 2014 [41]	DTI, sMRI	21 AD, 15 HC	Diff: FA sMRI: GMV	SVM	**Tract-Based FA + GMV**	**94.3**	**95.0**	**93.3**
					Tract-based FA	~89.0	90.5	86.7
					Voxel-based FA	~83.0	90.5	80.0
					GMV	~88.0	85.0	93.0
Dyrba et al., 2015 [42]	DTI, sMRI, rs-fMRI	28 AD, 25 HC	Diff. FA, MD, MO sMRI: GMV Rs-fMRI: local clustering coefficient, shortest path length	SVM MK-SVM	**DTI measures (SVM)**	**85.0**	**86.0**	**84.0**
					Rs-fMRI measures (SM)	74.0	82.0	64.0
					GMV (SVM)	81.0	82.0	80.0
					Rs-fMRI + DTI + GMV (SVM)	79.0	82.0	86.0
					DTI + GMV (SVM)	**85.0**	**79.0**	**92.0**
Chen et al., 2017 [43]	DTI, DKI	27 AD, 26 HC	Diff: FA, MD, DA, DR Kur: MK, AK, RK	SVM	**ALL-DKI** **RFE**	**96.2**	**100**	**92.8**
					ALL-DKI MMSE	90.6	100	83.9
					Diff-DKI RFE	92.5	100	86.7
					Diff-DKI MMSE	90.6	100	83.3
					Diff-DTI RFE	81.1	72.9	100
					Diff-DTI MMSE	86.8	81.3	95.2
					Kur-DKI RFE	86.8	83.3	91.3
					Kur-DKI MMSE	83.0	79.3	86.9

Table 1. *Cont.*

Article	Neuroimaging Technique	Subjects	Measures	Classifier	Classification Results			
					Feature Set/Method	ACC%	SEN%	SPE%
Multimodal analysis								
Cai et al., 2019 [44]	DTI, sMRI	165 AD, 165 HC	BC, connection strength	LDA	**BC (AAI)**	**84.6**	-	-
					CN (AAI)	73.0	-	-
					BC + CN (AAI)	79.8	-	-
					Hippocampal volume (AAI)	68.1	-	-
					MMSE (AAI)	70.2	-	-
					Hippocampal volume + MMSE (AAI)	71.1	-	-
					BC (HOA)	75.0	-	-
					CN (HOA)	71.1	-	-
					BC + CN (HOA)	72.2	-	-
					Hippocampal volume (HOA)	61.5	-	-
					MMSE (HOA)	70.2	-	-
					Hippocampal volume + MMSE (HOA)	66.6	-	-
Tang et al., 2016 [45]	DTI, sMRI	29 AD, 23 HC	Volume, deformation, FA, MD	LDA, SVM	Results reported for Right hippocampus with SVM Volume	78.4	63.6	100.0
					Shape			
					original	78.4	72.7	76.7
					PCA	70.3	63.6	80.0
					PCA + ttest	86.5	81.8	93.3
					DTI	83.8	86.4	80.0
					Volume + Shape			
					original	78.4	72.7	86.7
					PCA	73.0	68.2	80.0
					PCA + ttest	89.2	86.4	93.3
					DTI + Shape			
					original	81.8	72.7	93.3
					PCA	83.8	86.4	80.0
					PCA + ttest	**94.6**	**95.5**	**93.3**

Table 2. Studies that use machine learning to classify AD and MCI patients (bold classification methods indicate the preferred ones based on highest performances).

Article	Neuroimaging Technique	Subjects	Measures	Classifier	Classification Results				
					Task	Feature Set/Method	ACC%	SEN%	SPE%
Shao et al., 2012 [46]	DTI	17 AD, 21 HC, 23 MCI	FA, MD, FD	SVM, k-NN, NB	AD/HC (SVM)	**FD**	**100.0**	-	-
						FA	92.1	-	-
						MD	100.0	-	-
					MCI/HC (SVM)	**FD**	**97.7**	-	-
						FA	84.1	-	-
						MD	93.2	-	-
					MCI/AD (SVM)	**FD**	**85.0**	-	-
						FA	82.5	-	-
						MD	85.0	-	-
Nir et al., 2015 [47]	DTI	37 AD, 50 HC, 113 MCI	FA, MD	SVM	AD/HC	**MD-fdr cva (n = 641)**	**84.9**	**84.4**	**85.7**
						FA-fdr cva (n = 214)	77.8	78.2	77.3
						FA (n = 1080)	74.5	75.0	73.9
						MD (n = 1080)	80.6	79..2	82.4
					MCI/HC	**MD-fdr cvl (n = 12)**	**79.0**	**76.9**	**81.5**
						MD (n = 1080)	68.3	69.8	66.4
Demirhan et al., 2015 [48]	DTI	43 AD, 70 HC, 114 MCI	FA	SVM	AD/HC	Whole WM	80.8	-	-
						Relieff1500	87.8	-	-
					MCI/HC	Whole WM	63.6	-	-
						Relieff1500	78.5	-	-
					AD/MCI	Whole WM	73.9	-	-
						ReliefF1500	85.3	-	-
Prasad et al., 2015 [49]	DTI	38 AD, 50 HC, 38 lMCI, 74 eMCI	Measures of connectivity	SVM	AD/HC	FI(N) + FL(N)	78.2	-	-
					eMCI/HC	FI(N+M)	59.2	-	-
					lMCI/HC	FL(N)	62.8	-	-
					eMCI/lMCI	FI(N)+ FL(N)	63.4	-	-
Ebadi et al., 2017 [50]	DTI	15 AD, 15 HC, 15 MCI	FA	Logistic regression, random forest, NB, k-NN and SVM, ensemble	AD/HC (Ensemble)	No Feat. selection	73.3	-	-
						Feat. selection	**80.0**	-	-
					MCI/HC (Ensemble)	No Feat. selection	50.0	-	-
						Feat. selection	**70.0**	-	-
					AD/MCI (Ensemble)	No Feat. selection	73.3	-	-
						Feat. selection	**80.0**	-	-

Table 2. *Cont.*

Article	Neuroimaging Technique	Subjects	Measures	Classifier	Classification Results				
					Task	Feature Set/Method	ACC%	SEN%	SPE%
Maggipinto et al., 2017 [51]	DTI	89 AD, 90 HCI, 90 MCI	FA, MD	Random forest	AD/HC	**FA, non-nested**	**87.0**	-	-
						FA, nested	75.0	-	-
						MD, non- nested	83.0	-	-
						MD, nested	76.0	-	-
					MCI/HC	**FA, non-nested**	**81.0**	-	-
						FA, nested	59.0	-	-
						MD, non-nested	79.0	-	-
						MD, nested	60.0	-	-
Eldeeb et al., 2018 [52]	DTI	35 AD, 31 HC, 30 MCI	FA, MD	SVM	AD/HC	**MD-SIFT**	**98.3**	**97.0**	**100.0**
						MD-SURF	74.3	100	55.0
						FA-SIFT	95.5	98.0	95.0
						FA-SURF	62.0	92.0	20.0
					MCI/HC	**MD-SIFT**	**93.6**	**89.0**	**97.0**
						MD-SURF	83.0	82.3	92.0
						FA-SIFT	92.0	95.0	87.08
						FA-SURF	58.0	49.0	77.0
					AD/MCI	**MD-SIFT**	**92.0**	**98.0**	**91.0**
						MD-SURF	58.0	94.0	41.0
						FA-SIFT	92.0	98.0	87.0
						FA-SURF	56.0	100.0	20.0
					Multiclass	**MD-SIFT**	**89.0**	-	-
						MD-SURF	55.0	-	-
						FA-SIFT	87.0	-	-
						FA-SURF	43.0	-	-
Ye et al., 2019 [53]	DTI	40 AD, 27 cMCI, 48 sMCI, 46 HC	Connectivity strength	PLS-DA	AD/HC	Whole-brain	78.5 *	71.9	70.1
						MDMR selected	**81.7 ***	**67.0**	**76.2**
					cMCI/HC	Whole-brain	78.3 *	54.7	85.0
						MDMR selected	**86.2 ***	**71.3**	**79.3**

Table 2. *Cont.*

Article	Neuroimaging Technique	Subjects	Measures	Classifier	Classification Results				
					Task	Feature Set/Method	ACC%	SEN%	SPE%
Dalboni da Rocha et al., 2020 [54]	DTI	15 AD, 15 MCI, 15 HC	FA	SVM	AD/HC	Whole-brain	80	-	-
						Hippocampal Cingulum	**87**	**-**	**-**
						Parahippocampal Gyrus	83	-	-
					MCI/HC	**Whole-brain**	**60**	**-**	**-**
						Parahippocampal Cingulum	57	-	-
						Parahippocampal Gyrus	47	-	-
					AD/MCI	Whole-brain	77	-	-
						Hippocampal Cingulum	**83**	**-**	**-**
						Parahippocampal Gyrus	67	-	-
Dou et al., 2020 [55]	DTI	89 AD, 71 aMCI, 82 HC	FA, MD, DR, DA	SVM, LDA, XGB	AD/HC (SVM)	**Dataset 1**	**82.5**	**85.1**	**79.4**
						Dataset 2	82.3	80.9	82.3
					aMCI/HC (SVM)	**Dataset 1**	**52.0**	**24.7**	**74.6**
						Dataset 2	51.2	24.3	74.4
					AD/aMCI (SVM)	**Dataset 1**	**77.7**	**89.3**	**61.7**
						Dataset 2	82.2	83.3	81.0

* Area under Receiver Operating Characteristic (ROC).

3. Results

The 21 articles selected (Figure 2) are separated in two groups: classification considering only AD patients and healthy controls (HC) (n = 11) and classification including MCI patients (n = 10). For each article, when multiple classification approaches were tested, the best performance is reported in bold. Since some studies did not provide all the exact values of accuracy, sensitivity or specificity, these values have been deduced from plots.

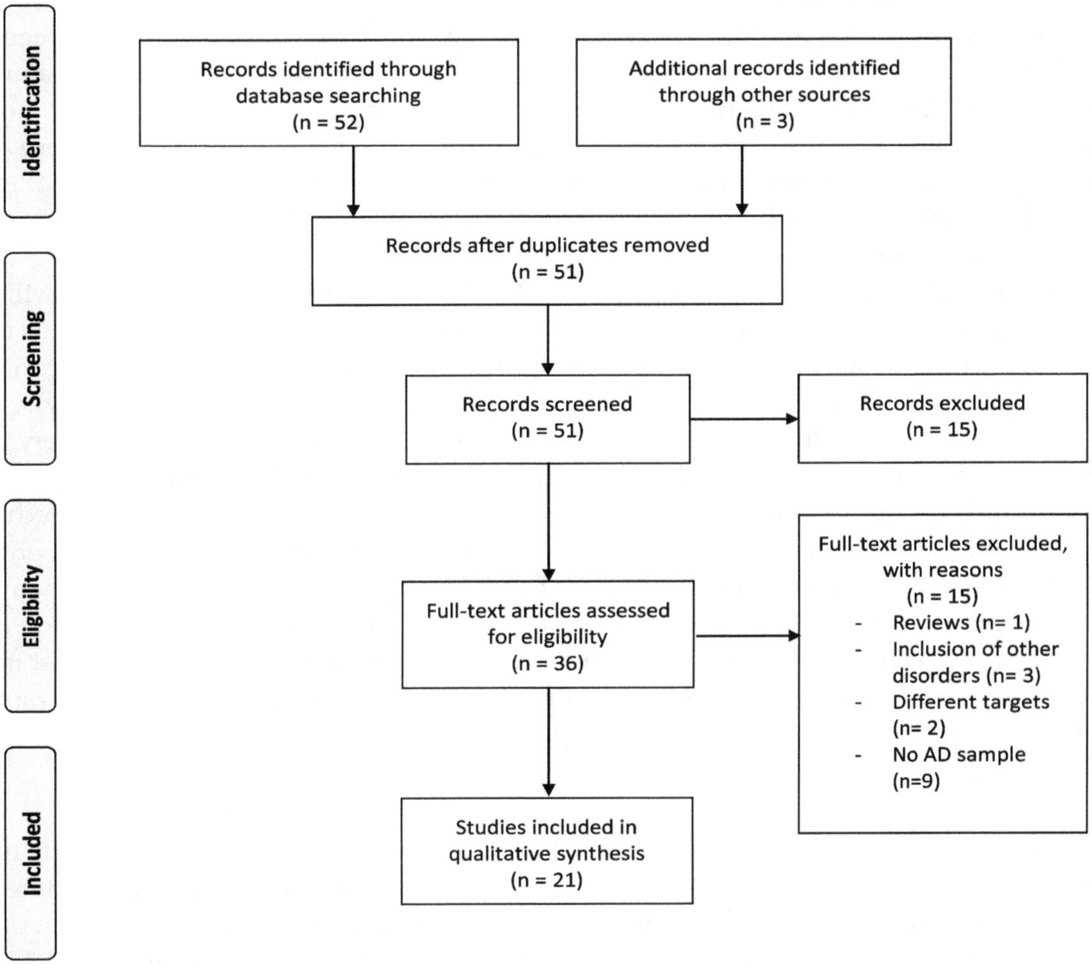

Figure 2. The four phases—identification, screening, eligibility and inclusion—of the process for the selection of the studies in this systematic review.

3.1. *AD/HC Classification*

The articles included in this review have been further classified depending on the type of neuroimaging technique used. Information extracted is showed in Table 1. Among the eleven studies of Table 1, four of them analyzed only DTI scans (DTI analysis), while the remaining seven also involved other neuroimaging modalities such as sMRI and rs-fMRI (multimodal analysis).

3.1.1. DTI Analysis

Graña et al. [35] trained an SVM using DTI measures to classify AD patients and HC. Images from DTI scans were preprocessed, in order to extract FA and MD. Different methods of cross-validation were employed, and the most accurate prediction was obtained by the leave-one-out method: with FA features, a 100% accuracy, sensitivity and specificity were achieved, while MD features achieved lower values.

Patil et al. [36] identified specific white matter regions which might represent AD markers. Classification between AD and HC was performed by the Adaptive Boosting (AdaBoost) algorithm. Considering FA measures and a set of 10 features, selected by a genetic algorithm, the accuracy, sensitivity and specificity scores were, respectively, 84.5%, 80.2% and 85.2%. If the feature set is not reduced, these values decreased due to overfitting (ACC = 75.3%), thus proving that features' reduction improves classification accuracy by removing redundancy. It can be noticed that, considering MD in place of FA, no significant changes in accuracy were observed, suggesting that FA is an effective parameter for AD/HC classification.

Patil and Ramakrishnan, in a successive study [37], focused on the correlation between the DTI indices and the mini-mental state examination (MMSE) score. FA, MD, DR and DA measures were obtained from DTI images of AD-damaged cerebral areas and then fed singularly or along with MMSE as inputs of an SVM, decision stumps and a simple logistic. The best results were achieved by considering the feature combination of FA and MMSE score (ACC = 94.2%) with SVM. Although there was not a significant correlation between DTI indices and MMSE score, the latter improved classification accuracy for each parameter.

Schouten et al. [38] differentiated between AD and HC through four DTI measures: FA, MD, DR and DA. As a first step, voxel-wise measures (FA, MD, DR, DA) were extracted via TBSS; these voxel measures were then separately clustered with independent component analysis (ICA). Then, probabilistic tractography applied on the clustering results allowed to determine a structural connectivity network and graph measures. Using TBSS, best accuracy was reached by RD (ACC = 84.8%), closely followed by the other DTI measures. ICA reached an accuracy of 85.1% with FA, while other performance scores were not dissimilar to those of TBSS. The ICA method allowed a significant reduction of features, while structural connectivity-based classification showed best results on the connectivity graph (ACC = 85.0) compared to other measures. Lastly, the Sparse Group Lasso (SGL) was used to assess the performance of parameters' combination: although reaching good classification accuracy, the best values were achieved by single parameters. Nevertheless, SGL shows that the most important contribution is given by TBSS and ICA's measures, connectivity graph and strength parameters. This finding suggests that DTI and graph theory provide complementary information.

3.1.2. Multimodal Analysis

Mesrob et al. [39] developed a multimodal method to classify AD and HC based on data from both DTI and structural MRI (sMRI). The model identified 73 anatomical cerebral regions of interest (ROIs) and the extraction of different parameters concerning them. Most distinctive regions for discrimination between subjects were selected using both univariate (t-test) and multivariate (SVM-based recursive feature elimination (SVM-RFE)) methods and then used to train an SVM for classification. FA and MD from DTI were considered, while gray matter concentration (GMC) was obtained from sMRI. Moreover, two multimodal parameters were used: MD/GMC and MD/FA. The best accuracy value (ACC = 99.6%) was achieved by the multimodal parameter MD/GMC on the 15 regions chosen through the multivariate feature selection method. Interestingly, the GMC parameter alone obtained higher accuracy value (76.5%) than any other accuracy obtained by other single parameters. However, classification with the multimodal parameter in the selected regions outperformed all other parameters combined.

Dyrba et al. [40], combined data originating from different kinds of scanners to classify AD patients and controls by considering FA and MD from DTI and the densities of white matter and gray matter (WMD, GMD) from sMRI. Such processed data served as the training set for an SVM and a naïve Bayes (NB) classifier. Furthermore, two different methods of cross-validation (CV) were employed: pooled CV and scanner-specific CV. Entropy-based information gain (IG) criterion, which allows to identify the more useful features for data separation, was used for feature selection. As expected, the SVM was more accurate than the NB classifier: best results were achieved by SVM using a pooled CV method on GMD data, with an accuracy of 89.3%. Interestingly, DTI data yielded inferior accuracy compared to GMD data.

Li et al. [41], combined DTI and sMRI indices to assess their discriminatory power in AD/HC classification. FA was measured from both tract- and voxel-based DTI, while gray matter volume (GMV) was obtained from sMRI. The best classification outcome resulted in the combination of tract-based FA and GMV (ACC = 94.3%). Considering only DTI indices, it was observed that tract-based FA yielded better accuracy than voxel-based FA.

Dyrba et al. [42] compared data derived from three different neuroimaging techniques: DTI, sMRI and resting-state functional MRI (rs-fMRI). The selected diffusion indexes were FA, MD and mode of anisotropy (MO). GMV was obtained from sMRI, while two parameters were extracted from rs-fMRI: "local clustering coefficient" and "shortest path length". Both single and multimodal parameters were used to train and test an SVM. A multiple kernel SVM (MK-SVM) was also tested, which allows for the combination of different imaging modalities. High accuracy values were reached using singular DTI indices (ACC= 85.0%) and GMV alone (ACC= 81.0%) as inputs for SVM, while for multimodal analysis, accuracy was 85.0% combining DTI measures and GMV. The multimodal results did not differ significantly from the results of the single modalities. In addition, the MK-SVM did not improve the results.

Chen et al. [43], assumed that combining DTI and DKI (diffusion kurtosis imaging) data could improve Alzheimer's detection compared to single modalities. Diffusion indices (FA, MD, DA, DR) were measured from both DTI and DKI, while kurtosis indices (mean kurtosis—MK, axial kurtosis—AK, radial kurtosis—RK) were obtained from DKI. Two different methods of features selection were employed: SVM-RFE and correlation coefficients with MMSE score (CORR-MMSE). SVM-RFE ranking led to high scores in the occipital white matter, whereas the scores from CORR-MMSE ranking selected the splenium of the corpus callosum and the posterior limb of the internal capsule, which were omitted in the scoring of diffusivity indices. According to these results, different regions are more predictive of the condition in different parametric maps and this presented a different sensitivity effect of matrices in pathological detection. The results show that DKI-diffusion indices (Diff-DKI) yielded a better performance than DTI-diffusion indices (Diff-DTI) (ACC = 92.4% vs. ACC = 81.1%). Moreover, the highest performance (ACC = 96.2%) resulted from the combination of kurtosis and diffusion indices from DKI (ALL-DKI), highlighting that kurtosis provided additional information in the detection of abnormalities.

Cai et al. [44] selected 330 participants from the ADNI (Alzheimer's Disease Neuroimaging Initiative) database and developed a classifier based on structural brain network modeling through the rich-club hierarchical network paradigm. Both the Automated Anatomical Labeling (AAL) and the Harvard-Oxford Atlas (HOA) were considered for the structural networks' construction, performed on DTI and b0 (sMRI) images, aligned with the PANDA pipeline tool, for each individual included in the study. The classification between AD and HC was performed through linear discriminant analysis (LDA) on the following topologic parameters extracted from the resulting structural brain networks: "betweenness centrality (BC)" and "connection strength". The classification accuracy of both BC and connections strength was compared with common measures in AD diagnosis: hippocampal volume and MMSE. The study findings reported significant difference in BC and connection strength between AD and controls for some brain regions, which were specific to each atlas (AAL or HOA). These relevant connections were considered as classification features to distinguish AD from controls. The best results were obtained using the AAL atlas, which achieved the best outcome in particular (ACC = 84.62%), with BC applied to the left putamen and left precuneus.

Tang et al. [45] closely examined the feasibility of AD/HC classification through volumetric, morphometric and DTI-based features specifically extracted from hippocampus and amygdala. T1 sMRI images of the participants were segmented with a two-level diffeomorphic multi-atlas likelihood-fusion algorithm and the help of an expert neuroanatomist, in order to calculate the volume of hippocampus and amygdala. The T1 images were also 3D segmented, creating triangulated surfaces of the regions of interest, and through large deformation diffeomorphic metric mapping (LDDMM), shrinking or expansion of local surface vertices, in relation to the adequate template, was estimated.

DTI images were processed and segmented to obtain FA and MD values of hippocampus and amygdala. The feature set thus included volumetric measures, DTI indices and the deformation degree at each vertex of the modeled surfaces. Given the high number of vertices (over 1200), feature reduction through principal component analysis (PCA, selecting 95% of variance) and t-test was explored. Classification was performed with both LDA and SVM, validated through leave-one-out cross-validation, with SVM achieving the best results, reaching an accuracy of 94.6% for the best-case scenario with the most significative feature set, for 37 total subjects. Even though the feature reduction process significantly improved the performance of the LDA classifier, while not substantially affecting SVM, the SVM classifier still outperformed the LDA. Given the complexity of results of this study in Table 1, we only reported the performance for the right hippocampus using SVM, for which the best performance was obtained, showing how the results change according to the combination of the image modalities used.

3.2. *AD/MCI/HC Classification*

In Table 2, ten articles that include MCI classification are summarized. All these studies employ only DTI analysis.

Shao et al. [46] proposed individual structural connectivity networks (ISCNs) to distinguish predementia and AD from healthy aging, in individual scans. For each connection, three attributes were calculated: fiber density (FD), the mean value of FA and mean value of MD across all voxels for all connection fibers. Once the structure of ISCNs was identified, three classifiers, namely, SVM, k-nearest neighbor (k-NN), NB were trained to classify subjects based on selected connections. Among the considered ML models, SVM yielded better accuracy. Patients with AD were distinguished from healthy control subjects with an accuracy of 100% using FD and MD, while patients with MCI were distinguished from healthy controls with an accuracy higher than 90%. This result is in line with previous findings of widely distributed FA decreases and MD increases in MCI. Furthermore, groups of MCI and AD patients were separated with an accuracy of about 85%, suggesting that ISCN alterations increase during the course of AD. These study findings suggested that ISCNs may have the potential of providing an imaging- and white matter-based biomarker for distinguishing between healthy subjects, aging subjects and patients with very early AD.

Nir et al. [47] investigated white matter integrity via a novel tract clustering and registration method that combines the strengths of voxel-wise and tractography-based methods, offering a compact representation of fiber bundles. In the proposed method, maximum density paths (MDP) was applied to whole-brain tractography. Differences in WM microstructure were determined by comparing FA and MD along each MDP. Significant MD and FA differences between AD patients and HC subjects were found, as well as MD differences between HC and late MCI subjects. Significant associations between FA, MD and MDP measures and cognitive deficits, as measured by MMSE scores, were also observed across all subjects. To discern between HC and AD groups, FA and MD values were tested along all the mean MDP points (1080 points). The subset of significant FA points (FAFDR CvA = 214 points) and the subset of significant MD points (MDFDR CvA = 641 points) was further tested: to distinguish between HC and MCI, all the MD values along all the MDP points (1080 points) were used, as well as the subset of significant MD points (MDFDR CvL = 12 points). Only MD measures were sensitive enough to detect MCI differences and revealed more profuse associations than FA in all analyses. The features interpolated along full mean MDPs were robust enough to reach high classification accuracies (~80%), so that reducing dimensionality by including only statistically significant MDP points did not dramatically increase classification accuracy (~85%).

Demirhan et al. [48] combined FA and MD measures from DTI to train an SVM classifier for the classification of HCs, AD and MCI patients. Good performances were reached by distinguishing AD from HC (87.8%), and MCI from HC (85.9%), while a lower value (78.4%) was obtained in separating MCI from AD subjects. Through ReliefF, an algorithm that makes it possible to identify the most discriminative voxels in white matter's map, a best feature set consisting of 1500 elements was extracted. Selecting a subset of these features did not provide a noticeable improvement in classification accuracy if the disease was at late stages. On the other hand, the selection of specific cerebral regions considerably improved the AD/MCI and MCI/HC classification.

Prasad et al. [49] compared an ensemble of different anatomical connectivity measures using both fiber and flow connectivity methods that may help in detecting AD patients. These features were fed into a repeated, stratified 10-fold cross-validation design, using SVMs to classify controls vs. AD, controls vs. early MCI (eMCI), controls vs. late MCI (L-MCI), and eMCI vs. L-MCI. The results exhibit a significant difference in the accuracy of the various feature sets used to distinguish between the various diagnostic groups. In each of these classification problems, nine different sets of features were used: the fiber connectivity matrix, (FI(M)), the flow connectivity matrix (FL(M)), the fiber network measures (FI(N)), the flow network measures (FL(M)), combinations of these sets as FI (N+M), FL(N+M), FI(N)+FL(N), FI(M)+FL(M) and FI(N+M)+FL(N+M). All of these connectivity measures were derived simply from diffusion images. The emphasis of the study was to explore and understand which diffusion-based network measures are predictive of Alzheimer's disease, in contrast to the optimization of classification accuracy, as in previous studies. In this way, the classification accuracy was adopted as the metric to evaluate different types of brain connectivity features, and to understand which ones may have an advantage in predicting MCI or AD insurgence.

Ebadi et al. [50] investigated the diagnostic potential of brain connectivity models regarding AD and MCI, applying graph theory to DTI measures. Graphs represented connections between different cerebral areas; once the graph measures were extracted, the best features were selected, in order to optimize the classifier's performance and reduce overfitting. Classification was conducted through different classification methods (logistic regression, random forest, NB, k-NN and SVM) and combining their output, to improve the performance of the whole model (Ensemble). They also tested a k-best feature selection method where the features are ranked based on their power in performing the classification, and then the top K features are selected for the given estimator. Ensemble with feature selection obtained the best performance. AD patients and HC were classified with an accuracy of 80.0%, while MCI patients were separated from controls with an accuracy of 66.7%; overall, the AD/MCI ratio reached an accuracy of 76.7%.

Maggipinto et al. [51] proved the effect of feature selection bias (FSB) occurring in DTI-based AD classification, leading to an overestimation of performance metrics. FA and MD maps were extracted and registered to the same reference, and the regions corresponding to white matter were isolated through the TBSS algorithm, extracting the skeleton of white fiber tracts for each patient. Feature selection was performed via Wilcoxon rank sum test and the ReliefF algorithm both in a "nested" (unbiased) and "non-nested" way: in the former, feature selection is done after training, while in the latter it is performed before the training (i.e., only once). The classification task was accomplished by a random forest with B = 300 learning trees trained with bootstrap aggregating. Performance was assessed with 100 rounds of 5-fold cross validation. The results showed that the performance diminished using a nested approach. For example, for FA accuracy, it dropped from a maximum mean value of 87% (non-nested) to 75% (nested) in AD/HC discrimination, while for MCI/HC accuracy dropped from 81% to 59%. The same behavior was observed considering MD, where ACC decreased from 83% to 76%, and from 79% to 66% for the AD/HC and MCI/HC classification, respectively.

Eldeeb et al. [52] proposed a novel method to extract relevant markers associated with FA and MD. After preprocessing of DTI-data, FA and MD maps of regions of interest were determined using a "bag-of-words" model. This model has been used to model the hippocampus diffusivity maps patterns, through clustering the extracted hippocampus features, where the number of features is changing from one slice to another. Both the speeded up robust features (SURF) and the scale invariant feature transform (SIFT) features were extracted. With these FA and MD maps, an SVM was then trained to classify the different groups of subjects. Classification was performed for each pair of groups, and then between all of the classes, solving a multiclass problem. The best accuracies were obtained with MD map using a SIFT features descriptor and are reported as follows: 98.3% AD/HC, 93.6% MCI/HC, 92.0% AD/MCI and 89.0% multiclass.

Ye et al. [53] conducted a connectome-wide association (CWAS) study on AD, stable MCI (sMCI), MCI converting to AD (cMCI) and healthy patients selected from the ADNI database to explore the alterations in structural connectivity networks of white matter without any a priori hypothesis on pathologic alterations. Whole-brain connectomes were generated through probabilistic fiber tracking of registered T1 images and DTI scans, separated in 90 regions according to the AAL atlas. Multivariate distance matrix regression (MDMR) paired with the delta method were applied to assess the variation of distance in connectivity patterns, highlighting the brain regions that displayed greater differences between the study groups. The discriminatory power of the connectivity features isolated by the MDMR analysis was tested by comparing the classification performance obtained with them against the whole-brain connectivity features, using a partial least squares discrimination analysis (PLS-DA) classifier with five-fold cross-validation on 161 subjects. For cMCI/HC classification, considering MDMR-selected features over whole-brain ones, the SEN score increased from 54.7% to 71.3%, while SPEC decreased from 85.0% to 79.3%; regarding AD/HC classification, SEN went from 71.9% to 67.0%, while SPEC grew from 70.1% to 76.2%.

Dalboni da Rocha et al. [54] classified AD, MCI and HC through an SVM applied to the patients' FA maps obtained through DTI, focusing on brain areas frequently associated with AD abnormalities. The analysis was repeated for the whole-brain and in specific brain areas both with and without a feature selection stage, based on the Fisher Score. As expected, results obtained without feature selection were lower. Among all the considered brain areas, two of them showed greater discriminatory power (consistently lower FA) between AD and HC: the bilateral cingulum in the hippocampal formation and the parahippocampal gyrus, in accordance with previous studies on AD indicating parahippocampal white matter modifications. Repeating the analysis of both regions by requiring the voxels to have a minimum Fisher Score (0.4/0.8) led to a maximum ACC of 93% in AD/HC classification considering the cingulum in the hippocampal formation and 90% for the parahippocampal gyrus. However, MCI/HC classification showed lower accuracy, in some cases close to chance level, possibly due to the inability to assess FA on a submillimeter scale.

Dou et al. [55] evaluated the integrity of whole-brain WM structure using automated fiber quantification (AFQ) for AD, amnestic MCI and healthy patients. The corrected, b0-aligned DTI images of the patients were processed with the AFQ toolkit in order to identify 20 major fiber tracts that have been shown to be relevant in AD progression, first by estimating the fiber tractography and then by segmenting the fiber tracts of interest. The FA, MD, DR, DA of each point was determined. Three classifiers were tested on a set of 1440 features per patient: SVM, LDA and extreme gradient boosting (XGB). Performance was evaluated both with 10-fold cross-validation and leave-one-out cross-validation. The results of this study summarized in Table 2 refer to SVM with leave-one-out cross validation for which the best results were obtained. Patients were divided into a discovery dataset and a replicated dataset and the statistical analysis, model learning and validation was repeated for both databases, obtaining agreeing results: ACC = 82.56–83.72% for AD/HC classification, 77.78%–82.28% for AD/aMCI classification and 52.02%–51.25% for aMCI/HC classification.

4. Discussion

In this review article, we identified twenty-two studies applying ML techniques for the classification of AD based on DTI imaging data, used alone or in combination with other imaging techniques. Some of the reviewed studies only differentiated between AD patients and healthy controls, while others also included a group of MCI patients for the identification and differentiation of the prodromal stage of the disease.

To the best of our knowledge, this is the first study that systematically reviewed classification approaches in AD with a focus on DTI. The attention to this specific technique is due to the fact that DTI is sensitive to microstructural white matter changes that are not visible with conventional volumetric techniques, and thus may contribute to the search for early biomarkers of the disease [56].

Studies discussed in this review have highlighted the role of DTI data as biomarkers of AD and MCI. Combining the application of ML approach with features extracted from DTI scans can provide a customized diagnosis for the early identification of AD, MCI and healthy subjects. Importantly, one of the great advantages of applying classification algorithms on neuroimaging data is the potential use for detecting AD at the prodromal stages, even well before clinical manifestation [57], which would have potential application in routine clinical settings in the future. In particular, the early detection of MCI is fundamental, since existing AD therapies show better results if the disease is still at earlier stages.

As regards the binary classification between AD and HC, very high performance in terms of accuracy (>90%) was achieved by several studies ([35,37,39,41,43,46,52]), among which, two even obtained 100% accuracy ([35,46]) (Figure 3). However, it should be noted that the sample size of these studies, in particular of the ones obtaining an accuracy of 100%, is quite limited (15–35 subjects per group), thus, the model could have been overfitted and could lack generalizability.

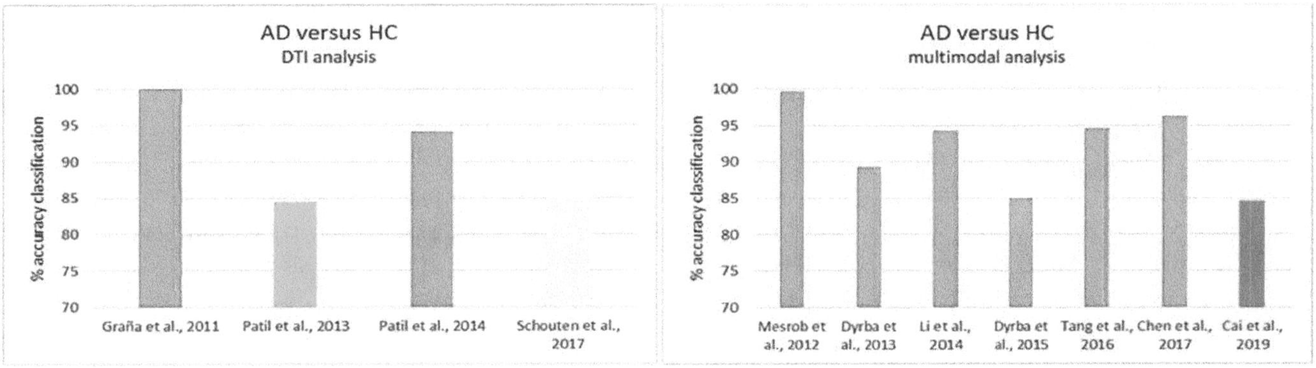

Figure 3. Distribution of the overall accuracy (%) reached by the studies about AD versus controls using DTI or multimodal analysis. Classifiers are reported with a different color bar: support vector machine (SVM) (**blue**), adaptive boosting (AdaBoost) (**green**), logistic elastic net regression (**yellow**), linear discriminant analysis (LDA) (**red**).

Studies reported in this review show evidence that automated DTI-based classifications of both MCI/HC and MCI/AD provide considerably inferior results than AD/HC separation (accuracy: ~80%). Only two studies obtained an accuracy higher than 90% [46,52], but also in this case, the limited sample size needs to be considered as a potential bias (Figure 4). Lower accuracy in these classifications is probably due to less marked differences between the features extracted. In addition, it is worth mentioning that, also from a clinical point of view, there is less confidence in the underlying pathology in MCI patients. Indeed, MCI itself is an heterogenous group, which is not always screened for primarily amnestic type or amyloid biomarkers that would increase the probability of prodromal AD.

Only one work [52] investigated the ternary problem: AD vs. MCI vs. HC and reached a good performance (accuracy = 89%). Thus, from this study, it seems that the integration of DTI with ML can be a variable instrument for the AD vs. MCI vs. HC classification also in clinical practice.

Interestingly, one study [49] also compared early MCI (eMCI) vs. late MCI (L-MCI), obtaining a quite low accuracy (63.4%). Thus, the problem of detecting subtle differences between subgroups needs to be further investigated.

Importantly, the reviewed studies differed by several factors including the sample sizes, the imaging analysis approach (i.e., voxel-based vs. tract-based), different features extracted, different feature selection methods and classification approaches. For this reason, it is difficult to quantitatively compare the different studies, while a qualitative analysis of the results can be performed.

Concerning the classification approach, it can be observed that SVM was the most frequently adopted method both for the classification of only AD [35,37,39–43,45] or also MCI [46–49,52,54,55] classification (Figures 3 and 4). Linear discriminant analysis [44,45,55] or naïve Bayes [40,46] were also sometimes used in AD classification. Other less common classification algorithms retrieved used

AdaBoost [36], extreme gradient boosting [55], Logistic elastic net regression [38], k-NN [46], Ensemble classification [50], random forest [51] and PLS-DA [53] (Figures 3 and 4).

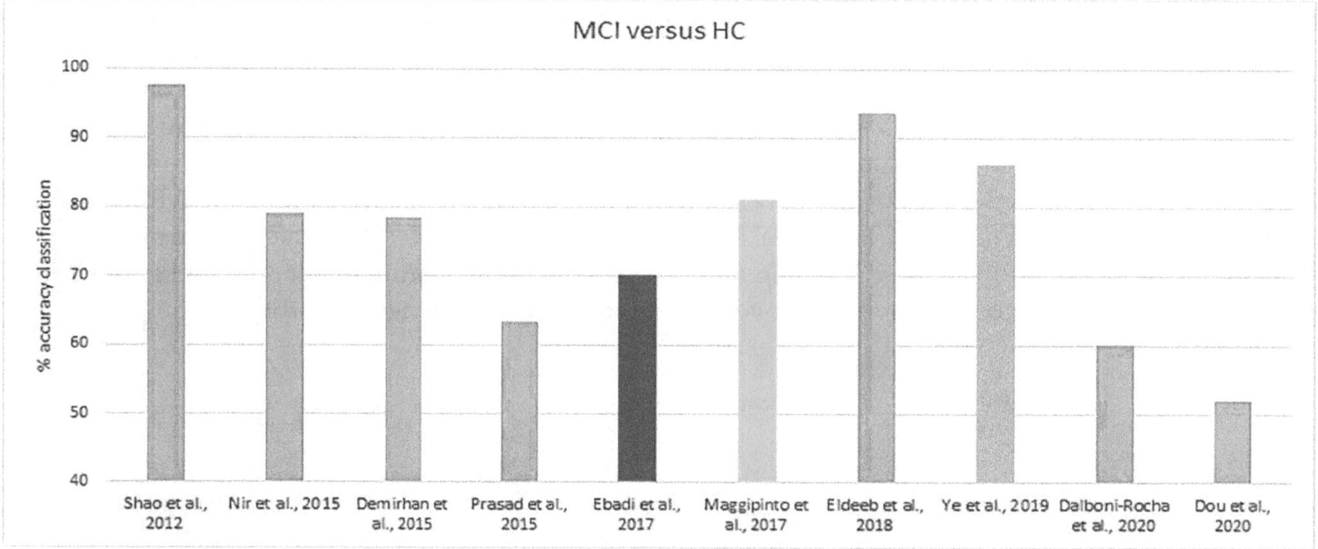

Figure 4. Distribution of the overall accuracy (%) reached by the studies about mild cognitive impairment (MCI) versus controls. Classifiers are reported with a different color bar: SVM (**blue**), Ensemble classification (**purple**), random forest (**green**), partial least squares discriminant analysis (PLS-DA) (**gray**).

Few studies have compared different classification approaches [40,45,46,55], all of them finding that SMV outperformed the other classifiers. However, in future studies, it would be useful to perform a more extensive comparison of the performance of diverse classification algorithms.

Another important factor that influences the performance concerns the extracted features. The first important distinction is between studies which computed voxel-based or ROI-based features (i.e., [35–37]) vs. studies relying on tract-based features (i.e., [38,49]). In the first case, diffusion features are computed in each voxel, or in specific ROIs, of the whole-brain, while in the second method, white matter fiber tracts are estimated and for each tract, the mean value of the desired diffusion feature is calculated. Then, while most of the studies computed quite common and simple diffusion features like fractional anisotropy, mean diffusivity, betweenness centrality, radial or axial diffusivity and connectivity strength (i.e., [35,37,44,51]), few studies extracted more complex features [38,49].

Most of these studies showed that FA represents the best diffusion feature for classification models and provides valuable information to distinguish between AD and healthy subjects [35,37,38,51], while others obtained better results using other features like MD [47,52]. Concerning MCI vs. HC classification, some studies [46,47,49,52] reached better performances using mean diffusivity and fiber density as features.

In one study [41], the performances using voxel- and tract-based features were compared. According to the result of this study, tract features seem to perform better in differentiating between AD and HC. This could be due to the fact that the clustering of voxel in the tracts reduces dimensionality by grouping voxels with similar anatomic and functional characteristics.

In addition, two studies [37,44] found that clinical parameters, such as MMSE score, can also improve classification performances, meaning that the inclusion of other types of features, like clinical scores, can improve the performance.

In addition to classification and feature extraction, feature selection is also important for identifying discriminating features. The selection of appropriate features not only removes the non-informative signal, but also reduces the computational time involved in classification. The two most adopted methods for feature selection are biologically informed and automated feature selection methods.

The former relies on prior biological knowledge about the discriminating ability of certain regions, generally obtained from existing literature, whereas the latter selects features based on general data characteristics, without prior knowledge.

The automated methods applied in the reviewed studies included genetic algorithm [36], t-test [39,45], recursive feature elimination [39,43], PCA [45], Wilcoxon rank sum test [51], ReliefF algorithm [48,51], multivariate distance matrix regression [53], false discovery rate [47] and k-best method [50]. Although it is difficult to say which is the best feature selection algorithm, since a comparison study is missing and several studies differentiate for multiple factors, it is evident from all these studies that selecting the most discriminant features improves the performance of the classifier by eliminating redundant or less useful features from the dataset. In particular, [51] shows that a feature selection which is blind to the t-test, leads to overoptimistic results (10% up to 30% relative increase in area under curve (AUC)).

Some studies applied a biologically informed selection method and focus only on regions, which are known to be compromised in AD, in particular hippocampus [44,45], parahippocampal gyrus and hippocampal cingulum [54] or amygdala [45]. Indeed, the hippocampus and the amygdala are among the anatomical structures of particular interest to the study of AD, mainly because of their active involvement in memory [58]. Both the global volume and the local shape of the hippocampus and the amygdala have been found to be compromised in AD [59,60]. The performance obtained by these studies are comparable to those obtained using automated methods. In particular, diffusion features from the right hippocampus [38,45] or from the parahippocampal gyrus [54] provided the best results in discriminating between AD/HC or AD/MCI. Indeed, it has previously been suggested that automated feature selection will not improve classification accuracy as compared to biologically informed feature selection, driven by prior biological knowledge of regions typically affected by AD, such as the hippocampus, amygdala, thalamus and caudate [61]. Notably, in the classification MCI/HC, whole-brain analysis performed better in [54], possibly due to the more subtle and sparse alterations in the prodromal stage of the disease.

The last important point to be considered when discussing the reviewed studies concerns the application of unimodal versus multimodal images. For AD/HC classification, five studies integrated DTI with sMRI [39–41,44,45], while only one also added fMRI [42]. One study also combined DTI with a more novel technique, which is DKI [43]. Notably, none of those studies applied a multimodal approach for the classification of MCI compared with AD.

All but one study [40] found that the results obtained using DTI measures outperformed those obtained with volumetric images. The contradictory results in [40] could be due to the advanced stage of the patient included in the study, so that the brain volume was highly compromised with cortical atrophy. Another possible explanation for this contradictory result could be represented by the multi-centric nature of the study. Indeed, it has been pointed out that DTI is more affected by site effects due to differences in acquisition parameters than volume measures [62]. For this reason, combining images of different sites could have mostly compromised the classification accuracy for DTI images.

In addition, most of these studies found that the combination of multimodal features outperformed the results obtained by using one single technique. Indeed, DTI-based features serve as a complementary tool to volume-based features, as the two imaging techniques reflect tissue changes associated with AD that correspond to pathological evidences in the gray matter and white matter, respectively. Thus, from the results of this review, it seems that combining several neuroimaging modalities is promising for further understanding the underlying disease mechanisms. However, it must be noted that [42] found that combining parameters from different neuroimaging modalities does not significantly improve AD/HC separation. Thus, future studies need to assess whether multimodal imaging, including functional (or metabolic) imaging methods, provides additional diagnostic accuracy for the classification of AD clinical labels, which could only be obtained from pathology.

In addition to the above-mentioned future lines of research, including the testing and fair comparison of different classifier and different feature extraction/selection approaches and a more systematic evaluation of the benefits of multimodal imaging compared with unimodal one, other future directions can be suggested. At first, it would be important to include larger samples of subjects since most of the reviewed study deals with quite low study groups. Larger samples from different sites, together with better pooling analysis methods, may improve the statistical power of the analysis, allowing to obtain more reliable information [63].

Then, future works should be more focused on the integration of heterogenous data sources, since promising results were obtained so far in this direction. Such data should importantly include physiological and functional parameters that can aid in constructing diagnostic tools with higher sensitivity and specificity, for more effective analysis of brain diseases [8]. Moreover, other miscellaneous data than neuroimaging could improve the classification of AD, including cognitive measures, risk factors associated with AD or cerebrospinal fluid measures [64].

Another important line of future direction consists in the implementation of longitudinal studies, which include different stages of AD for a better understanding of the progression of the disease, from the earliest to the most advanced stages. Indeed, a better understanding of the progression of neuronal deterioration and its correlation with psychological symptoms may help setting up new tailored treatments, such as real-time neurofeedback [65] and brain-computer interface training [66].

Finally, the application of deep learning methods and in their comparison with ML approaches should be better investigated in the future. With respect to conventional ML methods, deep learning algorithms require little or no image pre-processing, and can automatically infer an optimal representation of the data from the raw images without requiring prior feature selection, thus resulting in a more objective and less biased process [67]. Few papers on the application of deep learning approaches, and in particular convolutional neural networks, in the classification or prediction of AD using DTI imaging data have been recently published achieving good results [68,69]. More comprehensive studies are needed to evaluate the advantages of these methods compared with more traditional approaches.

5. Conclusions

To summarize, the results of this review showed that ML algorithms can be successfully applied to DTI or multimodal imaging data to deepen the current understanding of structural and functional connectivity mechanisms of AD and MCI, representing one of the ultimate goals of future AD-related research.

According to existing studies, the classification between AD and HC performs better than that between AD and MCI or MCI and HC, probably due to the less advanced study concerning MCI and to the heterogeneity of this group. Support vector machine appears to outperform the other classifiers, although in this domain other approaches (i.e., random forest) are promising. Regarding selected features, FA provided the most powerful results in AD/HC classification, possibly due to the high disruption of WM integrity, while in the detection of MCI, other features could be more reliable, in particular MD. Focusing on specific ROIs, in particular the hippocampus and the amygdala, which are known to be compromised in AD, might not decrease the performance compared with a whole-brain analysis, at least in the classification between AD and HC. Multimodal approaches that look for patterns of neurodegeneration across different kinds of bioimages are gaining increasing attention and seem to be promising for a better classification of AD or MCI. Multimodal imaging approaches, MCI-biomarkers, characterization of different stages of the disease, testing and comparing different types of classifiers, including deep learning algorithms, feature selection algorithms and bigger sample sizes, are important strategies that are likely to be emphasized in future studies.

Author Contributions: Conceptualization, L.B. (Lucia Billeci) and A.T.; methodology, A.B.; data curation, A.B., L.B. (Lorenzo Bachi); writing—original draft preparation, A.B.; writing—review and editing, L.B. (Lucia Billeci), L.B. (Lorenzo Bachi), A.T.; supervision, L.B. (Lucia Billeci). All authors have read and agreed to the published version of the manuscript.

Appendix A

List of Acronyms and Abbreviations

AAL	Automated Anatomical Labeling atlas
ACC	Accuracy
AD	Alzheimer's disease
ADNI	Alzheimer's Disease Neuroimaging Initiative
AFQ	Automated fiber quantification
AK	Axial kurtosis
AdaBoost	Adaptive boosting
ALL-DKI	Combination of kurtosis and diffusion indices from DKI
BC	Betweenness centrality
CAD	Computer-aided diagnosis
cMCI	MCI patients that eventually converts to AD
CORR-MMSE	Correlation coefficient with the MMSE score
CSF	Cerebrospinal fluid
CV	Cross-validation
CWAS	Connectome-wide association
DA	Axial diffusivity
Diff-DKI	DKI diffusion indices
Diff-DTI	DTI diffusion indices
DKI	Diffusion kurtosis imaging
DR	Radial diffusivity
DTI	Diffusion tensor imaging
eMCI	Early MCI patient
FA	Fractional anisotropy
FD	Fiber density
GMC	Grey matter concentration
GMD	Grey matter density
GMV	Grey matter volume
HC	Healthy control patient
HOA	Harvard-Oxford atlas
ICA	Independent component analysis
IG	Information gain
ISCN	Individual structural connectivity network
k-NN	*k*-nearest neighbors algorithm
LDA	Linear discriminant analysis
LDDMM	Large deformation diffeomorphic metric mapping
L-MCI	Late MCI patient
MCI	Mild cognitive impairment
MD	Mean diffusivity
MDMR	Multivariate distance matrix regression
MDP	Maximum density path
MK	Mean kurtosis
MK-SVM	Multiple-kernel SVM
ML	Machine learning
MMSE	Mini-mental state examination
MO	Mode of anisotropy
MRI	Magnetic resonance imaging
NB	Naïve Bayes classifier
PCA	Principal component analysis
PET	Positron mission tomography
PLS-DA	Partial least squares discrimination analysis

PRISMA	Preferred Reporting Items for Systematic Reviews and Meta-Analyses
RA	Relative anisotropy
rs-fMRI	Resting-state functional MRI
ROI	Region of interest
RK	Radial kurtosis
SEN	Sensitivity
SGL	Sparse group lasso
SIFT	Scale invariant feature transform
sMRI	Structural MRI
SPE	Specificity
SURF	Speed up robust features
SVM	Support vector machine
SVM-RFE	SVM-based feature recursive elimination
TBSS	Tract-based special statistics
WM	White matter
WMD	White matter density
XGB	Extreme gradient boosting

Appendix B

Appendix B.1. Machine Learning Overview

Machine learning (ML) is a broad term referring to an ensemble of computer algorithms that adapt their output through experience to match a desired outcome. Generally, an ML algorithm returns an output value determined by its input variables, called features, in order to refine the aptness of the computed output the program first learns on a training dataset, while evaluation of its performance is done on one or more validation datasets. The size of the data involved in both steps is crucial, as small samples could lead to unreliable results. ML models are most often grouped into three categories, depending on the nature of the learning process: in supervised learning, the program learns on a labelled dataset where the desired outcome is known, adjusting its output to replicate as best as possible the desired one; in unsupervised learning, the data is not labelled and the algorithm looks for similarities in the inputs by modeling their probability densities, highlighting the standing relations between them; in reinforcement learning, the algorithm discovers the desired outcome in a process of trial and error, and adapts its output to maximize the correct decisions that lead to it. The machine learning aspects of this review specifically concern one of the four kinds of learning problems, classification, where the output belongs to a discrete range (AD, HC and/or MCI) and with a supervised learning process. Consequently, these ML models are classifiers, i.e., objects that assign each feature vector x (a patient) to one of the c classes or groups. A brief description of each method mentioned in this paper follows. For additional background, see [70–72].

Appendix B.2. Support Vector Machine

The support vector machine (SVM) is a supervised, non-probabilistic linear classifier, meaning that it can learn to discriminate data belonging to two classes by searching for the linear boundary (called hyperplane) that maximizes the margin between the two known classes. If the input is an array x consisting of n features, meaning it is a point in a n-dimensional space, the SVM method finds a linear surface of dimension n-1 that divides the two clouds of n-dimensional points belonging to the two classes. That is, optimizing the hyperplane parameters in order to maximize its distance from the closest point, which is a problem that can be reduced to minimization of a quadratic error function. Although in its simplest definition SVM is a linear classifier, by employing the nonlinear kernel trick nonlinear classification can be performed. Moreover, the model can be adjusted if the two classes are not clearly separated in the n-dimensional space by relaxing the hard margin constraint in favor of a soft margin; SVM can also be adapted to resolve multiclass problems in various ways, generally by combining a bank of SVM classifiers.

Appendix B.3. Logistic Regression

Logistic regression, even if called "regression", is actually a classification model where the relationship between the features and the log-odds (the logarithm of the odds ratio) of the c classes is assumed to be linear. In other words, the posterior probability of each class is a logistic sigmoid function acting on a linear combination of the feature vector. The n parameters of the linear function are estimated for each class, so that for each datapoint x (consisting of n features), a score corresponding to each class is computed; the observation is then assigned to the class presenting the highest score. The parameters of the logistic regression can be determined by maximizing the log-likelihood of the data with a numerical optimization algorithm, typically with regularization of the coefficients (Maximum A Posteriori (MAP) estimation), such as the ridge regression (L2 penalty), the lasso regression (L1 penalty) or the elastic net regression (L1+L2 penalty). Regularization helps prevent excessive overfitting, reducing estimator variance whilst introducing a small bias. This model is usually formulated for a two-class problem, but can be extended to an arbitrary number of classes.

Appendix B.4. Naïve Bayes Classifier

The naïve Bayes classifier refers to a simple, yet robust family of models based on the assumption that the features x are independent. This assumption allows the posterior probability distribution for each class to depend merely on the product of n one-dimensional likelihoods, thus, not requiring estimation of conditional distributions. Parameters are learned with likelihood maximization, estimating the one-dimensional densities for each class and feature, which can be done in various ways, depending on the statistical hypotheses made on the data (the naïve Bayes event model). Usually, classification of data is done by choosing the most probable outcome, i.e., the class that exhibits the higher posterior probability for the observation.

Appendix B.5. Linear Discriminant Analysis

Linear discriminant analysis (LDA), derived from Fisher's discriminant analysis, is a classifier based on dimensionality reduction. The n-dimensional feature space is projected into one dimension with the weight array w: $y = w^{\mathrm{T}}x$. Each class is supposed to be distributed as a multivariate Gaussian, with all the covariance matrixes of the said class densities assumed to be equal (without this last assumption, the resulting model is the quadratic discriminant analysis). The log-odds of the classes posterior probability is then a linear function of x, and the decision boundary between any two classes is linear, resulting in a hyperplane in the feature space separating each pair of groups. Classification occurs by defining the thresholds over which the new data is assigned to one group instead of the others, in the projected one-dimensional space. Considering two classes 0 and 1, if $w^{\mathrm{T}}x > c$ x will be assigned to class 1, otherwise to class 0. Thus, learning for this model consists in defining the direction of projection that maximizes separation between the classes w and the decision threshold c by estimating the parameters of the multivariate of the classes' Gaussian distribution. Multiclass tasks can be performed either by combining several discriminants (one-versus-the-rest, one-versus-one) or by considering a single classifier with c linear discriminant functions.

Appendix B.6. Partial Least Squares Discriminant Analysis

Partial least squares discriminant analysis (PLS-DA) is a variant of the partial least squares regression, where the dependent variable y is converted to a categorical field. In a manner not dissimilar to principal component regression, partial least squares regression finds a set of linear combination of the inputs, selecting a subset of the components as regressors, but considering both

y and x for the projection into component space. This algorithm finds the latent variables with the maximum covariance with the y variable, instead of seeking directions that explain only the most variance. Considering all available directions would correspond to a conventional least square estimate, while selecting only a subset of them leads to a reduced regression with lower chances of overfitting. The conversion of the continuous value of y into its corresponding categorical value (i.e., turning a regressor into a classifier) can be done by comparing, for each new observation x, the c class values resulting from the PLS regression: the observation is then assigned to the class that showed the highest probability.

Appendix B.7. K-Nearest Neighbors

The nearest neighbor family of classifiers process new observations x depending on the outcome of the closest datapoints. On its most elementary form, the k-nearest neighbors (k-NN) classifier assigns the data x to the most popular class among its k neighbors, where k is a user-defined parameter. Distance can be determined with various metrics, the most common one being the Euclidean distance. Several versions of supervised k-NN exists, where the object of the learning process is usually the definition of the metric that better sorts the training inputs in their respective groups. This means finding the matrix M which, placed in $d(x_i, x_j) = (x_i - x_j)^T M(x_i - x_j)$ minimizes the classification error.

Appendix B.8. Random Forest

The random forest is a regression and classification technique based on bagging (bootstrap aggregating), by training a large ensemble of decision trees with low correlation between them, which are then averaged. A decision tree, often represented in their flowchart structure, is a model consisting of subsequent binary splits of the input space. A tree consists of its root, the first split; its branches, the next consecutive splits; the leaves, representing the predicted value (whether continuous or categorical). Building a tree corresponds to partitioning the input space in squares with lines that are parallel to coordinate axes. In a decision tree, leaning (growing) means deciding, at each node, the splitting threshold for the n-th input feature, which can be done by exhaustive research, minimizing an error function: for classification, two common measures are cross-entropy and the Gini index. After a sufficiently large tree is built it gets pruned, removing some of its branches by balancing the error function and a measure of model complexity (cost-complexity pruning). In a random forest, several trees are built, each time selecting a subset of the input variables. After the desired number of classification trees has been trained, the output classification is the result of a majority vote. By bagging the threes, instead of considering a single, larger tree, the overall variance of the model is decreased, although its bias is unchanged.

Appendix B.9. Boosting Techniques

The term boosting refers to a technique where several weak classifiers, with performance slightly above chance level, are combined to form a powerful committee, able to get very close to the target classification performance. Adaptive boosting (AdaBoost) is one of the most popular algorithms for boosting formulated for the two-class problem, where the weak classifiers are trained consequently, the performance of each one influencing the training of the next. Every one of the M training data points x is given a weight w_m, initially set to $1/M$. The first weak classifier is then trained, using the data to produce a class prediction $y \in \{-1, 1\}$. The next weak classifiers are trained after the weights are updated, giving more relevance to misclassified data. When the desired number of weak classifiers has been trained, the committee is formed: each one will contribute to the class prediction through a second set of weights a_j, one for each base classifier, determined by minimizing an exponential loss error function. One of the simplest forms of base learner that can be adopted is the decision stump, a single-level decision tree: the discrimination between two classes is done by comparing the features to a single threshold. Gradient boosting is a numerical development of the boosting method, often applied to decision trees. Through a differentiable loss function, the successive weak learners are trained in the gradient direction of minimal loss (gradient descent), fitting them to the negative gradient values of the chosen function. For classification, such loss function can consist in multinomial deviance, constructing at each iteration a number of trees equal to the total number of groups c, even though for binary classification a single tree for each iteration is sufficient.

References

1. Prince, M.; Bryce, R.; Albanese, E.; Wimo, A.; Ribeiro, W.; Ferri, C.P. The global prevalence of dementia: A systematic review and metaanalysis. *Alzheimers Dement.* **2013**, *9*, 63–75. [CrossRef]
2. Collie, A.; Maruff, P. The neuropsychology of preclinical Alzheimer's disease and mild cognitive impairment. *Neurosci. Biobehav. Rev.* **2000**, *24*, 365–374. [CrossRef]
3. Alzheimer's Association. 2019 Alzheimer's disease facts and figures. *Alzheimers Dement.* **2019**, *15*, 321–387. [CrossRef]
4. Jack, C.R.; Wiste, H.J.; Weigand, S.D.; Therneau, T.M.; Lowe, V.J.; Knopman, D.S.; Gunter, J.L.; Senjem, M.L.; Jones, D.T.; Kantarci, K.; et al. Defining imaging biomarker cut points for brain aging and Alzheimer's disease. *Alzheimers Dement.* **2017**, *13*, 205–216. [CrossRef] [PubMed]
5. Woolf, B.P. *Building Intelligent Interactive Tutors: Student-Centered Strategies for Revolutionizing E-Learning*; Morgan Kaufmann: Burlington, MA, USA, 2010.
6. Nayak, J.; Naik, B.; Behera, H.S. A Comprehensive Survey on Support Vector Machine in Data Mining Tasks: Applications & Challenges. *Int. J. Database Theory Appl.* **2015**, *8*, 169–186. [CrossRef]
7. Frisoni, G.B.; Fox, N.; Jack, C.R.; Scheltens, P.; Thompson, P. The clinical use of structural MRI in Alzheimer disease. *Nat. Rev. Neurol.* **2010**, *6*, 67–77. [CrossRef]
8. Greicius, M.D.; Srivastava, G.; Reiss, A.L.; Menon, V. Default-mode network activity distinguishes Alzheimer's disease from healthy aging: Evidence from functional MRI. *Proc. Natl. Acad. Sci. USA* **2004**, *101*, 4637–4642. [CrossRef] [PubMed]
9. Fripp, J.; Bourgeat, P.; Acosta, O.; Raniga, P.; Modat, M.; Pike, K.E.; Jones, G.; O'Keefe, G.; Masters, C.L.; Ames, D.; et al. Appearance modeling of 11C PiB PET images: Characterizing amyloid deposition in Alzheimer's disease, mild cognitive impairment and healthy aging. *NeuroImage* **2008**, *43*, 430–439. [CrossRef] [PubMed]
10. Cabral, C.; Silveira, M. Classification of Alzheimer's disease from FDG-PET images using favourite class ensembles. In Proceedings of the 2013 35th Annual International Conference of the IEEE Engineering in Medicine and Biology Society (EMBC), Osaka, Japan, 3–7 July 2013; Volume 2013, pp. 2477–2480. [CrossRef]
11. Szmuda, M.; Szmuda, T.; Springer, J.; Rogowska, M.; Sabisz, A.; Dubaniewicz, M.; Mazurkiewicz-Bełdzińska, M. Diffusion tensor tractography imaging in pediatric epilepsy—A systematic review. *Neurologia i Neurochirurgia Polska* **2016**, *50*, 1–6. [CrossRef] [PubMed]
12. Arab, A.; Wojna-Pelczar, A.; Khairnar, A.; Szabo, N.; Ruda-Kucerova, J. Principles of diffusion kurtosis imaging and its role in early diagnosis of neurodegenerative disorders. *Brain Res. Bull.* **2018**, *139*, 91–98. [CrossRef] [PubMed]
13. Billeci, L.; Calderoni, S.; Tosetti, M.; Catani, M.; Muratori, F. White matter connectivity in children with autism spectrum disorders: A tract-based spatial statistics study. *BMC Neurol.* **2012**, *12*, 148. [CrossRef]
14. Le Bihan, D.; Poupon, C.; Clark, C.A.; Pappata, S.; Molko, N.; Chabriat, H. Diffusion tensor imaging: Concepts and applications. *J. Magn. Reson. Imaging* **2001**, *13*, 534–546. [CrossRef] [PubMed]
15. Pierpaoli, C.; Jezzard, P.; Basser, P.J.; Barnett, A.; Di Chiro, G. Diffusion tensor MR imaging of the human brain. *Radiology* **1996**, *201*, 637–648. [CrossRef] [PubMed]
16. Alexander, A.L.; Lee, J.E.; Lazar, M.; Field, A.S. Diffusion tensor imaging of the brain. *Neurotherapeutics* **2007**, *4*, 316–329. [CrossRef] [PubMed]
17. Alves, G.S.; Knöchel, V.O.; Knöchel, C.; Carvalho, A.F.; Pantel, J.; Engelhardt, E.; Laks, J. Integrating Retrogenesis Theory to Alzheimer's Disease Pathology: Insight from DTI-TBSS Investigation of the White Matter Microstructural Integrity. *BioMed Res. Int.* **2015**, *2015*, 1–11. [CrossRef]
18. Smith, S.M.; Jenkinson, M.; Johansen-Berg, H.; Rueckert, D.; Nichols, T.E.; Mackay, C.E.; Watkins, K.E.; Ciccarelli, O.; Cader, M.Z.; Matthews, P.M.; et al. Tract-based spatial statistics: Voxelwise analysis of multi-subject diffusion data. *NeuroImage* **2006**, *31*, 1487–1505. [CrossRef]

19. Hagmann, P.; Cammoun, L.; Gigandet, X.; Meuli, R.; Honey, C.J.; Wedeen, V.J.; Sporns, O. Mapping the Structural Core of Human Cerebral Cortex. *PLoS Boil.* **2008**, *6*, e159. [CrossRef]
20. Xie, S.; Xiao, J.X.; Gong, G.L.; Zang, Y.-F.; Wang, Y.H.; Wu, H.K.; Jiang, X.X. Voxel-based detection of white matter abnormalities in mild Alzheimer disease. *Neurology* **2006**, *66*, 1845–1849. [CrossRef]
21. Ringman, J.M.; O'Neill, J.; Geschwind, D.; Medina, L.D.; Apostolova, L.G.; Rodriguez, Y.; Schaffer, B.; Varpetian, A.; Tseng, B.; Ortiz, F.; et al. Diffusion tensor imaging in preclinical and presymptomatic carriers of familial Alzheimer's disease mutations. *Brain* **2007**, *130*, 1767–1776. [CrossRef]
22. Cherubini, A.; Péran, P.; Spoletini, I.; Di Paola, M.; Di Iulio, F.; Hagberg, G.; Sancesario, G.; Gianni, W.; Bossù, P.; Caltagirone, C.; et al. Combined Volumetry and DTI in Subcortical Structures of Mild Cognitive Impairment and Alzheimer's Disease Patients. *J. Alzheimer's Dis.* **2010**, *19*, 1273–1282. [CrossRef]
23. Teipel, S.J.; Grothe, M.J.; Zhou, J.; Sepulcre, J.; Dyrba, M.; Sorg, C.; Babiloni, F. Measuring Cortical Connectivity in Alzheimer's Disease as a Brain Neural Network Pathology: Toward Clinical Applications. *J. Int. Neuropsychol. Soc.* **2016**, *22*, 138–163. [CrossRef] [PubMed]
24. Naggara, O.; Oppenheim, C.; Rieu, D.; Raoux, N.; Rodrigo, S.; Barba, G.D.; Meder, J.-F. Diffusion tensor imaging in early Alzheimer's disease. *Psychiatry Res. Neuroimaging* **2006**, *146*, 243–249. [CrossRef] [PubMed]
25. Zhang, Y.; Schuff, N.; Jahng, G.-H.; Bayne, W.; Mori, S.; Schad, L.; Mueller, S.; Du, A.-T.; Kramer, J.H.; Yaffe, K.; et al. Diffusion tensor imaging of cingulum fibers in mild cognitive impairment and Alzheimer disease. *Neurology* **2007**, *68*, 13–19. [CrossRef] [PubMed]
26. Medina, D.; Detoledo-Morrell, L.; Urresta, F.; Gabrieli, J.D.; Moseley, M.; Fleischman, D.; Bennett, D.A.; Leurgans, S.; Turner, D.A.; Stebbins, G.T. White matter changes in mild cognitive impairment and AD: A diffusion tensor imaging study. *Neurobiol. Aging* **2006**, *27*, 663–672. [CrossRef]
27. E Rose, S.; McMahon, K.L.; Janke, A.L.; O'Dowd, B.; De Zubicaray, G.I.; Strudwick, M.W.; Chalk, J.B. Diffusion indices on magnetic resonance imaging and neuropsychological performance in amnestic mild cognitive impairment. *J. Neurol. Neurosurg. Psychiatry* **2006**, *77*, 1122–1128. [CrossRef]
28. Fellgiebel, A.; Dellani, P.R.; Greverus, D.; Scheurich, A.; Stoeter, P.; Müller, M.J. Predicting conversion to dementia in mild cognitive impairment by volumetric and diffusivity measurements of the hippocampus. *Psychiatry Res. Neuroimaging* **2006**, *146*, 283–287. [CrossRef]
29. Müller, M.J.; Greverus, D.; Dellani, P.R.; Weibrich, C.; Wille, P.R.; Scheurich, A.; Stoeter, P.; Fellgiebel, A. Functional implications of hippocampal volume and diffusivity in mild cognitive impairment. *NeuroImage* **2005**, *28*, 1033–1042. [CrossRef]
30. Müller, M.J.; Greverus, D.; Weibrich, C.; Dellani, P.R.; Scheurich, A.; Stoeter, P.; Fellgiebel, A. Diagnostic utility of hippocampal size and mean diffusivity in amnestic MCI. *Neurobiol. Aging* **2007**, *28*, 398–403. [CrossRef]
31. Fellgiebel, A.; Müller, M.J.; Wille, P.; Dellani, P.R.; Scheurich, A.; Schmidt, L.G.; Stoeter, P. Color-coded diffusion-tensor-imaging of posterior cingulate fiber tracts in mild cognitive impairment. *Neurobiol. Aging* **2005**, *26*, 1193–1198. [CrossRef]
32. Choo, I.H.; Lee, N.Y.; Oh, J.-S.; Lee, J.S.; Lee, N.S.; Song, I.C.; Youn, J.C.; Kim, S.G.; Kim, K.W.; Jhoo, J.H.; et al. Posterior cingulate cortex atrophy and regional cingulum disruption in mild cognitive impairment and Alzheimer's disease. *Neurobiol. Aging* **2010**, *31*, 772–779. [CrossRef]
33. Selnes, P.; Aarsland, D.; Bjornerud, A.; Gjerstad, L.; Wallin, A.; Hessen, E.; Reinvang, I.; Grambaite, R.; Auning, E.; Kjærvik, V.K.; et al. Diffusion Tensor Imaging Surpasses Cerebrospinal Fluid as Predictor of Cognitive Decline and Medial Temporal Lobe Atrophy in Subjective Cognitive Impairment and Mild Cognitive Impairment. *J. Alzheimer's Dis.* **2013**, *33*, 723–736. [CrossRef] [PubMed]
34. Liberati, A.; Altman, D.G.; Tetzlaff, J.; Mulrow, C.; Gøtzsche, P.C.; Ioannidis, J.P.A.; Clarke, M.; Devereaux, P.J.; Kleijnen, J.; Moher, D. The PRISMA statement for reporting systematic reviews and meta-analyses of studies that evaluate health care interventions: Explanation and elaboration. *J. Clin. Epidemiol.* **2009**, *62*, e1–e34. [CrossRef] [PubMed]
35. Graña, M.; Termenon, M.; Savio, A.; González-Pinto, A.; Echeveste, J.; Perez, J.; Besga, A. Computer Aided Diagnosis system for Alzheimer Disease using brain Diffusion Tensor Imaging features selected by Pearson's correlation. *Neurosci. Lett.* **2011**, *502*, 225–229. [CrossRef] [PubMed]
36. Patil, R.B.; Piyush, R.; Ramakrishnan, S. Identification of brain white matter regions for diagnosis of Alzheimer using Diffusion Tensor Imaging. In Proceedings of the 2013 35th Annual International Conference of the IEEE Engineering in Medicine and Biology Society (EMBC), Osaka, Japan, 3–7 July 2013; pp. 6535–6538. [CrossRef]

37. Patil, R.B.; Ramakrishnan, S. Analysis of sub-anatomic diffusion tensor imaging indices in white matter regions of Alzheimer with MMSE score. *Comput. Methods Progr. Biomed.* **2014**, *117*, 13–19. [CrossRef] [PubMed]
38. Schouten, T.M.; Koini, M.; De Vos, F.; Seiler, S.; De Rooij, M.; Lechner, A.; Schmidt, R.; Heuvel, M.V.D.; Van Der Grond, J.; Rombouts, S.A. Individual classification of Alzheimer's disease with diffusion magnetic resonance imaging. *NeuroImage* **2017**, *152*, 476–481. [CrossRef] [PubMed]
39. Mesrob, L.; Sarazin, M.; Hahn-Barma, V.; De, S.L.C.; Dubois, B.; Gallinari, P.; Kinkingnéhun, S.; Mesrob, L.; Marie, S.; Valerie, H.-B.; et al. DTI and Structural MRI Classification in Alzheimer's Disease. *Adv. Mol. Imaging* **2012**, *2*, 12–20. [CrossRef]
40. Dyrba, M.; Ewers, M.; Wegrzyn, M.; Kilimann, I.; Plant, C.; Oswald, A.; Meindl, T.; Pievani, M.; Bokde, A.L.W.; Fellgiebel, A.; et al. Robust Automated Detection of Microstructural White Matter Degeneration in Alzheimer's Disease Using Machine Learning Classification of Multicenter DTI Data. *PLoS ONE* **2013**, *8*, e64925. [CrossRef]
41. Li, M.; Qin, Y.; Gao, F.; Zhu, W.; He, X. Discriminative analysis of multivariate features from structural MRI and diffusion tensor images. *Magn. Reson. Imaging* **2014**, *32*, 1043–1051. [CrossRef]
42. Dyrba, M.; Grothe, M.J.; Kirste, T.; Teipel, S.J. Multimodal analysis of functional and structural disconnection in Alzheimer's disease using multiple kernel SVM. *Hum. Brain Mapp.* **2015**, *36*, 2118–2131. [CrossRef]
43. Chen, Y.; Sha, M.; Zhao, X.; Ma, J.; Ni, H.; Gao, W.; Ming, N. Automated detection of pathologic white matter alterations in Alzheimer's disease using combined diffusivity and kurtosis method. *Psychiatry Res. Neuroimaging* **2017**, *264*, 35–45. [CrossRef]
44. Cai, S.; Huang, K.; Kang, Y.; Jiang, Y.; Von Deneen, K.M.; Huang, L. Potential biomarkers for distinguishing people with Alzheimer's disease from cognitively intact elderly based on the rich-club hierarchical structure of white matter networks. *Neurosci. Res.* **2019**, *144*, 56–66. [CrossRef] [PubMed]
45. Tang, X.; Qin, Y.; Wu, J.; Zhang, M.; Zhu, W.; Miller, M.I. Shape and diffusion tensor imaging based integrative analysis of the hippocampus and the amygdala in Alzheimer's disease. *Magn. Reson. Imaging* **2016**, *34*, 1087–1099. [CrossRef] [PubMed]
46. Shao, J.; Myers, N.; Yang, Q.; Feng, J.; Plant, C.; Böhm, C.; Förstl, H.; Kurz, A.; Zimmer, C.; Meng, C.; et al. Prediction of Alzheimer's disease using individual structural connectivity networks. *Neurobiol. Aging* **2012**, *33*, 2756–2765. [CrossRef] [PubMed]
47. Nir, T.M.; Villalon-Reina, J.E.; Prasad, G.; Jahanshad, N.; Joshi, S.H.; Toga, A.W.; Bernstein, M.A.; Jack, C.R.; Weiner, M.W.; Thompson, P.; et al. Diffusion weighted imaging-based maximum density path analysis and classification of Alzheimer's disease. *Neurobiol. Aging* **2015**, *36*, S132–S140. [CrossRef] [PubMed]
48. Demirhan, A.; Nir, T.M.; Zavaliangos-Petropulu, A.; Jack, C.R.; Weiner, M.W.; Bernstein, M.A.; Thompson, P.; Jahanshad, N. Feature selection improves the accuracy of classifying Alzheimer disease using diffusion tensor images. In Proceedings of the 2015 IEEE 12th International Symposium on Biomedical Imaging (ISBI), Brooklyn, NY, USA, 16–19 April 2015; pp. 126–130. [CrossRef]
49. Prasad, G.; Joshi, S.H.; Nir, T.M.; Toga, A.W.; Thompson, P.M.; Alzheimer's Disease Neuroimaging Initiative (ADNI). Brain connectivity and novel network measures for Alzheimer's disease classification. *Neurobiol. Aging* **2015**, *36*, S121–S131. [CrossRef] [PubMed]
50. Ebadi, A.; Da Rocha, J.L.D.; Nagaraju, D.B.; Tovar-Moll, F.; Bramati, I.; Coutinho, G.; Sitaram, R.; Rashidi, P. Ensemble Classification of Alzheimer's Disease and Mild Cognitive Impairment Based on Complex Graph Measures from Diffusion Tensor Images. *Front. Mol. Neurosci.* **2017**, *11*. [CrossRef] [PubMed]
51. Maggipinto, T.; Bellotti, R.; Amoroso, N.; Diacono, D.; Donvito, G.; Lella, E.; Monaco, A.; Scelsi, M.A.; Tangaro, S.; Initiative, A.D.N. DTI measurements for Alzheimer's classification. *Phys. Med. Boil.* **2017**, *62*, 2361–2375. [CrossRef] [PubMed]
52. Eldeeb, G.W.; Zayed, N.; Yassine, I.A. Alzheimer'S Disease Classification Using Bag-Of-Words Based on Visual Pattern of Diffusion Anisotropy for DTI Imaging. In Proceedings of the 2018 40th Annual International Conference of the IEEE Engineering in Medicine and Biology Society (EMBC), Honolulu, HI, USA, 17–21 July 2018; pp. 57–60.
53. Ye, C.; Mori, S.; Chan, P.; Ma, T. Connectome-wide network analysis of white matter connectivity in Alzheimer's disease. *NeuroImage Clin.* **2019**, *22*, 101690. [CrossRef]
54. Da Rocha, J.L.D.; Bramati, I.E.; Coutinho, G.; Moll, F.T.; Sitaram, R. Fractional Anisotropy changes in Parahippocampal Cingulum due to Alzheimer's Disease. *Sci. Rep.* **2020**, *10*, 1–8. [CrossRef]

55. Dou, X.; Yao, H.; Feng, F.; Wang, P.; Zhou, B.; Jin, D.; Yang, Z.; Li, J.; Zhao, C.; Wang, L.; et al. Characterizing white matter connectivity in Alzheimer's disease and mild cognitive impairment: An automated fiber quantification analysis with two independent datasets. *Cortex* **2020**, *129*, 390–405. [CrossRef]
56. Weston, P.S.; Simpson, I.J.; Ryan, N.S.; Ourselin, S.; Fox, N. Diffusion imaging changes in grey matter in Alzheimer's disease: A potential marker of early neurodegeneration. *Alzheimer's Res. Ther.* **2015**, *7*, 47. [CrossRef] [PubMed]
57. Misra, C.; Fan, Y.; Davatzikos, C. Baseline and longitudinal patterns of brain atrophy in MCI patients, and their use in prediction of short-term conversion to AD: Results from ADNI. *NeuroImage* **2009**, *44*, 1415–1422. [CrossRef] [PubMed]
58. A Phelps, E.; Phelps, E. Human emotion and memory: Interactions of the amygdala and hippocampal complex. *Curr. Opin. Neurobiol.* **2004**, *14*, 198–202. [CrossRef] [PubMed]
59. Laakso, M.; Soininen, H.; Partanen, K.; Helkala, E.-L.; Hartikainen, P.; Vainio, P.; Hallikainen, M.; Hänninen, T.; Sr, P.J.R. Volumes of hippocampus, amygdala and frontal lobes in the MRI-based diagnosis of early Alzheimer's disease: Correlation with memory functions. *J. Neural Transm.* **1995**, *9*, 73–86. [CrossRef] [PubMed]
60. Lehéricy, S.; Baulac, M.; Chiras, J.; Piérot, L.; Martin, N.; Pillon, B.; Deweer, B.; Dubois, B.; Marsault, C. Amygdalohippocampal MR volume measurements in the early stages of Alzheimer disease. *Am. J. Neuroradiol.* **1994**, *15*, 929–937.
61. Chu, C.; Hsu, A.-L.; Chou, K.-H.; Bandettini, P.; Lin, C. Does feature selection improve classification accuracy? Impact of sample size and feature selection on classification using anatomical magnetic resonance images. *NeuroImage* **2012**, *60*, 59–70. [CrossRef] [PubMed]
62. Teipel, S.J.; Reuter, S.; Stieltjes, B.; Acosta-Cabronero, J.; Ernemann, U.; Fellgiebel, A.; Filippi, M.; Frisoni, G.B.; Hentschel, F.; Jessen, F.; et al. Multicenter stability of diffusion tensor imaging measures: A European clinical and physical phantom study. *Psychiatry Res. Neuroimaging* **2011**, *194*, 363–371. [CrossRef]
63. Woo, C.-W.; Chang, L.J.; A Lindquist, M.; Wager, T.D. Building better biomarkers: Brain models in translational neuroimaging. *Nat. Neurosci.* **2017**, *20*, 365–377. [CrossRef]
64. Cohen, D.S.; Carpenter, K.A.; Jarrell, J.T.; Huang, X. Deep learning-based classification of multi-categorical Alzheimer's disease data. *Curr. Neurobiol.* **2019**, *10*, 141–147.
65. Rana, M.; Gupta, N.; Da Rocha, J.L.D.; Lee, S.; Sitaram, R. A toolbox for real-time subject-independent and subject-dependent classification of brain states from fMRI signals. *Front. Mol. Neurosci.* **2013**, *7*. [CrossRef]
66. Liberati, G.; Da Rocha, J.L.D.; Van Der Heiden, L.; Raffone, A.; Birbaumer, N.; Belardinelli, M.O.; Sitaram, R. Toward a Brain-Computer Interface for Alzheimer's Disease Patients by Combining Classical Conditioning and Brain State Classification. *J. Alzheimer's Dis.* **2012**, *31*, S211–S220. [CrossRef] [PubMed]
67. Vieira, S.; Pinaya, W.H.L.; Mechelli, A. Using deep learning to investigate the neuroimaging correlates of psychiatric and neurological disorders: Methods and applications. *Neurosci. Biobehav. Rev.* **2017**, *74*, 58–75. [CrossRef] [PubMed]
68. Liu, Y.; Li, Z.; Ge, Q.; Lin, N.; Xiong, M. Deep Feature Selection and Causal Analysis of Alzheimer's Disease. *Front. Mol. Neurosci.* **2019**, *13*. [CrossRef] [PubMed]
69. Marzban, E.N.; Eldeib, A.M.; Yassine, I.A.; Kadah, Y.M.; Initiative, F.T.A.D.N. Alzheimer's disease diagnosis from diffusion tensor images using convolutional neural networks. *PLoS ONE* **2020**, *15*, e0230409. [CrossRef]
70. Bishop, C. *Pattern Recognition and Machine Learning*; Springer-Verlag: New York, NY, USA, 2006.
71. Hastie, T.; Tibshirani, R.; Friedman, J. *The Elements of Statistical Learning: Data Mining, Inference, and Prediction*, 2nd ed.; Springer: Berlin/Heidelberg, Germany, 2009.
72. Ballabio, D.; Consonni, V. Classification tools in chemistry. Part 1: Linear models. PLS-DA. *Anal. Methods* **2013**, *5*, 3790–3798. [CrossRef]

4

Analyzing Age-Related Macular Degeneration Progression in Patients with Geographic Atrophy using Joint Autoencoders for Unsupervised Change Detection

Guillaume Dupont [1], **Ekaterina Kalinicheva** [1], **Jérémie Sublime** [1,2,*], **Florence Rossant** [1,*] and **Michel Pâques** [3]

[1] ISEP, DaSSIP Team, 92130 Issy-Les-Moulineaux, France; guillaume.dupont@isep.fr (G.D.); ekaterina.kalinicheva@isep.fr (E.K.)

[2] Université Paris 13, LIPN - CNRS UMR 7030, 93430 Villetaneuse, France

[3] Clinical Imaging Center 1423, Quinze-Vingts Hospital, INSERM-DGOS Clinical Investigation Center, 75012 Paris, France; mpaques@15-20.fr

* Correspondence: jeremie.sublime@isep.fr or sublime@lipn.univ-paris13.fr (J.S.); florence.rossant@isep.fr (F.R.);

Abstract: Age-Related Macular Degeneration (ARMD) is a progressive eye disease that slowly causes patients to go blind. For several years now, it has been an important research field to try to understand how the disease progresses and find effective medical treatments. Researchers have been mostly interested in studying the evolution of the lesions using different techniques ranging from manual annotation to mathematical models of the disease. However, artificial intelligence for ARMD image analysis has become one of the main research focuses to study the progression of the disease, as accurate manual annotation of its evolution has proved difficult using traditional methods even for experienced practicians. In this paper, we propose a deep learning architecture that can detect changes in the eye fundus images and assess the progression of the disease. Our method is based on joint autoencoders and is fully unsupervised. Our algorithm has been applied to pairs of images from different eye fundus images time series of 24 ARMD patients. Our method has been shown to be quite effective when compared with other methods from the literature, including non-neural network based algorithms that still are the current standard to follow the disease progression and change detection methods from other fields.

Keywords: ARMD; change detection; unsupervised learning; medical imaging

---

1. Introduction

Dry age-related macular degeneration (ARMD or sometimes AMD), a degenerative disease affecting the retina, is a leading cause of intractable visual loss. It is characterized by a centrifugal progression of atrophy of the retinal pigment epithelium (RPE), a cellular layer playing a key role in the maintenance of the photoreceptors. Blindness may occur when the central part of the eye, the fovea, is involved. The disease may be diagnosed and monitored using fundus photographs: ophthalmologists can observe pathologic features such as drusen that occur in the early stages of the ARMD, and evaluate the geographic atrophic (GA) progression in the late stages of degeneration (Figure 1).

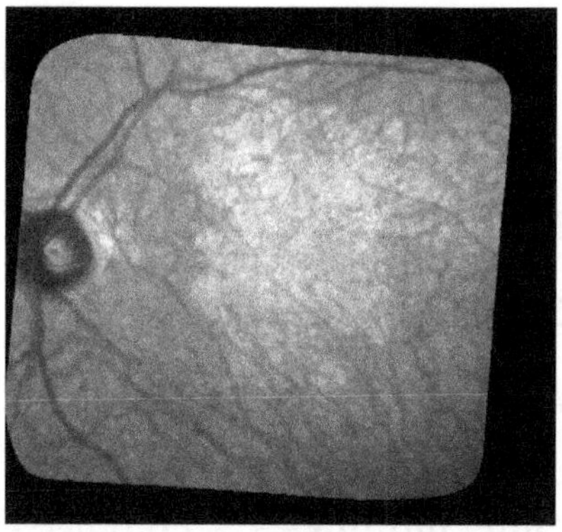

(**a**) Pair 1: before

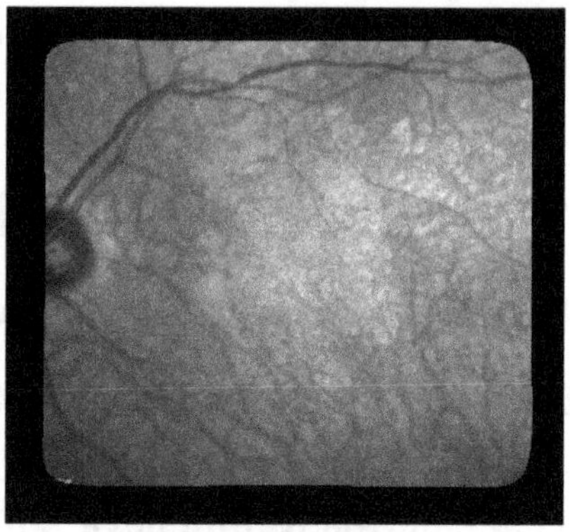

(**b**) Pair 1: after

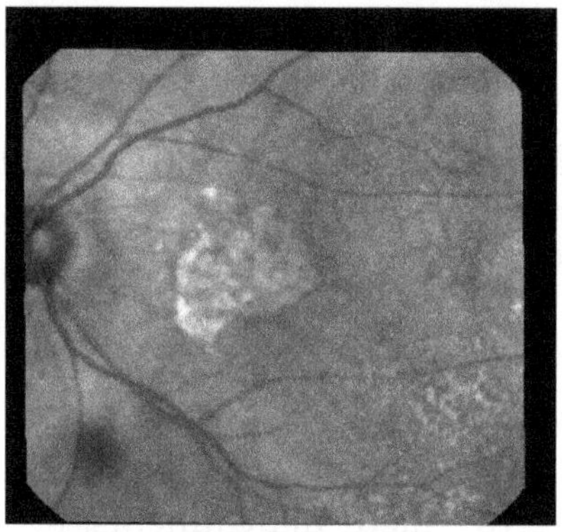

(**c**) Pair 2: before

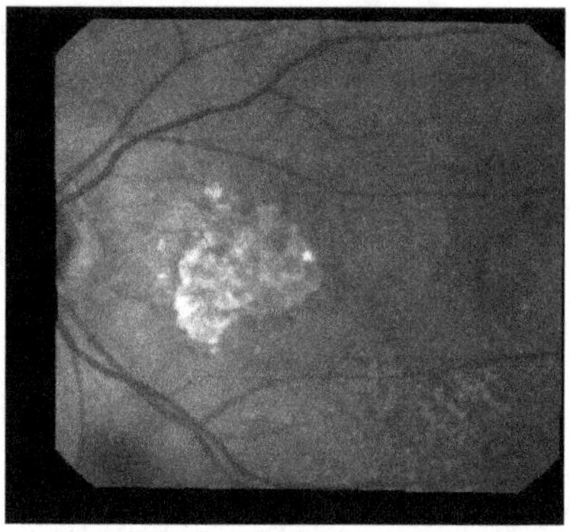

(**d**) Pair 2: after

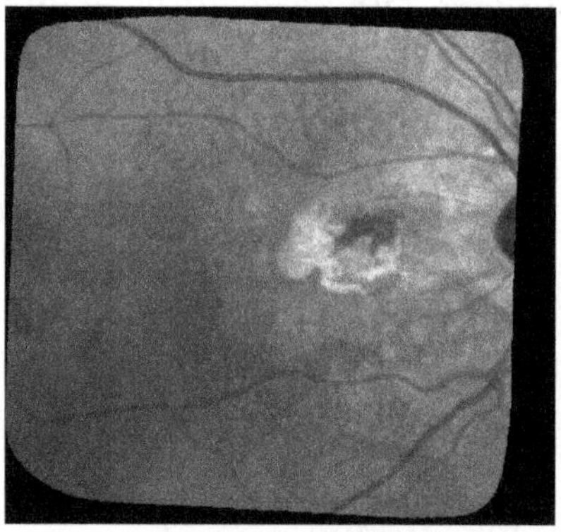

(**e**) Pair 3: before

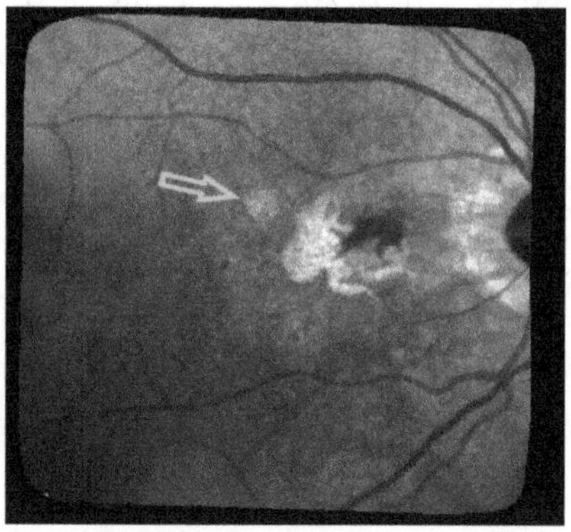

(**f**) Pair 3: after

Figure 1. 3 of pairs of images acquired six months apart, the GA corresponds to the bright areas. The green arrow in (**f**) shows a new lesion.

Automatic analysis of fundus images with dry ARMD is of high medical interest [1] and this has been an important research field for two decades, for diagnosis [2] or follow up [3,4] purposes. Imaging modalities are most often color eye fundus images [5–7], fundus autofluorescence (FAF) [4,8,9], and, to a lesser extent, confocal scanning laser ophthalmoscopy (cSLO) in infrared (IR), or optical coherence tomography (OCT) [10]. In this work, we process cSLO images in IR: this modality is comfortable for the patient, and it has higher resolution and higher contrast than color imaging, an older technology. Our goal is to detect the appearance of new atrophic areas and quantify the growth of GA from pairs of images acquired at regular time intervals to ultimately propose predictive models of the disease progress.

Figure 1 shows three pairs of consecutive images, taken at 6-month intervals. The lesions (GA) are the brighter regions in the fundus and around the optical disk. Automatic processing to follow up these areas is obviously very challenging given the quality of the images: uneven illumination, saturation issues, illumination distortion between images, GA poorly contrasted with retinal structures interfering (vessel, optical disk), blur, etc. The difficulty also lies in the high variability of the lesions in terms of shape, size, and number. The lesion boundary is quite smooth in some cases (c and d) and very irregular in others (a and b). At any time, new spots can appear (as shown by the green arrow between e and f) and older lesions can merge. All these features make the segmentation task very difficult, and especially long and tedious to perform manually. It is worth noting that even experts cannot be sure of their manual delineation in all cases.

Modeling ARMD evolution from a series of eye fundus images requires segmenting the GA in each image and/or to perform a differential analysis between consecutive images to get the lesion growth. In this paper, we propose a differential analysis method based on a joint convolutional fully convolutional autoencoder. Our model is fully unsupervised and does not require labeled images that are difficult to come by in quantity and quality high enough to train a supervised neural network. Our method is applied to pairs of images of a patient eye fundus time series and aims at efficiently segmenting medically significant changes between the two images: meaningless differences caused by image quality or lighting issues are ignored while changes related to GA lesion evolution are extracted.

The remainder of the paper is organized as follows: In Section 2, we review works dedicated to automated processing of images of eye fundus with ARMD and we present approaches for change detection applied to medical image analysis as well as other fields. In Section 3, we present briefly our data and the way we process our images. Then, we detail our proposed method and the architecture of our neural network (Section 4). Section 5 shows our experimental results. Finally, we draw some conclusions in Section 6 and give some possible future perspectives of this work.

2. Related Works

This state-of-the-art section is split into three sections presenting methods closest to this work and also based on the differential approach first. Then, we will introduce a few methods also developed for the study of ARMD or other eye diseases but that rely on a segmentation based approach on individual images. In addition, we will finish this state of the art with some examples of other change detection methods from outside the field of medical imaging.

Before we start, we remind our readers that this work introduces a fully unsupervised method for change detection in ARMD images. The main difference between supervised and unsupervised learning is the following:

- In supervised learning, Machine Learning algorithms are trained using data that have been pre-classified or annotated by human with the goal of building a model based on these data. This model is then applied to new data with the goal of providing a classification for them. While this type of Machine Learning is considered to be the most powerful, its main weakness is that it cannot be used if no or not enough annotated data are available.
- In unsupervised learning, on the other hand, all data are provided raw and without any annotation or classification, and the algorithm must find by itself different classes called clusters of elements that are similar. Since the process is not guided, hence the name "unsupervised", the cluster found using this process may or may not match the classes expected by the users, and the performances of unsupervised learning are expected to be lower than these of supervised learning. Unsupervised Learning is usually used as an exploratory task or when there are no available annotated data (or not enough), both of which are the case for our application to ARMD image time series.

With this related work section, we hope to demonstrate that providing fully automated tools reaching the required level of performance for medical application is a difficult task, especially in an unsupervised context with few annotated images.

2.1. *Differential Approaches Applied to ARMD*

The following works are most related to our proposed algorithm as they are unsupervised algorithms applied to various eye disease images, including ARMD: In [11], Troglio et al. published an improvement of their previous works realized with Nappo [12] where they use the Kittler and Illingworth (K&I) thresholding method. Their method consists of applying the K&I algorithm on random sub-images of the difference image obtained between two consecutive eye fundus images of a patient with retinopathy. By doing so, they obtain multiple predictions for each pixel and can then make a vote to decide the final class. This approach has the advantage that it compensates for the non-uniform illumination across the image; however, it is rather primitive since it does not actually use any Machine Learning and rely on different parameters of the thresholding method to then make a vote. To its credit, even if it achieves a relatively weak precision, it is fully unsupervised like our method. In [6], the authors tackle a similar problematic to ours where they correct eye fundus images by pairs, by multiplying the second image by a polynomial surface whose parameters are estimated in the least-squares sense. In this way, illumination distortion is lessened and the image difference enhances the areas of changes. However, the statistical test applied locally at each pixel is not reliable enough to get an accurate map of structural changes.

2.2. *Segmentation First Approaches Applied to ARMD and Other Eye Diseases*

Other works related with eye diseases take the different approach of segmenting lesions in individual images instead of looking for changes in pairs of images. In [5], Köse et al. proposed an approach where they first segment all healthy regions to get the lesions as the remaining areas. This approach also requires segmenting separately the blood vessels, which is known to be a difficult task. This method involves many steps and parameters that need to be supervised by the user. In [4], Ramsey et al. proposed a similar but unsupervised method for the identification of ARMD lesions in individual images: They use an unsupervised algorithm based on fuzzy c-means clustering. Their method achieves good performances for FAF images, but it performs less well for color fundus photographs. We can also mention the work of Hussain et al. [13] in which the authors are proposing another supervised algorithm to track the progression of drusen for ARMD follow-up. They first use U-Nets to segment vessels and detect the optic disc with the goal of reducing the region of interest for drusen detection. After this step, they track the drusen using intensity ratio between neighbor pixels.

Using the same approach of segmenting the lesions first and then tracking the changes, there are a few supervised methods available. We can, for instance, mention [14] in which the authors propose another related work in which they use a pre-trained supervised neural network to detect ARMD lesions with good results. In addition, in [15], the same team uses another supervised convolutional neural network (CNN) to assess the stage of ARMD based on the lesions.

Other traditional more machine learning approaches have also been used for GA segmentation such as the k-nearest neighbor classifiers [9], random forests [7], as well as combinations of Support Vector Machines and Random Forests [16]. Feature vectors for these approaches typically include intensity values, local energy, texture descriptors, values derived from multi-scale analysis and distance to the image center. Nevertheless, these algorithms are supervised: they require training the classifier from annotated data, which brings us back to the difficulty of manually segmenting GA areas.

Related to other medical images, in [17], the authors show that the quantization error (QE) of the output obtained with the application of Self Organized Maps [18] is an indicator of small local changes in medical images. This work is also unsupervised but has the defaults that the SOM algorithm cannot provide a clustering on its own and must be coupled with another algorithm such as K-Means to do so. Furthermore, since there is no feature extraction done, this algorithm would most likely be very sensitive to the lighting and contrast issues that are present in most eye fundus time series. Lastly, the use of SOM based methods on monochromatic images is discouraged since no interesting topology may be found from a single attribute.

Finally, the literature also contains a few user-guided segmentation frameworks [19,20] that are valuable when it is possible to get a user input.

2.3. *Change Detection Methods from Other Fields*

Apart from medicine, change detection algorithms have been proposed for many different applications such as remote sensing or video analysis. In [21], the authors reveal a method combining principal component analysis (PCA) and K-means algorithm on the difference image. In [22], an architecture relying on joint auto-encoders and convolutional neural networks is proposed to detect non-trivial changes between two images. In [23], the authors propose an autoencoder architecture for anomaly detection in videos.

Finally, as we have seen that quite a few methods rely on segmentation first and change detection after, we can also mention a few noteworthy unsupervised segmentation algorithms used outside the field of medicine: Kanezaki et al. [24] used CNN to group similar pixels together with consideration of spatial continuity as a basis of their segmentation method. In addition, Xia and Kulis [25] developed W-Net using a combination of two U-Nets with a soft Normalized-Cut Loss.

In Table 1, we sum up the main methods presented in this related work section. The first column specifies if the method is supervised or unsupervised. The second column indicates if the method uses the directly pairs of images (or their difference), or if it uses individual images to segment them first and then compare the segmentations. The "Algorithm" column details which algorithm is used. The last column gives the application field.

Table 1. Summary of the state-of-the-art methods for change detection that are mentioned in this work.

Authors	Supervised	Images Used	Algorithm	Application
Troglio, Napo et al. [11,12]	No	Pairs	K&I Thresholding	ARMD
Marrugo et al. [6]	No	Pairs	Image correction	ARMD
Köse et al. [5]	semi	Individual	Raw segmentation	ARMD
Ramsey et al. [4]	No	Individual	Fuzzy C-Means	ARMD
Hussain et al. [13]	Yes	Individual	U-Nets	ARMD
Burlina et al. [14,15]	Yes	Individual	pre-trained CNN	ARMD
Kanezaki et al. [24]	No	Individual	CNN	Image Processing
Sublime et al. [26]	No	Pairs	Joint-AE & KMeans	Remote Sensing
Celik et al. [21]	No	Pairs	PCA & KMeans	Remote Sensing
Our Method	No	Pairs	Joint-AE	ARMD

3. Dataset Presentation

In this section, we will provide some details on the image time series used in this work in terms of their characteristics, flaws, and how we pre-processed them before comparing different methods for change detection on them.

Our images whose main characteristics can be found in Table 2 were all acquired at the Quinze–Vingts National Ophthalmology Hospital in Paris, in cSLO with IR illumination. This modality has the advantage of being one of the most common and cheapest legacy method of image acquisition for eye fundus images, thus allowing to have lots of images and to follow the patients for several years. However, it is infrared only and therefore all images are monochromatic and may contain less information than images acquired from other techniques with multiple channels (that are less common for this type of exam and more difficult to find in numbers).

Table 2. Description of the data.

Number of patients	15
Number of image time series	18
Average number of images per series	13
Total number of images	336
Acquisition period	2007–2019
Average time between two images	6 months

While some 3D OCT and 2D FAF images were available, the infrared light penetrates better than blue light through media opacities and requires pupil dilation hence IR imaging is more robust (and better supported by patients). Although OCT is becoming the preferred imaging modality to appreciate the progression of GA, it requires a standard acquisition modality at each exam to ensure comparability, hence a lot of data acquired during routine follow-up cannot be used. On the other hand, the 30° IR imaging is the default mode of fundus image acquisition and hence most patients have such image taken whatever the OCT protocol has been done. Thus, we stick to cSLO with infrared only so that we could have longer and more homogeneous series, and therefore all images are monochromatic and may contain less information than images acquired from other techniques with multiple channels (that are less common for this type of exam and more difficult to find in numbers).

Patients have been followed-up during a few years, hence we have a series of retinal fundus images, sometimes for both eyes (hence the number of series and patients being different in Table 2), showing the progression of the GA. The average number of images in each series is 13. The images are dated from 2007 for the oldest to 2019 for the most recent. All pictures are in grayscale and vary greatly in size, but the most common size is 650 $\times$ 650 pixels.

As mentioned previously, we notice many imperfections such as blur, artifacts and, above all, non-uniform illumination inside the images and between them (see Figure 2). All images were spatially aligned with i2k software (https://www.dualalign.com/retinal/image-registration-montage-software-overview.php). In every image, the area of useful data does not fill the entire image and is surrounded by black borders. The automatic detection of these black zones in each image gives a mask of the useful data, and the intersection of all masks the common retinal region where changes can be searched for.

We also designed a new method to compensate for illumination distortion between the images (not published yet). This algorithm is based on an illumination/reflectance model and corrects all images of a series with respect to a common reference image. Uneven illumination generally remains present in every processed image (Figure 2), but the smooth illumination distortions are compensated. The calculus of the absolute value of the difference between two consecutive images demonstrates the benefit of this algorithm (Figure 2, last column).

We used five different series of images to evaluate quantitatively our method of change detection: they feature different characteristics in terms of disease progress, lesion shape and size. We developed several user-guided segmentation tools to make the ground truth, based on classical segmentation algorithms: thresholding applied locally on a rectangle defined by the user, parametric active contour model initialized by the user, and simple linear interpolation between points entered by the user. The user can use the most appropriate tool to locally delimit the lesion border, and thus progresses step by step. Local thresholding or active contour algorithm makes it possible to obtain segmentations that depend less on the user than the use of interpolation, which is applied when the two previous methods fail. However, the segmentation remains mostly manual, user-dependent, and tedious. An ophthalmologist realized all segmentation used in our experiments. Finally, the binary change mask between two consecutive images was obtained by subtraction of the segmentation masks.

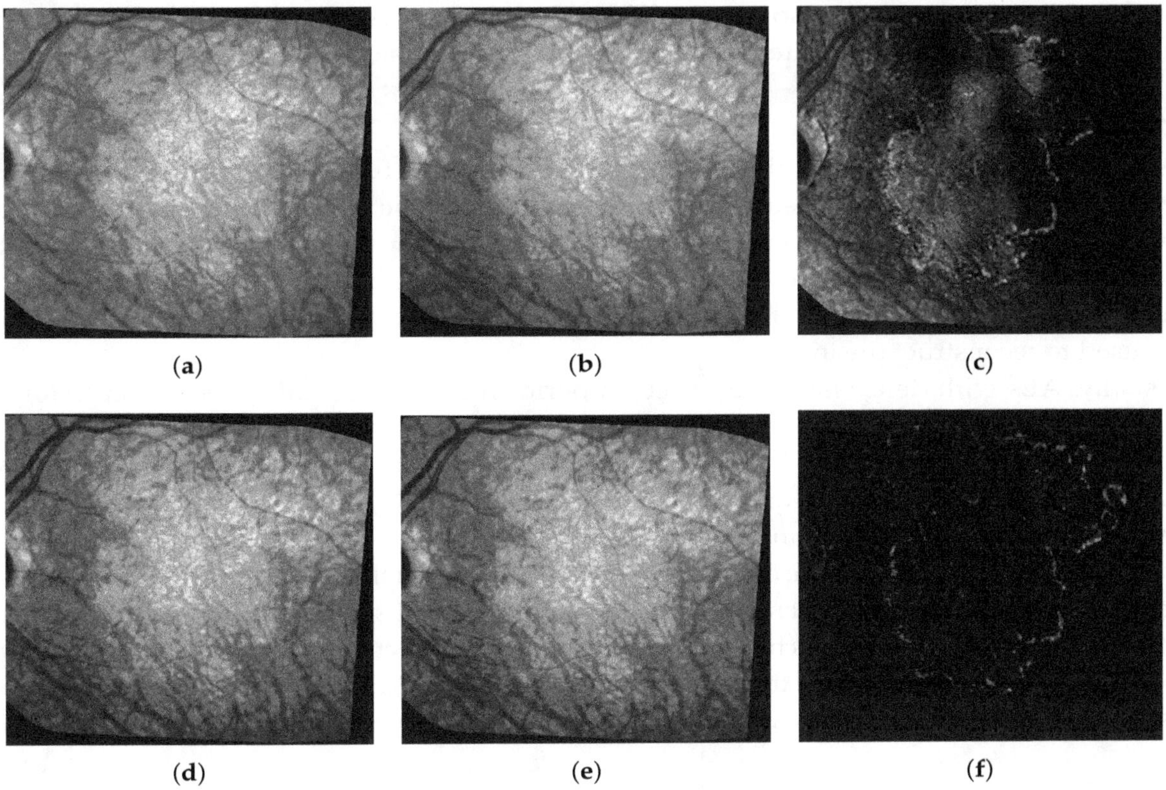

Figure 2. Example of Illumination correction. The three images on the top row represent the two original consecutive images (**a**,**b**), and their raw difference in absolute value (**c**); on the bottom row: the same images after illumination correction (**d**,**e**), and the new difference (**f**).

It is worth noting that the manual segmentation of a single image by expert ophthalmologists takes on average 13 min for a single image, and that many disagreements as to what the ideal segmentation should be arise when comparing the segmentations made by different experts for the same image: In particular, many doctors disagree on which internal changes are interesting or not (and therefore should or should not be in the ground truth), and they may also have different advice for the borders of particularly difficult lesions. For these reasons, and because we kept the results of only a single ophthalmologist, the ground-truth provided for our images have to be taken with caution as they are not always reliable, and, as we will see in later sections, they may feature defects that will affect dices' indexes computed based on them. Furthermore, for the same reason that it takes a lot of time to produce reliable change maps, our test set is relatively small in size compared to other applications that features much larger data sets, and in particular larger test sets.

4. Description of Our Proposed Architecture

Our algorithm is inspired from earlier works from remote sensing [22,26], where the authors applied an unsupervised deep autoencoder to automatically map non-trivial changes between pairs of satellite images to detect meaningful evolutions such as new constructions or changes in landcover while discarding trivial seasonal changes.

In our paper, we use the similarities between satellite images and our medical ARMD eye fundus to adapt their method: both types of images may suffer from lighting issues, noise issues, blurry elements, complex objects present in the images, various time gaps between two images of the same series, and most importantly the common goal of detecting meaningful changes despite all these issues.

While they share similarities, our medical images and satellite images are also quite different: they do not have the same number of channels, they have very different sizes, and the nature of the objects and changes to detect is also quite different. For these reasons, the following subsection will detail how we modified their architecture, and it will explain all steps of our algorithm.

4.1. *Joint Autoencoder Architecture*

As mentioned earlier, in this research, we use a fully convolutional autoencoder. Autoencoders [27] are a type of neural networks whose purpose is to make the output as close as possible to the input. During the learning process, the encoder learns some meaningful representation of the initial data that is transformed back with the decoder. Hence, in a fully convolutional AE, a stack of convolutive layers is applied to the input image in order to extract feature maps (FM) which will then be used to reconstruct the input image.

Usually, AEs with dense layers are used to perform a dimensionality reduction followed by a clustering or segmentation. However, in computer vision, fully convolutional AEs are preferred for their ability to extract textures. Examples of such networks include fully convolutional networks (FCNs) [28] or U-Nets [29]. However, in our case, we do not use Max-pooling layers, and so we keep the same dimensions as the input and only the depth increases.

Our network (Figure 3) is made of four convolutional layers in the encoder of size 16, 16, 32, and 32, respectively, and in the same way as four convolutional layers of size 32, 32, 16, and 16, respectively, in the decoder side. We apply a batch normalization and a ReLU activation function at each step of the network except for the last layer of the encoder where we only add the L2 normalization, and also for the last layer of the decoder where we apply a Sigmoid function (see in Figure 3).

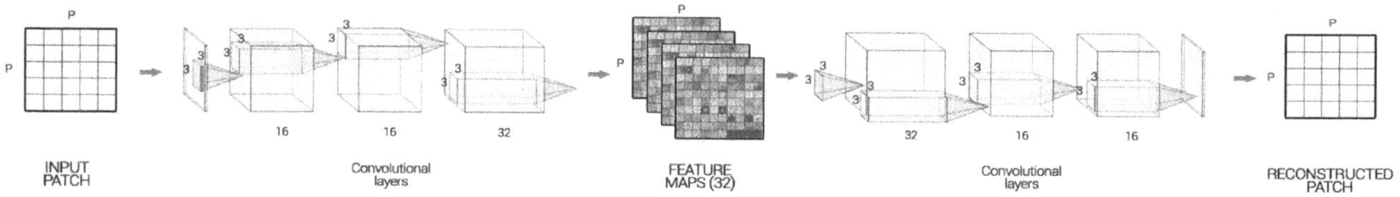

Figure 3. Autoencoder architecture for our algorithm.

4.2. *Algorithm Steps*

Our algorithm is made of four steps. We start by dividing the images into several patches. Then, we build the joint autoencoder where it learns how to reconstruct the images, and after we tweak the method by learning the autoencoder to reconstruct not the image itself but the precedent or the future image. The neural networks will learn easily the changes due to the non-uniform illumination or noise but will fail on ARMD progression generating a high reconstruction error (RE), consequently making it possible to detect them. The next subsections will detail some of these steps:

4.2.1. Patches Construction

One of the issues with the retinal fundus images we have is their shape. Indeed, our images are not necessarily square and differ from one set to another. This is why we use an approach based on patches that allows us to manage several sizes of images but also several forms of useful areas thanks to a simple manipulation that we explain right away.

As mentioned in Section 3, the area of useful data are not rectangular and is generally surrounded by black borders, which can be detected by a simple logic test. As can be seen in Figure 4, we solve this problem by using the Inpainting function of the library *scikit-image* [30] to complete this background. This inpainting function is based on the biharmonic equation [31,32], and it exploits the information in the connected regions to fill the black zones with consistent gray level values. Let us denote by $P \times P$ the size of the patches. The image is also padded with $\frac{P}{2}$ pixels along all dimensions and directions before applying the inpainting. Thanks to this operation, we can extract patches from the whole image, i.e., patches centered on every useful pixel, without any cropping, and so we can exploit all our available data without border effects.

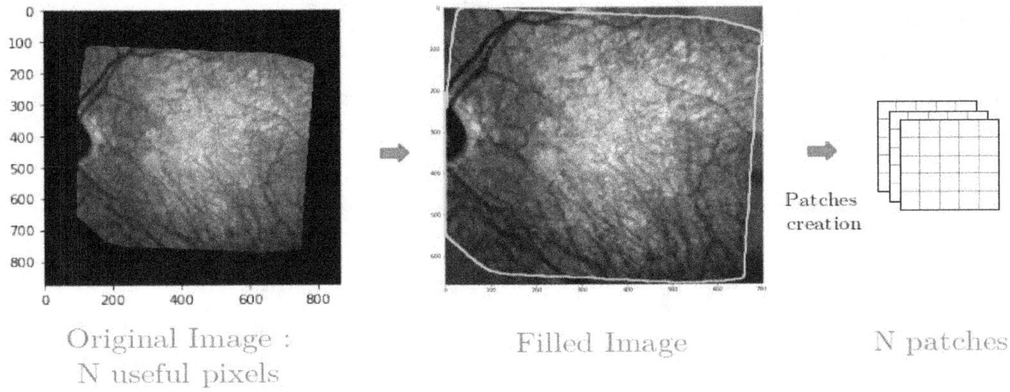

Figure 4. Patches construction,useful pixels are inside the green area.

4.2.2. Pre-Training

Let us consider a series of M images representing the progression of ARMD in a patient's eye. After the pre-processing and once the images have been aligned and cropped, all images from the same series have the same number of N useful patches. From there, to pre-train or network, we sample $\left\lfloor \frac{N}{M} \right\rfloor$ of the patches for every image hence, regardless of the size of the series, we use a total of N patches. This allows us to build a unique autoencoder AE that works for all pairs in the series, and to prevent overfitting.

As an example, for a series of 16 images and 600×600 useful patches per image, we would randomly sample $\frac{1}{16}$ of the patches for each image of the series (22,500 patches per image), and use a total of 360,000 patches to pre-train our network.

When processing the patches, our network applies a Gaussian filter in order to weight the pixels by giving more importance to the center of the patch in the RE calculus.

During the encoding pass of the AE, the model extracts feature maps of N patches of chosen samples with convolutional layers (Figure 5), and then, during the decoding pass, it reconstructs them back to the initial ones.

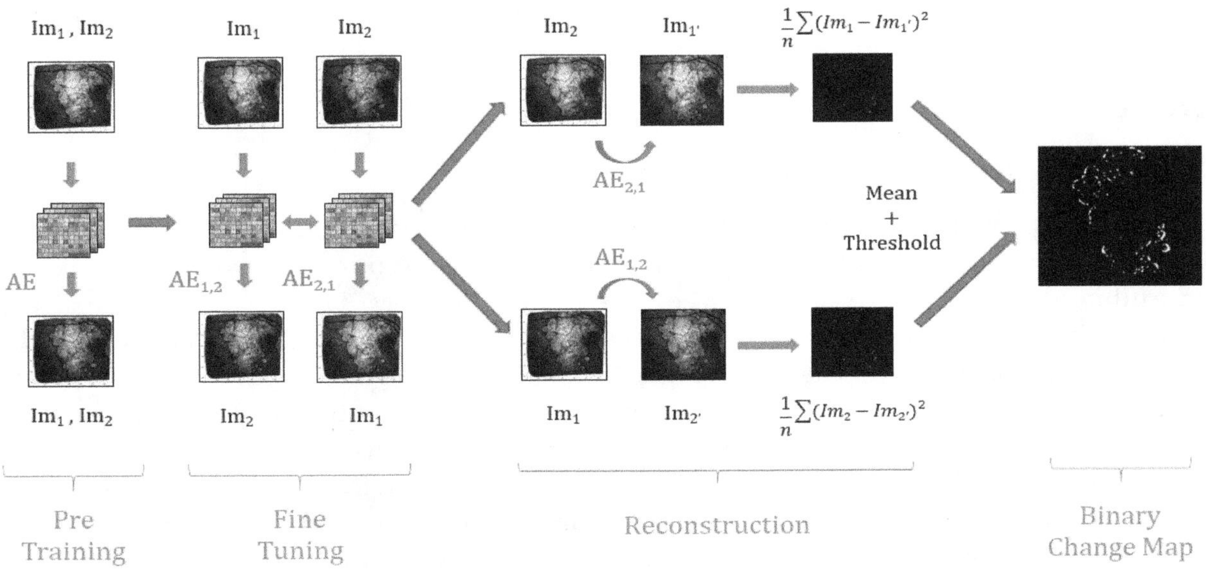

Figure 5. Structure of the algorithm. Example for set of two images Im_1 and Im_2 and n the number of patches.

4.2.3. Fine-Tuning

For every consecutive pair $i, i+1$ with $i \in [\![1; M-1]\!]$ of images, we are going to build two autoencoders initialized with the weights found in the pre-training part. On one hand, $AE_{i,i+1}$ aims to reconstruct patches of Im_{i+1} from patches of Im_i and, on the other hand, $AE_{i+1,i}$ is going to reconstruct patches of Im_i from patches of Im_{i+1}.

The whole model is trained to minimize the difference between: the decoded output of $AE_{i,i+1}$ and Im_{i+1}, the decoded output of $AE_{i+1,i}$ and Im_i, and the encoded outputs of $AE_{i,i+1}$ and $AE_{i+1,i}$, see Figure 5.

This joint configuration where the learning is done in both temporal directions, using joint backpropagation, has empirically proven to be much more robust than using a regular one-way autoencoder. To optimize the parameters of the model, we use the mean squared error (MSE) of the reconstructed patches.

For the fine-tuning, we stop iterating and running epochs when the MSE of the reconstructed patches stabilizes, as is standard for the training of Deep Learning networks.

4.2.4. Reconstruction and Thresholding

Once the models are trained and stabilized, we perform the image reconstruction. For each pair, we note $Im_{i+1'}$ the reconstruction of Im_{i+1} from Im_i with $AE_{i,i+1}$ and likewise we note $Im_{i'}$ the reconstruction of Im_i from Im_{i+1} with $AE_{i+1,i}$. Then, we calculate the reconstruction error RE for every patch between Im_i and $Im_{i'}$ on one side and between Im_{i+1} and $Im_{i+1'}$ on another side. This gives us two images for each pair representing the average REs for $Im_{i'}$ and $Im_{i+1'}$ that we average to get only one. The model will easily learn the transformation of unchanged areas from one image to the other: changes in luminosity and blurring effects. At the same time, because the changes caused by the disease progression are unique, they will be considered as outliers by the model, and thus will have a high RE. Hence, we apply Otsu's thresholding [33] that requires no parameters and enables us to produce a binary change map (BCM).

If we sum up, our algorithm uses the strengths of joint auto-encoders to map the light changes, contrast defects, and texture changes from one image to another. This way, most of the image defects and noise issues will be removed. In addition, then, we use the inability of the auto-encoder to predict structural changes in the lesions through time (this algorithm is not designed to do this), as is the inability of the algorithm to generate a high reconstruction error in areas where the lesions have progressed when comparing the encoded reconstructed images with the real images. This way, we have a fully unsupervised way to remove noise and detect changes in the lesions. The full process is explained in Figure 5.

5. Experimental Results

5.1. Experimental Setting

We chose to compare our methods presented in Section 4.1 with three other methods, all on the preprocessed images. We applied all the methods to three of our series for which we have a ground truth.

The following parameters were chosen for all convolutional layers of our method: kernel size to 3, stride to 1, and padding to 1. The Adam algorithm was used to optimize the models. We set the number of epochs to 8 for the pre-training phase and just 1 for the fine-tuning phase. These parameters were chosen as they are the limit after which the reconstruction error generally does not improve anymore. More epochs during the pre-training phase led to more required epochs to adjust the model to each couple during the fine-tuning phase without much improvements on the results. In addition, more epochs on the fine-tuning phase did not lead to any significant improvement in the results and sometimes resulted in overfitting. Therefore, we fix these parameters both to ensure quality results and to avoid running extra unneeded epochs for both the pre-training and fine-tuning phase.

For both phases, the learning rate was set to 0.0001 and the batch size to 100.

The first method that we use for comparison is a simple subtraction of two consecutive images with an application of Otsu's thresholding on the result. The second comparison is a combination of principal component analysis (PCA) and K-means algorithm on the difference image proposed by Celik et al. in [21], and we apply it to medical images with blocks of size 5. To finish, we take a Deep-Learning based approach [24] which uses CNN to group similar pixels together with consideration of spatial continuity. This work by Kanezaki et al. was initially made for unsupervised segmentation; consequently, we apply the algorithm to our images and then do the segmentation substractions to get binary change maps. The convolution layers have the same configuration than for our network and we set the parameter for the *minimum number of labels* to 3.

As it is common practice, even for unsupervised algorithms, we assess the results of the different methods using classical binary indexes intended for supervised classification: accuracy, precision, recall, and F1-Score. All formulas are given in Equations (1)–(4), where we used the change areas as the positive class and no change as the negative class. The notations "TP", "TN", "FP", and "FN" are used for true positive, true negative, false positive, and false negative, respectively.

Accuracy refers to the proportion of correct predictions made by the model. It is sensitive to class imbalance:

$$Accuracy = \frac{TP + TN}{TP + TN + FP + FN} \tag{1}$$

Precision is the proportion of identifications classified as positive by the model that is actually correct:

$$Precision = \frac{TP}{TP + FP}. \tag{2}$$

Recall is the proportion of positive results that are correctly identified. It can be thought of as the proportion of progression of the lesion correctly identified:

$$Recall = \frac{TP}{TP + FN}. \tag{3}$$

F1-Score also known as the F-Measure, or balanced F Score, is the harmonic mean between the precision and the recall and is computed as follows:

$$F1 = \frac{2 \times precision \times recall}{precision + recall} \tag{4}$$

5.2. Parameters' Fine-Tuning

The fully convolutional AE model for change detection is presented in Section 4.1.

There are two main parameters in our algorithm. The first one is the the patch size P. As we can see in Figure 6, a smaller value of P will increase our precision and, on the contrary, a high value of P will increase our recall. Thus, the challenge is to find a trade-off value between both scores in order to get the best F1 score possible. In order to improve the performances, we decided to introduce a second parameter: sigma σ. This one refers to Gaussian weights which are applied to the patches to give more importance to central pixels and less to pixels closer to the sides of the patches during the RE loss computation. For each series, we did experiments such as the one shown in Figure 7 to find the best patch size P and value σ. In general, we got that a high size of the patch gave us a relatively good recall and the Gaussian weights allow us to regain precision. Two pairs of values came up more often: patch size $P = 13$ and a value $\sigma = 12$ for patients with larger lesions, and patch size $P = 7$ and a value $\sigma = 5$ for patients with smaller lesions.

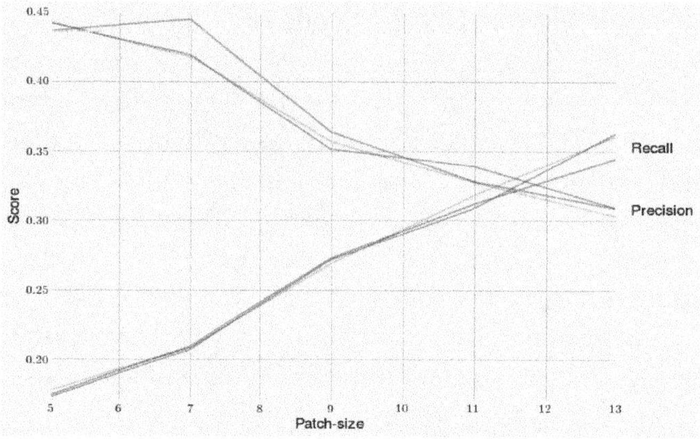

(**a**)

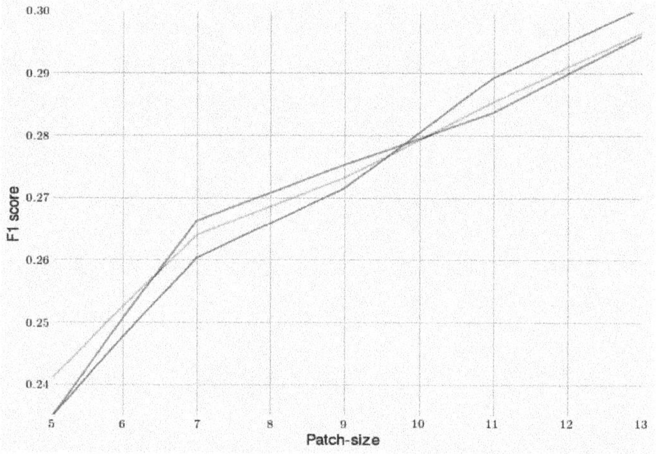

(**b**)

Figure 6. Average recall, Precision, and F1 Score depending on the patch size and sigma: $\sigma = 5$ *in red* $\sigma = 7$ *in green* $\sigma = 9$ *in blue.* (**a**) Recall and Precision depending on the patch size; (**b**) F1 Score depending on the Patch size.

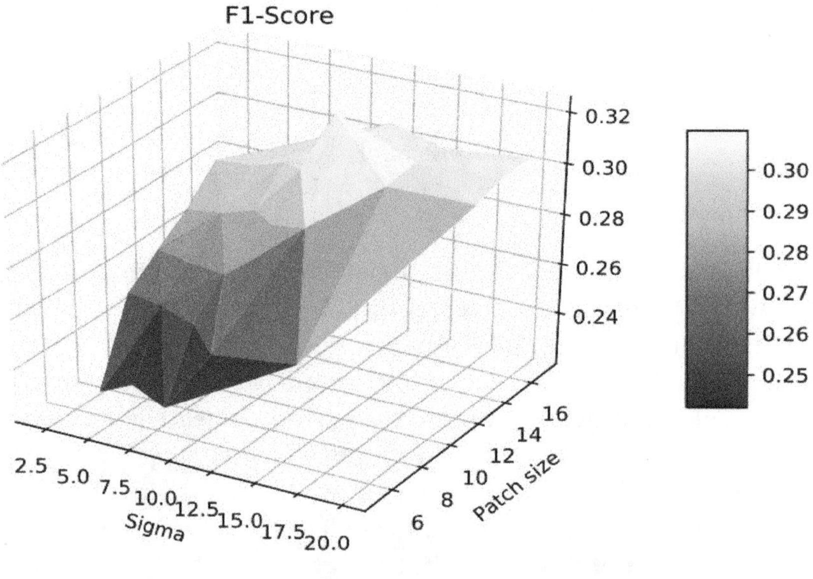

Figure 7. F1-Score as a function of the patch size and the value of sigma σ on patient 005.

All of the algorithm steps were executed on an Nvidia GPU (RTX TITAN) with 64 GB of RAM and an Intel 9900 k. It took about 20 min for a series of 8 frames with a patch size P of 13, with the execution time increasing with it.

5.3. Results

The results for patients 1, 3, 5, 10, and 115 are shown in Table 3, as well as Figures 8–11 that we added for visual inspection purposes. Additional images for patient 18 are available in some of the figures. Other patients were not added to Table 3 or the figures because we do not have reliable enough change map ground-truths to compute the dice indexes, or because we do not have them at all. Note that the scores presented in Table 3 are for the complete series (15 to 20 pairs per patient), while the scores shown in the figures are for the individual couples of images used in each example. The bottom line of Table 3 shows the weighted mean values for all indexes and all methods for all series.

When looking at Table 3, we can see that the simple difference coupled with Otsu thresholding achieves the best recall results on average that there is no clear winner for the Precision, and that our proposed method on average has the best F1 Score.

Please note that we did not display the Accuracy because of the strong class imbalance, with a large majority of "no change class" pixels leading to results over 85% for Kanezaki's approach and the simple differentiating with Otsu thresholding, and over 95% for our approach and Celik approach. Since these figures are obviously very biased and given that we are more interested in "change" pixels than "no change" pixels, we did not report them in Table 3 and preferred to focus on commenting on the Precision, Recall, and F1-score that are less affected by class imbalance.

Table 3. Results and comparison of the different approaches. It contains the means of the recall, the precision, and the F1 score for each time series. For each patient, the best dice results are in bold.

Patient ID	Method	Authors	Recall	Precision	F1 Score
	Diff + Otsu	-	**0.68**	0.11	0.16
001	CNN	Kanezaki et al.	0.32	**0.29**	0.18
15 images	PCA + KMeans	Celik et al.	0.48	0.28	**0.3**
	Joint-AE	Our method	0.44	0.21	0.26
	Diff + Otsu	-	**0.55**	0.1	0.17
003	CNN	Kanezaki et al.	0.2	0.27	0.07
5 images	PCA + KMeans	Celik et al.	0.24	**0.33**	0.27
	Joint-AE	Our method	0.29	0.28	**0.28**
	Diff + Otsu	-	**0.46**	0.2	0.26
005	CNN	Kanezaki et al.	0.2	**0.43**	0.21
8 images	PCA + KMeans	Celik et al.	0.26	0.37	0.28
	Joint-FCAE	Our method	0.33	0.34	**0.32**
	Diff + Otsu	-	**0.68**	0.06	0.10
010	CNN	Kanezaki et al.	0.32	0.03	0.05
6 images	PCA + KMeans	Celik et al.	0.47	0.23	0.29
	Joint-FCAE	Our method	0.38	**0.35**	**0.36**
	Diff + Otsu	-	**0.53**	0.25	0.29
115	CNN	Kanezaki et al.	0.33	0.15	0.16
9 images	PCA + KMeans	Celik et al.	0.24	0.38	0.25
	Joint-FCAE	Our method	0.33	**0.39**	**0.34**
Total	Diff + Otsu	-	**0.58**	0.16	0.20
(patients'	CNN	Kanezaki et al.	0.27	0.27	0.14
mean—43	PCA + KMeans	Celik et al.	0.33	**0.32**	0.27
images)	Joint-AE	Our method	0.35	**0.32**	**0.31**

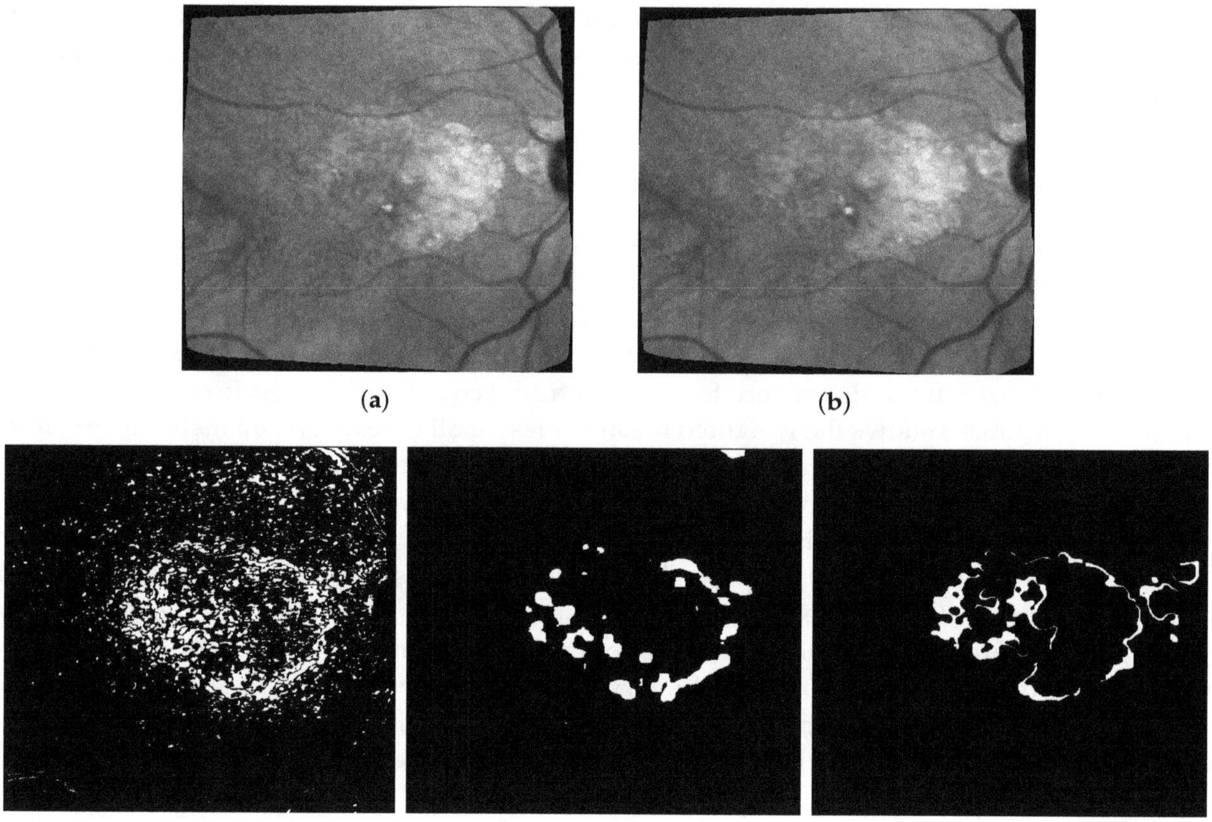

(a) (b)

(c) (d) (e)

Figure 8. Difference + Otsu thresholding vs. our approach (AE) on patient 003. (**a**) Image at $t = 0$; (**b**) Image at $t + 3$ months; (**c**) Raw difference and Otsu thresholding, F1 score = 0.26; (**d**) Our method, F1 score = 0.36; (**e**) Proposed ground truth.

Our interpretation of these results is the following: Otsu thresholding applied to the difference between two images has the best recalls because it detects most real change pixels. However, the binary change map is also very noisy, corresponding to a high number of false positives (wrongly detected changes), which is confirmed by the very low precision score. This can also be observed in Figures 8c and 11d, which are examples of the high number of false positives detected using Otsu thresholding compared with the ground truth in Figure 8c, or our method results in Figure 8e.

In Figures 9–11, we compare our approach with the two other algorithms relying on more advanced Machine Learning techniques. First, we can see that, like in Table 3, our approach gets the best F1-score for both patients and pairs of images. Then, we can see that the Kanezaki et al. approach achieves over-segmentation in Figure 9d and under-segmentation in Figure 10d, which highlights that it is more difficult to parametrize properly and may require different parameters for each pair of image, which is not the case for both our approach and the Celik et al. approach. Finally, regarding the comparison between the Celik et al. approach and our proposed method, we can see from Figures 9e,f, 10e,f, and 11e,f that also, like in Table 3, the Celik et al. approach achieves overall good results that are comparable to the ones of our method. However, in the same way that we have better F1-score and accuracy results, the visual results for our methods are also better as the changes we detect in the lesions are cleaner and overall less fragmented into very small elements compared with the ones found by the Celik et al. approach.

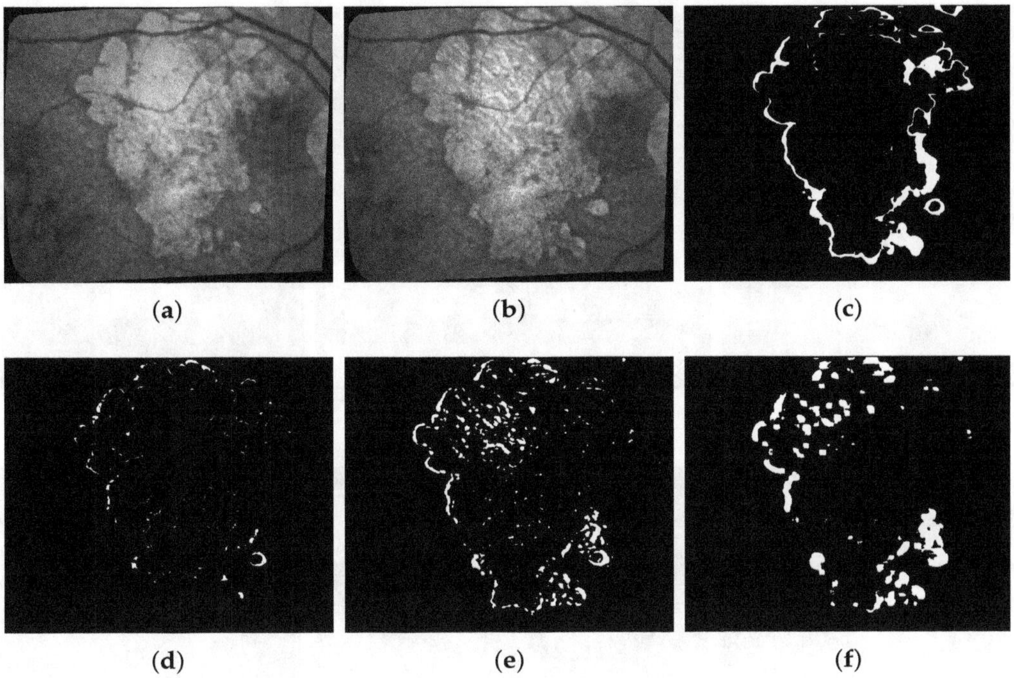

Figure 9. Comparison example of the three methods on patient 005. (**a**) Corrected Image from October 2017; (**b**) Corrected Image from June 2018; (**c**) Proposed ground truth; (**d**) Asako Kanezaki's approach, F1 score = 0.15; (**e**) Turgay Celik's approach, F1 score = 0.35; (**f**) Our Fully Convolutional AE, F1 score = 0.4.

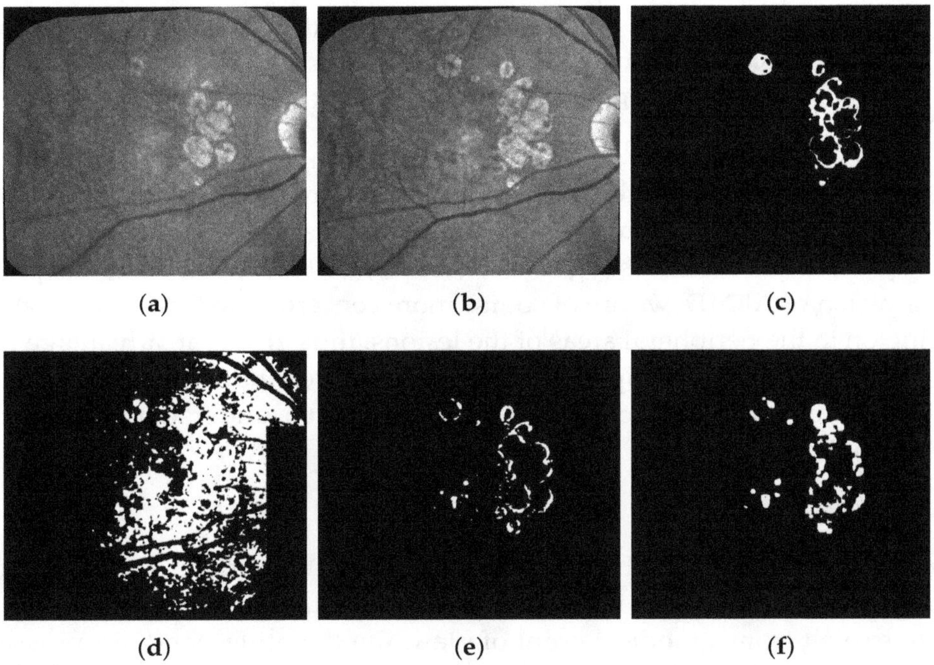

Figure 10. Comparison example of the three methods on patient 001. (**a**) Corrected Image from April 2017; (**b**) Corrected Image from October 2017; (**c**) Proposed ground truth; (**d**) Asano Kanezaki's approach, F1 score = 0.17; (**e**) Turgay Celik's approach, F1 score = 0.43; (**f**) Our Fully convolutional AE, F1 score = 0.43.

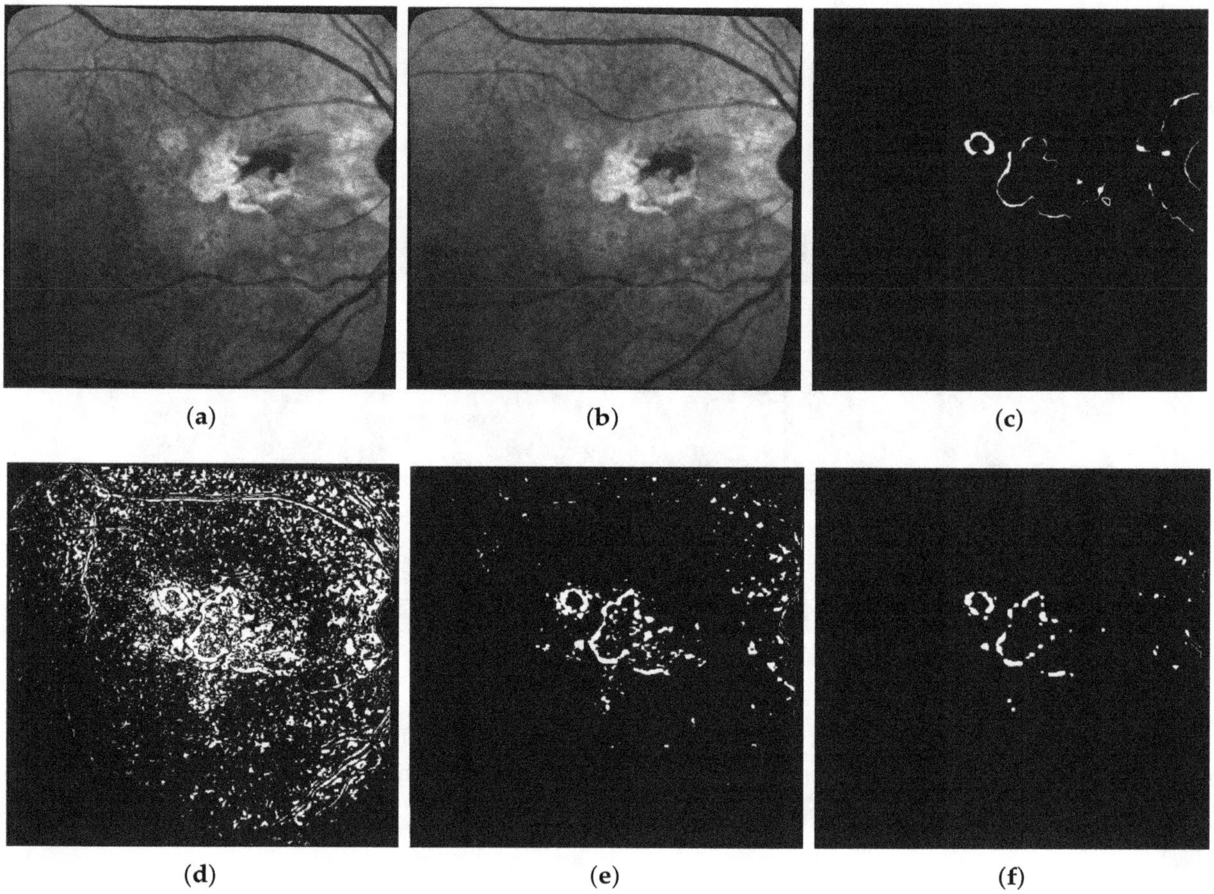

Figure 11. Comparison example of the three methods on patient 010. (a) Corrected Image from November 2017; (b) Corrected Image from May 2018; (c) Proposed ground truth; (d) Otsu thresholding, F1 score = 0.05; (e) Turgay Celik's approach, F1 score = 0.253; (f) Our Fully convolutional AE, F1 score = 0.38.

When looking at the figures and areas where the changes are detected, we can see that our method finds changes that are more in the peripheral areas of the lesions, while the Celik et al. approach tends to find lots of noisy elements inside existing lesions (see Figure 10e). From a medical point of view and to study the progression of ARMD, we are of course more concerned with lesion growth and therefore with what is going on in the peripheral areas of the lesions, thus giving an advantage to our methods, since it is better at capturing these peripheral changes. However, it does not mean that changes deep inside the lesions have no values and could not be used to better understand the mechanisms of the disease in another study.

5.4. Discussion

Overall, we can conclude that both Otsu thresholding and Kanezaki's approach suffer from risks of over-segmentation detecting a lot of noise, or under-segmentation detecting nothing, both of which are impossible to exploit from a medical point of view. On the other hand, despite somewhat mild recall and precision scores, the Celik approach and our method are visually much better at detecting meaningful changes in ARMD lesions' structures. Moreover, we can see that, despite the strong class imbalance that we mentioned earlier, our proposed method has a slightly higher F1-Score and finds structures that are visually better and more interesting from a medical point of view since they tend to be more on the outside and at the limits of existing lesions instead of inside them, and are also less fragmented.

To conclude this experimental section, we would like to discuss some of the main weaknesses and limitations of our proposed approach and of this study overall.

The first limitation that is not inherent to our approach is the difficulty to get accurate ground-truths to assess the quality of the results (hence why unsupervised learning should be preferred). In particular, all the ground-truths we have completely ignore possible textural changes within existing areas of geographic atrophy, and they don't always have the level of accuracy we hope for when it comes to subtle small changes in the lesions. This is due to the fact that most of these ground truths are built by subtracting masks of segmented lesions during two consecutive exams as shown in Figure 12: Doing so results in ground-truths that ignore most of the changes happening inside the lesions. It is worth mentioning that series with larger lesions are more affected by this issue as these lesions are more likely to have internal changes.

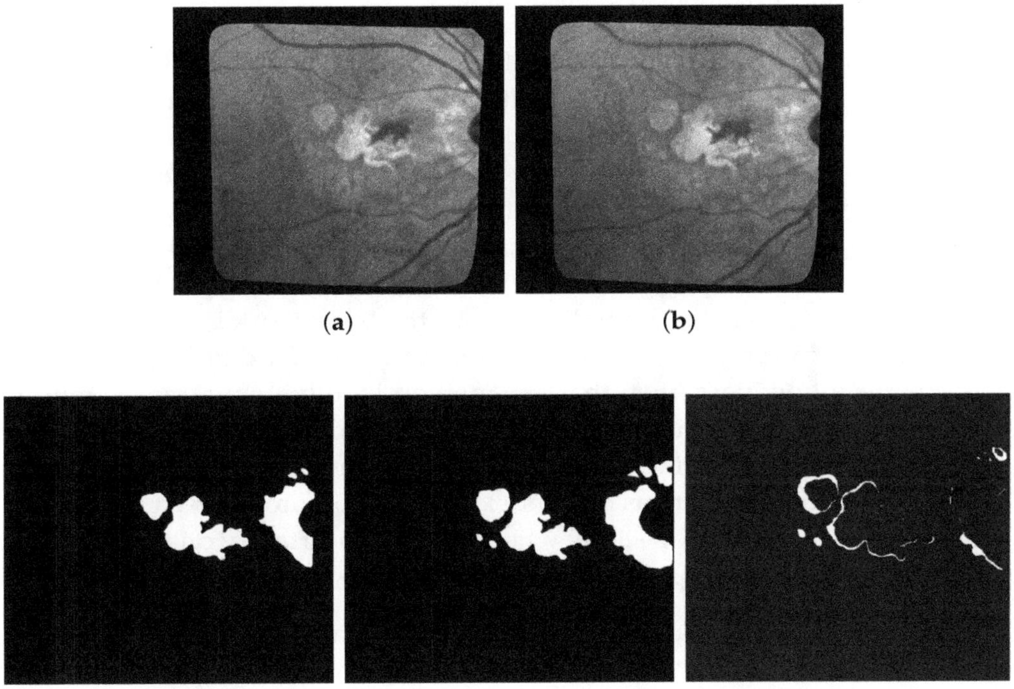

(a) (b)

(c) (d) (e)

Figure 12. Example of ground-truth build for patient 010 based on two consecutive masks of segmented lesions at time t and $t + 1$: All changes inside the lesions, textural or otherwise, are ignored. (**a**) Image t; (**b**) Image $t + 1$; (**c**) segmentation mask t; (**d**) segmentation mask $t + 1$; (**e**) Ground truth built from Mask t and $t + 1$.

This explains some of the low dice scores from Table 3 since in many cases there are internal changes (textural, structural, or both) happening within ARMD lesions, and some of them will be detected by the algorithms used in this paper. However, almost all of these changes detected inside the lesions will be classified as false positive since they are not present on the ground truth. One example of such issue is shown in Figure 13 where all pixels in red in sub-figure (d) will be classified as false positive despite some of them being actual changes (seeing some internal structural changes is possible by zooming in on sub-figures a and b).

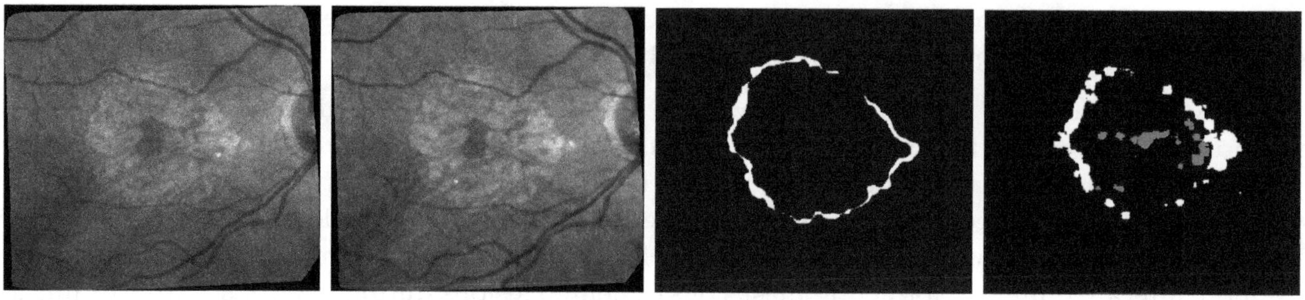

(a) (b) (c) (d)

Figure 13. Example of a segmentation in (d) where all changes detected in red will be considered false positive since the ground truth does not consider changes within existing lesions regardless of if they are structural of textural. (**a**) Image of patient 018 at time t; (**b**) Image of patient 018 at time $t + 1$; (**c**) Proposed Ground truth; (**d**) Proposed segmentation.

The second obvious weakness of our approach is also related to the difficulty of finding reliably annotated data and ground-truth. Because it is difficult to find them, we propose an unsupervised approach. In addition, unfortunately, unsupervised approaches are known to produce results that are less impressive than their supervised counterparts. A fully unsupervised framework which has the advantage that it does not require any annotated data to be trained—which is a real strength when very few are available—but has the weakness that its performances are weaker. In future works, we hope to refine our method so that we can improve the quality indexes a bit, but, even with better ground-truths, we expect the performances to remain limited so long as the framework is fully unsupervised.

A third limitation that can be mentioned and comes more from the data and experimental protocol than the methods is the following: Given that our method is fully unsupervised, and since we use change maps made by experts ophthalmologists that are not always reliable due to disagreements between experts on what is an interesting change or not, we have both a test set problem (as mentioned before), and a choice of metric problem as dice indexes while commonly used are probably not ideal to evaluate unsupervised methods, especially when there is uncertainty on the quality of the expert change maps. Two solutions that we plan to use on our future works are the following:

- To have several experts rating the proposed change maps, and use the average mark as a quality index. This method has the advantage that it is the fairest, but it is inconvenient that it is very time consuming and does not scale with large datasets as it takes on average 13 min for an ophthalmologist to do a quality segmentation on a single image.
- Using unsupervised quality indexes alongside the accuracy and the three dice indexes that we already use, so that we have a more fair evaluation of all methods. While this has the advantage of scaling well, it is probably a weaker quality argument than supervised indexes and experts' ratings for an application in the field of medicine.

The fourth limitation of our method that can be pointed out is that, as it stands, our algorithm does not yet achieve the goal of predicting how the pathology evolves: Our method detects changes and how the ARMD lesions evolved from one image to the next, but it does not provide any growth model or any interpretation of why it grew this way. Furthermore, while our algorithm detects changes fairly well, it is yet unable to predict future changes and therefore to tell in advance how the lesions might evolve on the short or long term for a given patient. While prediction was not the goal of the method proposed in this paper, it is certainly a future evolution that we are interested in. In fact, we hope that we will be able to use the results provided by our method on how the lesions grow and change from one image to the next to build predictive models based on this information. Some leads on approaches with which to combine our algorithm include other deep learning approaches such as long short term memory [34], gated recurrent units [35], or generative adversarial networks [36], all of which have shown to be useful for time series prediction or long term predictions.

Finally, even if our work does not lead to a huge leap forward in result quality due to various issues that we previously mentioned, the fact that we proposed a deep learning architecture will make it a lot easier in the future to couple our approach with predicting architectures such as the ones we just mentioned.

6. Conclusions

In this paper, we have presented a new fully unsupervised deep learning architecture based on a joint autoencoder that detects the evolution of ARMD lesions in an eye fundus series of images. With a pre-cleaning of the series to remove as many lighting issues as possible, our proposed method is based on an auto-encoder architecture that can detect non-trivial changes between pairs of images, such as the evolution of a lesion, while discarding more trivial changes such as lighting problems or slight texture changes due to different image angles. Our proposed method was applied to three real sets of images, and was compared with three methods from the state of the art. Despite mild F1-Score results due to various issues, our method has been shown to give good enough results for a fully unsupervised algorithm and to perform better than the other methods from the state of the art, and may prove useful to assist doctors in properly detecting the evolution of ARMD lesions by proposing a first raw segmentation of the evolution.

While our results are not perfect and cannot yet be used for a fully automated diagnosis, it is obvious to us that our proposed algorithm may prove useful to assist doctors in properly detecting the evolution of ARMD lesions by proposing a first raw segmentation of the evolution that is a lot better than what can be done with the existing methods.

In our future works, our priority will be to solve our ground-truth and test set issues by trying to have more experts producing and rating our results. This is an important pre-requisite as we plan on working on approaches that can work on full time series rather than pairs of images. This would also require both better lighting correction algorithms but may lead to more interesting models to predict the evolution of ARMD. Developing long-term prediction algorithms is another goal of ours that could be achieved using a combination of this work on longer series with other deep approaches that are more adapted for prediction.

Finally, as there are other modalities of images available to study ARMD, some of which have colors, but with different resolutions, one of our other goals would be to combine several of these types of images to globally improve our prediction scores. This future work of combining images with different scales, alignments, and color bands shall prove to be very challenging and will hopefully yield more interesting results while still using a fully unsupervised approach.

Author Contributions: M.P. and the Clinical Imaging Center of Paris Quinze-Vingts hospital provided the data after a first preprocessing step. M.P. also provided the medical knowledge necessary to interpret our algorithm's results. F.R. and M.P. worked together to produce and validate ground truths as reliable as possible. F.R. worked on data curation and the preprocessing algorithm for lighting correction. Most of the software programming, investigation, and experiments, as well as the result visualization were done by G.D. during his internship. J.S. and E.K. worked on the problem analysis and conceptualization, as well as domain adaptation from Remote Sensing to Medical Imaging. All authors participated in the validation of the experimental results. G.D. and E.K. wrote the original manuscript draft. J.S. revised and edited the manuscript. F.R. and J.S. conducted the project and were G.D. advisors for his internship. All authors have read and agreed to the published version of the manuscript.

Acknowledgments: This study has been approved by a French ethical committee (Comité de Protection des Personnes) and all participants gave informed consent. The authors would like to thank M. Clément Royer who helped us during the revision phase of this paper.

Abbreviations

The following abbreviations are used in this manuscript:

AE	Autoencoder
ARMD or AMD	Age Related Macular Degeneration
BCM	Binary Change Map
CNN	Convolutional Neural Networks
cSLO	confocal Scanning Laser Ophthalmoscopy
FAF	Fundus Autofluorescence
GA	Geographic Atrophy
IR	Infrared
OCT	Optical Coherence Tomography
PCA	Principal Component Analysis
RE	Reconstruction Error
RPE	Retinal Pigment Epithelium

References

1. Kanagasingam, Y.; Bhuiyan, A.; Abràmoff, M.D.; Smith, R.T.; Goldschmidt, L.; Wong, T.Y. Progress on retinal image analysis for age related macular degeneration. *Prog. Retin. Eye Res.* **2014**, *38*, 20–42. [CrossRef]
2. Priya, R.; Aruna, P. Automated diagnosis of Age-related macular degeneration from color retinal fundus images. In Proceedings of the 2011 3rd International Conference on Electronics Computer Technology, Kanyakumari, India, 8–10 April 2011; Volume 2, pp. 227–230.
3. Köse, C.; Sevik, U.; Gençalioglu, O. Automatic segmentation of age-related macular degeneration in retinal fundus images. *Comput. Biol. Med.* **2008**, *38*, 611–619. [CrossRef]
4. Ramsey, D.J.; Sunness, J.S.; Malviya, P.; Applegate, C.; Hager, G.D.; Handa, J.T. Automated image alignment and segmentation to follow progression of geographic atrophy in age-related macular degeneration. *Retina* **2014**, *34*, 1296–1307. [CrossRef]
5. Köse, C.; Sevik, U.; Gençalioğlu, O.; Ikibaş, C.; Kayikiçioğlu, T. A Statistical Segmentation Method for Measuring Age-Related Macular Degeneration in Retinal Fundus Images. *J. Med. Syst.* **2010**, *34*, 1–13. [CrossRef]
6. Marrugo, A.G.; Millan, M.S.; Sorel, M.; Sroubek, F. Retinal image restoration by means of blind deconvolution. *J. Biomed. Opt.* **2011**, *16*, 116016. [CrossRef]
7. Feeny, A.K.; Tadarati, M.; Freund, D.E.; Bressler, N.M.; Burlina, P. Automated segmentation of geographic atrophy of the retinal epithelium via random forests in AREDS color fundus images. *Comput. Biol. Med.* **2015**, *65*, 124–136. [CrossRef]
8. Lee, N.; Laine, A.F.; Smith, R.T. A hybrid segmentation approach for geographic atrophy in fundus auto-fluorescence images for diagnosis of age-related macular degeneration. In Proceedings of the 2007 29th Annual International Conference of the IEEE Engineering in Medicine and Biology Society, Lyon, France, 22–26 August 2007; pp. 4965–4968.
9. Hu, Z.; Medioni, G.G.; Hernandez, M.; Sadda, S.R. Automated segmentation of geographic atrophy in fundus autofluorescence images using supervised pixel classification. *J. Med. Imaging* **2015**, *2*, 014501. [CrossRef]
10. Hu, Z.; Medioni, G.G.; Hernandez, M.; Hariri, A.; Wu, X.; Sadda, S.R. Segmentation of the geographic atrophy in spectral-domain optical coherence tomography and fundus autofluorescence images. *Investig. Ophthalmol. Vis. Sci.* **2013**, *54*, 8375–8383. [CrossRef]
11. Troglio, G.; Alberti, M.; Benediktsson, J.; Moser, G.; Serpico, S.; Stefánsson, E. Unsupervised Change-Detection in Retinal Images by a Multiple-Classifier Approach. In *International Workshop on Multiple Classifier Systems*; Springer: Berlin/Heidelberg, Germany, 2010; pp. 94–103.
12. Troglio, G.; Nappo, A.; Benediktsson, J.; Moser, G.; Serpico, S.; Stefánsson, E. Automatic Change Detection of Retinal Images. In Proceedings of the World Congress on Medical Physics and Biomedical Engineering, Munich, Germany, 7–12 September 2009; Volume 25, pp. 281–284.

13. Hussain, M.A.; Govindaiah, A.; Souied, E.; Smith, R.; Bhuiyan, A. Automated tracking and change detection for Age-related Macular Degeneration Progression using retinal fundus imaging. In Proceedings of the 2018 Joint 7th International Conference on Informatics, Electronics & Vision (ICIEV) and 2018 2nd International Conference on Imaging, Vision & Pattern Recognition (icIVPR), Kitakyushu, Japan, 25–29 June 2018; pp. 394–398. [CrossRef]
14. Burlina, P.; Freund, D.E.; Joshi, N.; Wolfson, Y.; Bressler, N.M. Detection of age-related macular degeneration via deep learning. In Proceedings of the 2016 IEEE 13th International Symposium on Biomedical Imaging (ISBI), Prague, Czech Republic, 13–16 April 2016; pp. 184–188.
15. Burlina, P.M.; Joshi, N.; Pekala, M.; Pacheco, K.D.; Freund, D.E.; Bressler, N.M. Automated Grading of Age-Related Macular Degeneration From Color Fundus Images Using Deep Convolutional Neural Networks. *JAMA Ophthalmol.* **2017**, *135*, 1170–1176. [CrossRef]
16. Phan, T.V.; Seoud, L.; Cheriet, F. Automatic Screening and Grading of Age-Related Macular Degeneration from Texture Analysis of Fundus Images. *J. Ophthalmol.* **2016**, *2016*, 5893601. [CrossRef]
17. Wandeto, J.; Nyongesa, H.; Rémond, Y.; Dresp, B. Detection of small changes in medical and random-dot images comparing self-organizing map performance to human detection. *Inform. Med. Unlocked* **2017**, *7*, 39–45. [CrossRef]
18. Kohonen, T. (Ed.) *Self-Organizing Maps*; Springer: Berlin/Heidelberg, Germany, 1997.
19. Lee, N.; Smith, R.T.; Laine, A.F. Interactive segmentation for geographic atrophy in retinal fundus images. In Proceedings of the 2008 42nd Asilomar Conference on Signals, Systems and Computers, Pacific Grove, CA, USA, 26–29 October 2008; pp. 655–658.
20. Deckert, A.; Schmitz-Valckenberg, S.; Jorzik, J.; Bindewald, A.; Holz, F.; Mansmann, U. Automated analysis of digital fundus autofluorescence images of geographic atrophy in advanced age-related macular degeneration using confocal scanning laser ophthalmoscopy (cSLO). *BMC Ophthalmol.* **2005**, *5*, 8. [CrossRef]
21. Celik, T. Unsupervised change detection in satellite images using principal component analysis and *k*-means clustering. *IEEE Geosci. Remote Sens. Lett.* **2009**, *6*, 772–776. [CrossRef]
22. Kalinicheva, E.; Sublime, J.; Trocan, M. Change Detection in Satellite Images Using Reconstruction Errors of Joint Autoencoders. In *Artificial Neural Networks and Machine Learning—ICANN 2019: Image, Processings of the 8th International Conference on Artificial Neural Networks, Munich, Germany, 17–19 September 2019*; Proceedings, Part III; Lecture Notes in Computer Science 11729; Springer: Cham, Switzerland, 2019; pp. 637–648, ISBN 978-3-030-30507-9. [CrossRef]
23. Chong, Y.S.; Tay, Y.H. Abnormal Event Detection in Videos Using Spatiotemporal Autoencoder. In *Advances in Neural Networks—ISNN 2017, Proceedings of the 14th International Symposium, ISNN 2017, Sapporo, Hakodate, and Muroran, Hokkaido, Japan, 21–26 June 2017*; Proceedings, Part II; Cong, F., Leung, A.C., Wei, Q., Eds.; Springer: Berlin/Heidelberg, Germany, 2017; Volume 10262, pp. 189–196. [CrossRef]
24. Kanezaki, A. Unsupervised Image Segmentation by Backpropagation. In Proceedings of IEEE International Conference on Acoustics, Speech, and Signal Processing (ICASSP), Calgary, AB, Canada, 15–20 April 2018 .
25. Xia, X.; Kulis, B. W-Net: A Deep Model for Fully Unsupervised Image Segmentation. *arXiv* **2017**, arXiv:1711.08506.
26. Sublime, J.; Kalinicheva, E. Automatic Post-Disaster Damage Mapping Using Deep-Learning Techniques for Change Detection: Case Study of the Tohoku Tsunami. *Remote Sens.* **2019**, *11*, 1123. [CrossRef]
27. Hinton, G.E.; Salakhutdinov, R.R. Reducing the Dimensionality of Data with Neural Networks. *Science* **2006**, *313*, 504–507. [CrossRef]
28. Long, J.; Shelhamer, E.; Darrell, T. Fully Convolutional Networks for Semantic Segmentation. *arXiv* **2014**, arXiv:1411.4038.
29. Ronneberger, O.; Fischer, P.; Brox, T. U-net: Convolutional networks for biomedical image segmentation. In *International Conference on Medical Image Computing and Computer-Assisted Intervention*; Springer: Berlin/Heidelberg, Germany, 2015; pp. 234–241.
30. Van der Walt, S.; Schönberger, J.L.; Nunez-Iglesias, J.; Boulogne, F.; Warner, J.D.; Yager, N.; Gouillart, E.; Yu, T. scikit-image: Image processing in Python. *PeerJ* **2014**, *2*, e453. [CrossRef] [PubMed]
31. Chui, C.; Mhaskar, H. MRA contextual-recovery extension of smooth functions on manifolds. *Appl. Comput. Harmon. Anal.* **2010**, *28*, 104–113. [CrossRef]
32. Damelin, S.B.; Hoang, N.S. On Surface Completion and Image Inpainting by Biharmonic Functions: Numerical Aspects. *Int. J. Math. Math. Sci.* **2018**, *2018*, 1–8. [CrossRef]

33. Otsu, N. A Threshold Selection Method from Gray-Level Histograms. *IEEE Trans. Syst. Man Cybern.* **1979**, *9*, 62–66. [CrossRef]
34. Gers, F.A.; Schmidhuber, J.; Cummins, F.A. Learning to Forget: Continual Prediction with LSTM. *Neural Comput.* **2000**, *12*, 2451–2471. [CrossRef] [PubMed]
35. Cho, K.; van Merrienboer, B.; Gülçehre, Ç.; Bahdanau, D.; Bougares, F.; Schwenk, H.; Bengio, Y. Learning Phrase Representations using RNN Encoder-Decoder for Statistical Machine Translation. In Proceedings of the 2014 Conference on Empirical Methods in Natural Language Processing, EMNLP 2014, Doha, Qatar, 25–29 October 2014; pp. 1724–1734. [CrossRef]
36. Goodfellow, I.J.; Pouget-Abadie, J.; Mirza, M.; Xu, B.; Warde-Farley, D.; Ozair, S.; Courville, A.C.; Bengio, Y. Generative Adversarial Nets. In *Advances in Neural Information Processing Systems 27, Proceedings of the Annual Conference on Neural Information Processing Systems 2014, Montreal, QC, Canada, 8–13 December 2014*; Ghahramani, Z., Welling, M., Cortes, C., Lawrence, N.D., Weinberger, K.Q., Eds.; 2014; pp. 2672–2680.

5

Explainable Deep Learning Models in Medical Image Analysis

Amitojdeep Singh [1,2,*], Sourya Sengupta [1,2] and Vasudevan Lakshminarayanan [1,2]

1 Theoretical and Experimental Epistemology Laboratory, School of Optometry and Vision Science, University of Waterloo, Waterloo, ON N2L 3G1, Canada; sourya.sengupta@uwaterloo.ca (S.S.); vengulak@uwaterloo.ca (V.L.)

2 Department of Systems Design Engineering, University of Waterloo, Waterloo, ON N2L 3G1, Canada

* Correspondence: amitojdeep.singh@uwaterloo.ca

Abstract: Deep learning methods have been very effective for a variety of medical diagnostic tasks and have even outperformed human experts on some of those. However, the black-box nature of the algorithms has restricted their clinical use. Recent explainability studies aim to show the features that influence the decision of a model the most. The majority of literature reviews of this area have focused on taxonomy, ethics, and the need for explanations. A review of the current applications of explainable deep learning for different medical imaging tasks is presented here. The various approaches, challenges for clinical deployment, and the areas requiring further research are discussed here from a practical standpoint of a deep learning researcher designing a system for the clinical end-users.

Keywords: explainability; explainable AI; XAI; deep learning; medical imaging; diagnosis

1. Introduction

Computer-aided diagnostics (CAD) using artificial intelligence (AI) provides a promising way to make the diagnosis process more efficient and available to the masses. Deep learning is the leading artificial intelligence (AI) method for a wide range of tasks including medical imaging problems. It is the state of the art for several computer vision tasks and has been used for medical imaging tasks like the classification of Alzheimer's [1], lung cancer detection [2], retinal disease detection [3,4], etc. Despite achieving remarkable results in the medical domain, AI-based methods have not achieved a significant deployment in the clinics. This is due to the underlying black-box nature of the deep learning algorithms along with other reasons like computational costs. It arises from the fact that, despite having the underlying statistical principles, there is a lack of ability to explicitly represent the knowledge for a given task performed by a deep neural network. Simpler AI methods like linear regression and decision trees are self-explanatory as the decision boundary used for classification can be visualized in a few dimensions using the model parameters. However, these lack the complexity required for tasks such as classification of 3D and most 2D medical images. The lack of tools to inspect the behavior of black-box models affects the use of deep learning in all domains including finance and autonomous driving where explainability and reliability are the key elements for trust by the end-user. A schematic explaining the relationship between deep learning and the need for explanations is shown in Figure 1.

A medical diagnosis system needs to be transparent, understandable, and explainable to gain the trust of physicians, regulators as well as the patients. Ideally, it should be able to explain the complete logic of making a certain decision to all the parties involved. Newer regulations like the European General Data Protection Regulation (GDPR) are making it harder for the use of black-box models in all businesses including healthcare because retraceability of the decisions is now a requirement [5].

An artificial intelligence (AI) system to complement medical professionals should have a certain amount of explainability and allow the human expert to retrace the decisions and use their judgment. Some researchers also emphasize that even humans are not always able to or even willing to explain their decisions [5]. Explainability is the key to safe, ethical, fair, and trust-able use of artificial intelligence (AI) and a key enabler for its deployment in the real world. Breaking myths about artificial intelligence (AI) by showing what a model looked at while making the decision can inculcate trust among the end-users. It is even more important to show the domain-specific features used in the decision for non-deep learning users like most medical professionals.

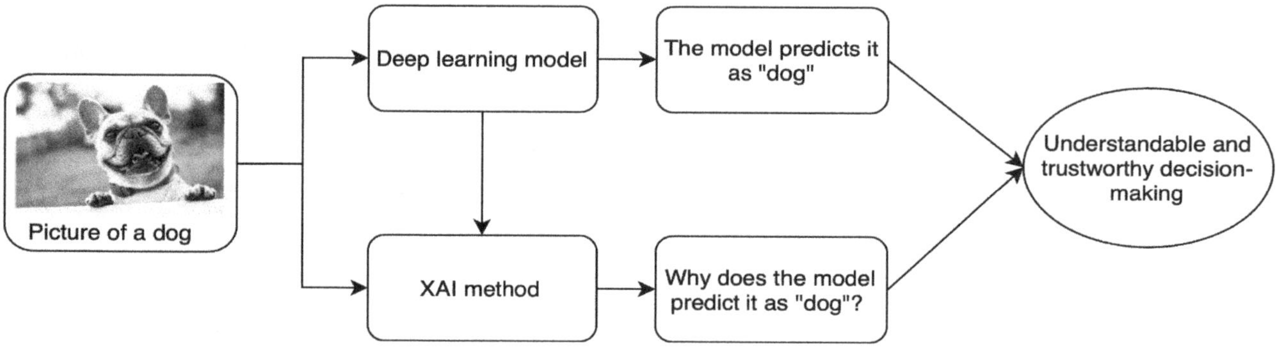

Figure 1. A brief schematic of basics of XAI methods.

The terms explainability and interpretability are often used interchangeably in the literature. A distinction between these was provided in [6] where interpretation was defined as mapping an abstract concept like the output class into a domain example, while explanation was defined as a set of domain features such as pixels of an image the contribute to the output decision of the model. A related term to this concept is the uncertainty associated with the decision of a model. Deep learning classifiers are usually not able to say "I don't know" in situations with ambiguity and instead return the class with the highest probability, even if by a narrow margin, making uncertainty a crucial topic. Lately, uncertainty has been analyzed along with the problem of explainability in many studies to highlight the cases where a model is unsure and in turn, make the models more acceptable to non-deep learning users. There have been studies about the uncertainty of machine learning algorithms which include those for endoscopic videos [7] and tissue parameter estimation [8]. We limit the scope of this paper to explainability methods and discuss uncertainty if a study used it along with explainability. The topic of uncertainty in deep learning models can be itself a subject of a future review. As noted earlier, deep learning models are considered as non-transparent as the weights of the neurons can not be understood as knowledge directly. [9] showed that neither the magnitude or the selectivity of the activations, nor the impact on network decisions is sufficient for deciding the importance of a neuron for a given task. A detailed analysis of the terminologies, concepts and, use cases of explainable artificial intelligence (AI) is provided in [10].

This paper describes the studies related to the explainability of deep learning models in the context of medical imaging. A general taxonomy of explainability approaches is described briefly in the next section and a comparison of various attribution based methods is performed in Section 3. Section 4 reviews various explainability methods applied to different medical imaging modalities. The analysis is broken down into Sections 4.1 and 4.2 depending upon the use of attributions or other methods of explainability. The evolution, current trends, and some future possibilities of the explainable deep learning models in medical image analysis are summarized in Section 5.

2. Taxonomy of Explainability Approaches

Several taxonomies have been proposed in the literature to classify different explainability methods [11,12]. Generally, the classification techniques are not absolute, it can vary widely depending upon the characteristics of the methods and can be classified into many overlapping or non-overlapping classes simultaneously. Different kinds of taxonomies and classification methods are discussed briefly here and a detailed analysis of the taxonomies can be found in [10,11] and a flow chart for them is shown in Figure 2.

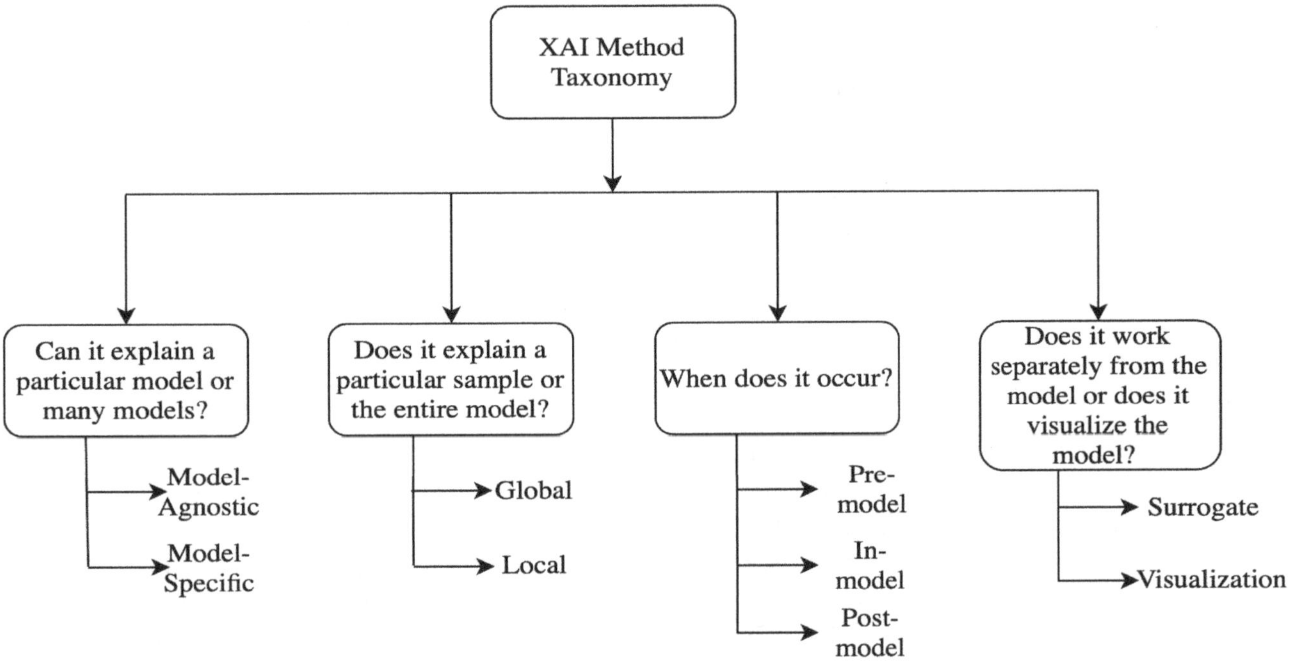

Figure 2. Taxonomy of XAI methods.

2.1. *Model Specific vs. Model Agnostic*

Model-specific interpretation methods are based on the parameters of the individual models. The graph neural network explainer (GNNExplainer) [13] is a special type of model-specific interpretability where the complexity of data representation needs specifically the graph neural network (GNN). Model Agnostic methods are mainly applicable in post-hoc analysis and not limited to specified model architecture. These methods do not have direct access to the internal model weights or structural parameters.

2.2. *Global Methods vs. Local Methods*

Local interpretable methods are applicable to a single outcome of the model. This can be done by designing methods that can explain the reason for a particular prediction or outcome. For example, it is interested in specific features and their characteristics. On the contrary, global methods concentrate on the inside of a model by exploiting the overall knowledge about the model, the training, and the associated data. It tries to explain the behavior of the model in general. Feature importance is a good example of this method, which tries to figure out the features which are in general responsible for better performance of the model among all different features.

2.3. *Pre-Model vs. In-Model vs. Post-Model*

Pre-model methods are independent and do not depend on a particular model architecture to use it on. Principal component analysis (PCA) [14], t-Distributed Stochastic Neighbor Embedding (t-SNE) [15] are some common examples of these methods. Interpretability methods, integrated into the model itself, are called as in-model methods. Some methods are implemented after building a model and hence these methods are termed as post model and these methods can potentially develop meaningful insights about what exactly a model learned during the training.

2.4. Surrogate Methods vs. Visualization Methods

Surrogate methods consist of different models as an ensemble which are used to analyze other black-box models. The black box models can be understood better by interpreting the surrogate model's decisions by comparing the black-box model's decision and surrogate model's decision. The decision tree [16] is an example of surrogate methods. The visualization methods are not a different model, but it helps to explain some parts of the models by visual understanding like activation maps.

It is to be noted that these classification methods are non-exclusive, these are built upon different logical intuitions and hence have significant overlaps. For example, most of the post-hoc models like attributions can also be seen as model agnostic as these methods are typically not dependent upon the structure of a model. However, some requirements regarding the limitations on model layers or the activation functions do exist for some of the attribution methods. The next section describes the basic concept and subtle difference between various attribution methods to facilitate a comparative discussion of the applications in Section 4.

3. Explainability Methods—Attribution Based

There are broadly two types of approaches to explain the results of deep neural networks (DNN) in medical imaging—those using standard attribution based methods and those using novel, often architecture, or domain-specific techniques. A majority of the papers for explaining deep learning in medical image diagnosis use attribution based methods. Their model agnostic plug and play nature along with readily available open-source implementations make them a convenient solution. The deep learning practitioners can, therefore, focus on designing a model optimal for a given task and use these easy to generate explanations for understanding the model better. Since attribution based studies are a majority (with many of them using multiple attribution based methods), we discuss them beforehand. The applications for those methods are ordered according to the anatomical districts, i.e., organ groups for the diagnosed diseases in Section 4.1. Other methods are used in only a few studies each which typically uses a single method and are hence discussed along with their applications in Section 4.2 which is ordered by the explainability method used.

The problem of assigning an attribution value or contribution or relevance to each input feature of a network led to the development of several attribution methods. The goal of an attribution method is to determine the contribution of an input feature to the target neuron which is usually the output neuron of the correct class for a classification problem. The arrangement of the attributions of all the input features in the shape of the input sample forms heatmaps known as the attribution maps. Some examples of attribution maps for different images are shown in Figure 3. The features with a positive contribution to the activation of the target neuron are typically marked in red while those negatively affecting the activation are marked in blue. These are the features or pixels in case of images providing positive and negative evidence of different magnitudes, respectively.

The commonly used attribution methods are discussed in this section and the applications in the next section. It must be noted that some of the approaches like DeepTaylor [17] provide only positive evidence and can be useful for a certain set of tasks. The attribution methods can be applied on a black box convolutional neural network (CNN) without any modification to the underlying architecture making them a convenient yet powerful XAI tool. An empirical comparison of some of the methods discussed in this section and a unified framework called DeepExplain is available in [18]. Most of the methods discussed here apart from the newer Deep Learning Important FeaTures (LIFT) and Deep SHapley Additive exPlanations (SHAP) are implemented in the iNNvestigate toolbox [19].

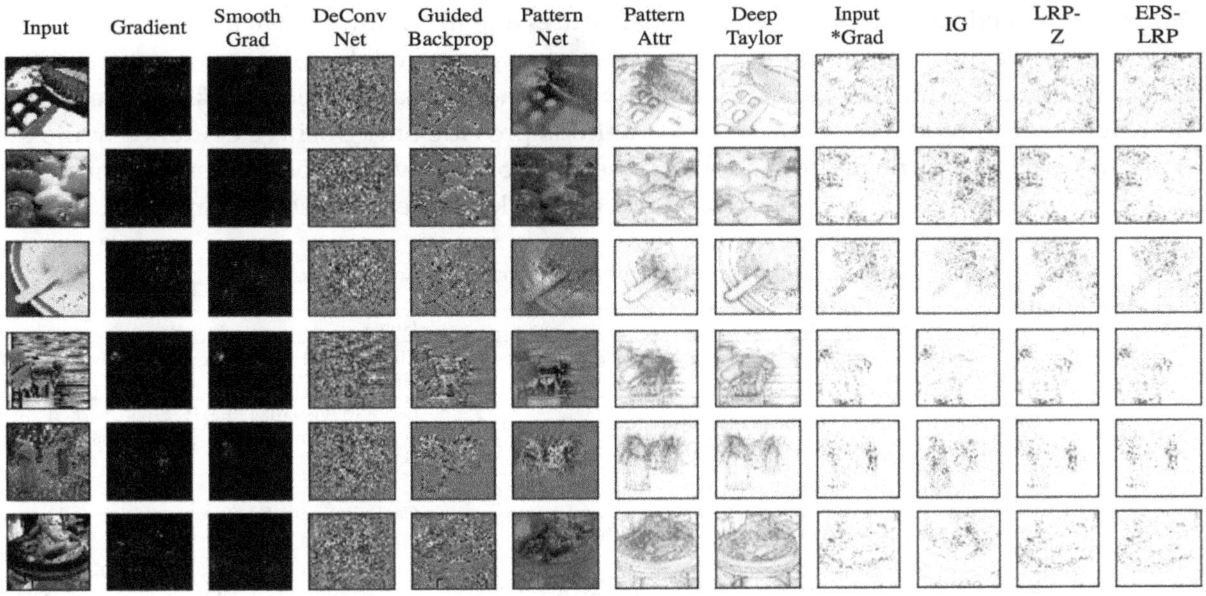

Figure 3. Attributions of VGG-16 with images from Imagenet using the methods implemented in [19].

3.1. Perturbation Based Methods—Occlusion

Perturbation is the simplest way to analyze the effect of changing the input features on the output of an AI model. This can be implemented by removing, masking, or modifying certain input features, and running the forward pass (output computation), and measuring the difference from the original output. This is similar to the sensitivity analysis performed in parametric control system models. The input features affecting the output the most are ranked as the most important. It is computationally expensive as a forward pass needs to be run after perturbing each group of features of the input. In the case of image data the perturbation is performed by covering parts of an image with a grey patch and hence occluding them from the system's view. It can provide both positive and negative evidence by highlighting the responsible features.

This technique was applied by Zeiler and Fergus [20] to the convolutional neural network (CNN) for the image classification task. Occlusion is the benchmark for any attribution study as it is a simple to perform model agnostic approach which reveals the feature importance of a model. It can reveal if a model is overfitting and learning irrelevant features as in the case of adversarial examples [21]. The adversarial examples are the inputs designed to cause the model to make a false decision and are like optical illusions for the models. In that case, the model misclassifies the image (say a cat as a dog) despite the presence of discriminating feature

Occluding all features (pixels) one-by-one and running the forward pass each time can be computationally expensive and can take several hours per image [18]. It is common to use patches of sizes such as 5×5, 10×10, or even larger depending on the size of the target features and computational resources available.

Another perturbation based approach is Shapley value sampling which computes approximate Shapely Values by taking each input feature for a sample number of times. It a method from the coalitional game theory which describes the fair distribution of the gains and losses among the input features. It was originally proposed for the analysis of regression [22]. It is slower than all other approaches as the network has to be run samples $\times$ number of features times. As a result it is not a practical method in its original form but has led to the development of game theory-based methods like Deep SHapley Additive exPlanations (SHAP) as discussed in the next subsection.

3.2. Backpropagation Based Methods

These methods compute the attribution for all the input features with a single forward and backward pass through the network. In some of the methods these steps need to be repeated multiple times but it is independent of the number of input features and much lower than for perturbation-based methods. The faster run-time comes at the expense of a weaker relationship between the outcome and the variation of the output. Various backpropagation based attribution methods are described in Table 1. It must be noted that some of these methods provide only positive evidence while others provide both positive and negative evidence. The methods providing both positive and negative evidence tend to have high-frequency noise which can make the results seem spurious. [18].

Table 1. Backpropagation based attribution methods.

Method	Description	Notes
Gradient	Computes the gradient of the output of the **target neuron** with respect to the input.	The **simplest** approach but is usually not the most effective.
DeConvNet [20]	Applies the **ReLU to the gradient computation instead** of the gradient of a neuron with ReLU activation.	Used to **visualize the features** learned by the layers. **Limited** to CNN models with **ReLU activation**.
Saliency Maps [23]	Takes the **absolute value of the partial derivative** of the target output neuron with respect to the input features to find the features which affect the output the most with least perturbation.	**Can't distinguish between positive and negative** evidence due to absolute values.
Guided backpropagation (GBP) [24]	Applies the **ReLU to the gradient computation in addition** to the gradient of a neuron with ReLU activation.	Like DeConvNet, it is textbflimited to CNN models with **ReLU activation**.
LRP [25]	**Redistributes the prediction score** layer by layer with a backward pass on the network using a particular rule like the **ϵ-rule** while ensuring numerical stability	There are alternative stability rules and **limited** to CNN models with **ReLU activation** when all activations are **ReLU**.
Gradient × input [26]	Initially proposed as a method to **improve sharpness of attribution maps** and is computed by multiplying the signed partial derivative of the output with the input.	It **can approximate occlusion** better than other methods in certain cases like multi layer perceptron (MLP) with Tanh on MNIST data [18] while being instant to compute.
GradCAM [27]	Produces **gradient-weighted class activation maps** using the gradients of the target concept as it flows to the final convolutional layer	Applicable to **only CNN** including those with fully connected layers, structured output (like captions) and reinforcement learning.
IG [28]	Computes the **average gradient** as the input is varied from the **baseline** (often zero) to the actual input value unlike the Gradient × input which uses a single derivative at the input.	It is **highly correlated with the rescale rule of DeepLIFT** discussed below which can act as a good and faster approximation.
DeepTaylor [17]	Finds a rootpoint near each neuron with a value close to the input but with output as 0 and uses it to recursively estimate the attribution of each neuron using **Taylor decomposition**	Provides **sparser explanations**, i.e., focuses on key features but provides **no negative evidence** due to its assumptions of only positive effect.
PatternNet [29]	Estimates the input signal of the output neuron using an **objective function**.	Proposed to counter the incorrect attributions of other methods on **linear systems** and generalized to deep networks.
Pattern Attribution [29]	Applies Deep Taylor decomposition by searching the **rootpoints in the signal direction** for each neuron	Proposed along with **PatternNet** and uses decomposition instead of signal visualization
DeepLIFT [30]	Uses a reference input and computes the reference values of all hidden units using a forward pass and then proceeds backward **like LRP**. It has two variants—**Rescale rule** and the one introduced later called **RevealCancel** which treats positive and negative contributions to a neuron separately.	Rescale is strongly related to and **equivalent in some cases to ϵ-LRP** but is **not applicable to models involving multiplicative rules. RevealCancel handles such cases** and using RevealCancel for convolutional and Rescale for fully connected layers reduces noise.
SmoothGrad [31]	An improvement on the gradient method which averages the gradient over multiple inputs with additional noise	Designed to visually sharpen the attributions produced by gradient method using class score function.
Deep SHAP [32]	It is a fast **approximation** algorithm to compute the game theory based **SHAP values**. It is connected to DeepLIFT and uses **multiple background samples** instead of one baseline.	Finds attributions for **non neural net models** like trees, support vector machines (SVM) and **ensemble** of those with a neural net using various tools in the the SHAP library.

An important property of attribution methods known as completeness was introduced in the DeepLIFT [30] paper. It states that the attributions for a given input add up to the target output minus the target output at the baseline input. It is satisfied by integrated gradients, DeepTaylor and Deep SHAP but not by DeepLIFT in its rescale rule. A measure generalizing this property is proposed in [18] for a quantitative comparison of various attribution methods. It is called sensitivity-n and involves comparing the sum of the attributions and the variation in the target output in terms of PCC. Occlusion is found to have a higher PCC than other methods as it finds a direct relationship between the variation in the input and that in the output.

The evaluation of attribution methods is complex as it is challenging to discern between the errors of the model and the attribution method explaining it. Measures like sensitivity-n reward the methods designed to reflect the network behavior closely. However, a more practically relevant measure of an attribution method is the similarity of attributions to a human observer's expectation. It needs to be performed with a human expert for a given task and carries an observer bias as the methods closer to the observer expectation can be favored at the cost of those explaining the model behavior. We underscore the argument that the ratings of different attribution methods by experts of a specific domain are potentially useful to develop explainable models which are more likely to be trusted by the end users and hence should be a critical part of the development of an XAI system.

4. Applications

The applications of explainability in medical imaging are reviewed here by categorizing them into two types—those using pre-existing attribution based methods and those using other, often specific methods. The methods are discussed according to the explainability method and the medical imaging application. Table 2 provides a brief overview of the methods.

4.1. Attribution Based

A majority of the medical imaging literature that studied interpretability of deep learning methods used attribution based methods due to their ease of use. Researchers can train a suitable neural network architecture without the added complexity of making it inherently explainable and use a readily available attribution model. This allows the use of either a pre-existing deep learning model or one with a custom architecture for the best performance on the given task. The former makes the implementation easier and allows one to leverage techniques like transfer learning [33,34] while the latter can be used to focus on specific data and avoid overfitting by using fewer parameters. Both approaches are beneficial for medical imaging datasets which tend to be relatively smaller than computer vision benchmarks like ImageNet [35].

Post-model analysis using attributions can reveal if the model is learning relevant features or if it is overfitting to the input by learning spurious features. This allows researchers to adjust the model architecture and hyperparameters to achieve better results on the test data and in turn a potential real-world setting. In this subsection, some recent studies using attribution methods across different medical imaging modalities are reviewed in the order of the anatomical districts from top to bottom of the human body. The reviewed tasks include explanations of deep learning for diagnosing conditions from brain MRI, retinal imaging, breast imaging, CT scans, chest X-ray as well as skin imaging.

4.1.1. Brain Imaging

A study comparing the robustness of various attribution based methods for convolutional neural network (CNN) in Alzheimer's classification using brain MRI [36] performed a quantitative analysis of different methods. Gradient $\times$ input, Guided backpropagation (GBP), LRP, and occlusion were the compared methods. The L2 norm between the average attribution maps of multiple runs for the same model to check the repeatability of heatmaps for identically trained models. It was found to be an order of magnitude lower for the first three methods compared to the baseline occlusion since occlusion covers a larger area. LRP performed the best overall indicating the superiority of a completely attribution based method over function and signal-based methods. The similarity between the sum, density, and gain (sum/density) for the top 10 regions of the attributions across the runs was also the highest for LRP. In another study [37] GradCAM and Guided backpropagation (GBP) were used to analyze the clinical coherence of the features learned by a CNN for automated grading of brain tumor from MRI. For the correctly graded cases, both the methods had the most activation in the tumor region while also activating the surrounding ventricles which can indicate malignancy as well. In some cases, this focus on non-tumor regions and some spurious patterns in Guided backpropagation (GBP) maps lead to errors indicating unreliability of the features.

4.1.2. Retinal Imaging

A system producing IG heatmaps along with model predictions was explored as a tool to assist diabetic retinopathy (DR) grading by ophthalmologists [38]. This assistance was found to increase the accuracy of the grading compared to that of an unassisted expert or with the model predictions alone. Initially, the system increased the grading time but with the user's experience, the grading time decreased and the grading confidence increased, especially when both predictions and heatmaps were used. Notably, the accuracy did reduce for patients without DR when model assistance was used and an option to toggle the assistance was provided. An extension of IG called Expressive gradients (EG) was proposed in [39] for weakly supervised segmentation of lesions for Age-related macular degeneration (AMD) diagnosis. A convolutional neural network (CNN) with a compact architecture outperformed larger existing convolutional neural network (CNN)s and Expressive gradients (EG) highlighted the regions of interest better than conventional IG and Guided backpropagation (GBP) methods. Expressive gradients (EG) extends IG by enriching input-level attribution map with high-level attribution maps. A comparative analysis of various explainability models including DeepDeep Learning Important FeaTures (LIFT), DeepSHapley Additive exPlanations (SHAP), IG, etc. was performed for on a model for detection of choroidal neovascularization (CNV), diabetic macular edema (DME), and drusens from optical coherence tomography (OCT) scans [40]. Figure 4 highlights better localization achieved by newer methods (e.g., DeepSHAP) in contrast to noisy results from older methods (e.g., saliency maps).

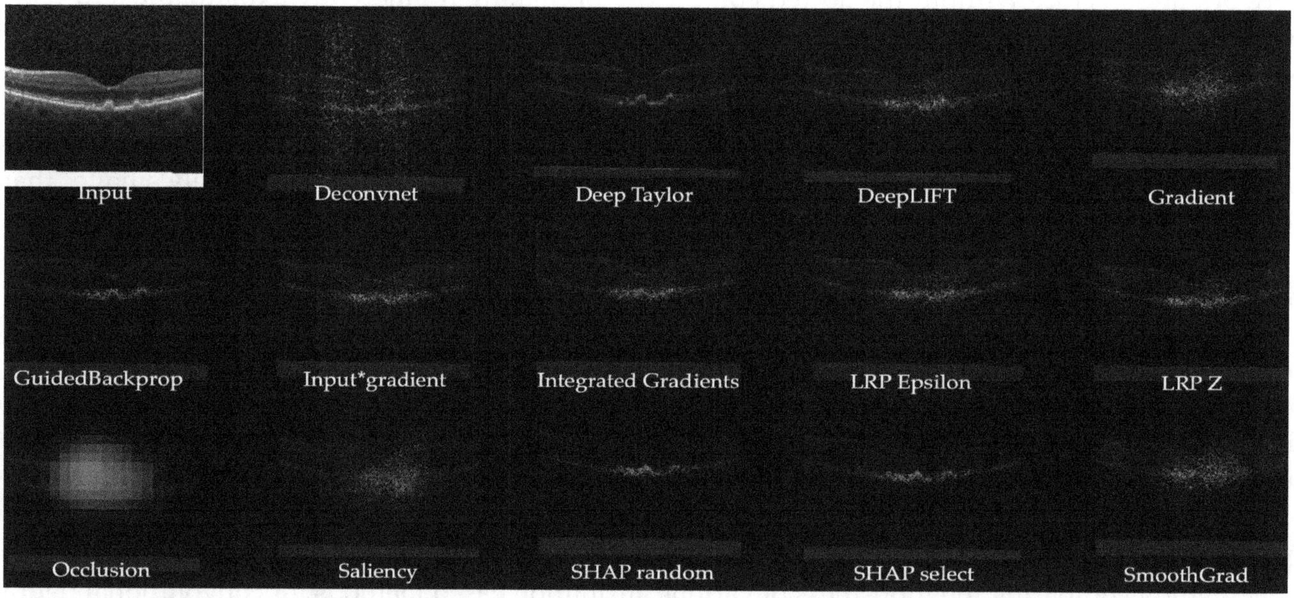

Figure 4. Example of heat maps from a retinal OCT image [40].

4.1.3. Breast Imaging

IG and SmoothGrad were used to visualize the features of a convolutional neural network (CNN) used for classifying estrogen receptor status from breast MRI [41]. The model was observed to have learned relevant features in both spatial and dynamic domains with different contributions from both. The visualizations revealed the learning of certain irrelevant features resulting from pre-processing artifacts. These observations led to changes in the pre-processing and training approaches. An earlier study for breast mass classification from mammograms [42] using two different convolutional neural network (CNN)s—AlexNet [43] and GoogleNet [44]—employed saliency maps to visualize the image features. Both the convolutional neural network (CNN)s were seen to learn the edges of the mass which are the main clinical criteria, while also being sensitive to the context.

4.1.4. CT Imaging

A DeepDreams [45] inspired attribution method was presented in [46] for explaining the segmentation of tumor from liver CT images. This novel method formulated using the concepts of DeapDreams, an image generation algorithm can be applied to a black-box neural network like other attribution methods discussed in Section 3. It performed a sensitivity analysis of the features by maximizing the activation of the target neuron by performing gradient ascent, i.e., finding the steepest slope of the function. A comparison between networks trained on real tumors and synthetic tumors revealed that the former was more sensitive to clinically relevant features and the latter was focusing on other features too. The network was found to be sensitive to intensity as well as sphericity in coherence with domain knowledge.

4.1.5. X-ray Imaging

In a recent study for detection of COVID-19 from chest X-ray images [47], a method called GSInquire was used to produce heatmaps for verifying the features learned by the proposed COVID-net model. GSInquire [48] was developed as an attribution method that outperformed prior methods like SHAP and Expected gradients in terms of the proposed new metrics—impact score and impact coverage. The impact score was defined as the percentage of features which impacted the model decision or confidence strongly. While impact coverage was defined in the context of the coverage of adversarially impacted factors in the input. Another study performed the analysis of uncertainty and interpretability for COVID-19 detection using chest X-rays. The heatmaps of the sample inputs for the trained model were generated using saliency maps, Guided GradCAM, GBP, and Class activation maps (CAM).

4.1.6. Skin Imaging

The features of a suite of 30 CNN models trained for melanoma detection [49] were compared using GradCAM and Kernel SHapley Additive exPlanations (SHAP). It was shown that even the models with high accuracy would occasionally focus on the features that were irrelevant for the diagnosis. There were differences in the explanations of the models that produced similar accuracy which was highlighted by the attribution maps of both the methods. This showed that distinct neural network architectures tend to learn different features. Another study [50] visualized the convolutional neural network (CNN) features for skin lesion classification. The features for the last two layers were visualized by rescaling the feature maps of the activations to the input size. The layers were observed to be looking at indicators like lesion borders and non-uniformity in color as well as risk factors like lighter skin color or pink texture. However, spurious features like artifacts and hair which have no significance were also learned indicating some extent of overfitting.

There are other studies using attribution based methods for diagnosis in addition to the more common imaging modalities discussed above. For example, a study performed uncertainty and interpretability analysis on CNNs for semantic segmentation of colorectal polyps, a precursor of rectal cancers [51]. Using GBP for heatmaps the convolutional neural network (CNN)s were found to be utilizing the edge and shape information to make predictions. Moreover, the uncertainty analysis revealed higher uncertainty in misclassified samples. There is plenty of opportunity for applying the explainability of deep learning methods to other modalities like laparoscopy and endoscopy e.g., [52]. An explainable model using SHapley Additive exPlanations (SHAP) attributions for hypoxemia, i.e., low blood oxygen tension prediction during surgery was presented in [53]. The study was performed for analyzing preoperative factors as well as in-surgery parameters. The resulting attributions were in line with known factors like BMI, physical status (ASA), tidal volume, inspired oxygen, etc.

The attribution based methods were one of the initial ways of visualizing neural networks and have since then evolved from simple class activation map and gradient-based methods to advanced techniques like Deep SHapley Additive exPlanations (SHAP). The better visualizations of these methods show that the models were learning relevant features in most of the cases. Any presence of spurious features was scrutinized, flagged to the readers, and brought adjustments to the model training methods. Smaller and task-specific models like [39] along with custom variants of the attribution methods can improve the identification of relevant features.

4.2. Non-Attribution Based

The studies discussed in this subsection approached the problem of explainability by developing a methodology and validating it on a given problem rather than performing a separate analysis using pre-existing attributions based methods like those previously discussed. These used approaches like attention maps, concept vectors, returning a similar image, text justifications, expert knowledge, generative modeling, combination with other machine learning methods, etc. It must be noted that the majority of these are still post-model but their implementation usually needs specific changes to the model structure such as in the attention maps or the addition of expert knowledge in case of rule-based methods. In this section, the studies are grouped by the explainability approach they took. Figure 5 shows a schematic of these methods according to the taxonomy discussed in Section 2. These are characterized in a hierarchical way using multiple taxonomies for a finer classification.

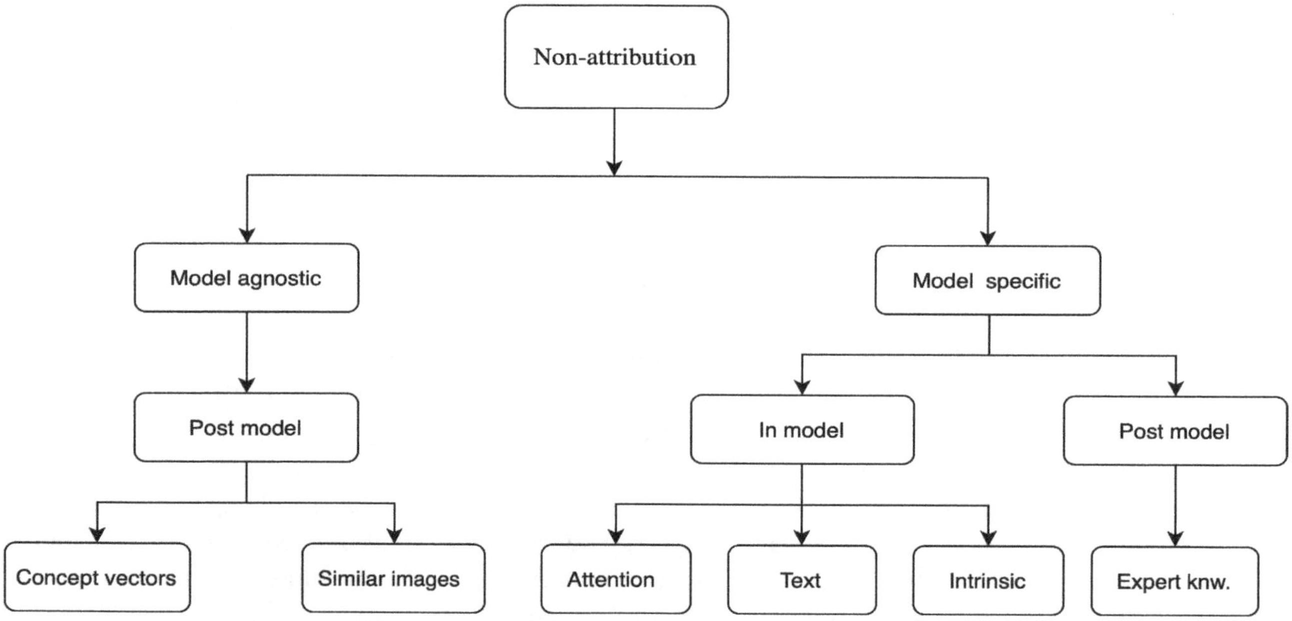

Figure 5. Classification of explainability methods that are not attribution based.

4.2.1. Attention Based

Attention is a popular and useful concept in deep learning. The basic idea of attention is inspired by the way humans pay attention to different parts of an image or other data sources to analyze them. More details about attention mechanisms in neural networks are discussed in [54]. An example of attention in medical diagnosis is given in [55]. Here, we discuss how attention-based methods can be used as an explainable deep learning tool for medical image analysis.

A network called MDNet was proposed [56] to perform a direct mapping between medical images and corresponding diagnostic reports. With an image model and a language model in it, the method used attention mechanisms to visualize the detection process. Using that attention mechanism, the language model found predominant and discriminatory features to learn the mapping between images and the diagnostic reports. This was the first work that exploited the attention mechanism to get insightful information from medical image dataset.

In [57] an interpretable version of U-Net [58] called SAUNet was proposed. It added a parallel secondary shape stream to capture important shape-based information along with the regular texture features of the images. The architecture used an attention module in the decoder part of the U-Net. The spatial and shape attention maps were generated using SmoothGrad to visualize the high activation region of the images.

4.2.2. Concept Vectors

A novel method called TCAV was proposed in [59] to explain the features learned by different layers to the domain experts without any deep learning expertise in terms of human-understandable concepts. It took the directional derivative of the network in the concept space much like that in the input feature space for saliency maps. It was tested to explain the predictions of diabetic retinopathy (DR) levels where it successfully detected the presence of microaneurysms and aneurysms in the retina. This provided justifications that were readily interpretable for the medical practitioners in terms of presence or absence of a given concept or physical structure in the image. However, many clinical concepts like the texture or the shape of a structure cannot be sufficiently described in terms of the presence or absence and need a continuous scale of measurement.

An extension of TCAV, which used the presence or absence of concepts, using Regression Concept Vectors (RCV) in the activation space of a layer was used to detect continuous concepts [60]. The task of the network was to detect tumors from breast lymph node samples. It was found that most of the relevant features like area and contrast were present in the early layers of the model. A further improvement over the TCAV used a new metric called Uniform unit Ball surface Sampling (UBS) [61] to provide layer-agnostic explanations for continuous and high dimensional features. It could explain high dimensional radiomics concepts across multiple layers which were validated using mammographic images. The model produced variations amongst the important concepts which were found to be lower across the layers of the SqueezeNet [62] compared to a baseline CNN with 3 dense layers explaining the better performance of the SqueezeNet.

4.2.3. Expert Knowledge

A vast majority of the research discussed in this review tried to correlate model features with expert knowledge using different approaches. Another approach was to use domain-specific knowledge to craft rules for prediction and explanation. An example of using task-specific knowledge to improve the results as well as the explanations were provided in [63] for brain midline shift (MLS) estimation using U-Net [58] based architecture and keypoints. It was reduced to the problem of detecting a midline using the model under domain constraints. The original midline was obtained using the endpoints and hence the shift from the predicted one was computed. The model also provided confidence intervals of the predictions making them more trustworthy for the end-user. Another study [64] used guidelines for rule-based segmentation of lung nodules followed by a perturbation analysis to compute the importance of features in each region. The explanations provided in terms of the regions already marked using rules were found to be more understandable for the users and showed the bias in data for improving the model. This method was then used to provide explanations at a global level for the entire dataset providing an overview of the relevant features.

4.2.4. Similar Images

Some studies provided similarly labeled images to the user as a reason for making a prediction for a given test image. A study [6] proposed analysis of layers of a 3D-convolutional neural network (CNN) using Gaussian mixture model (GMM) and binary encoding of training and test images based on their Gaussian mixture model (GMM) components for returning similar 3D images as explanations. The system returned activation wise similar training images using atlas as a clarification for its decision. It was demonstrated on 3D MNIST and an MRI dataset where it returned images with similar atrophy conditions. However, it was found that the activation similarity depended on the spatial orientation of images in certain cases which could affect the choice of the returned images.

In a study on dermoscopic images, a triplet-loss and k nearest neighbors (kNN) search-based learning strategy was used to learn convolutional neural network (CNN) feature embeddings for interpretable classification [65]. The evidence was provided as nearest neighbors and local image regions responsible for the lowest distance between the test image and those neighbors. Another approach used monotonic constraints to explain the predictions in terms of style and depth two datasets—dermoscopy images and post-surgical breast aesthetics [66]. It concatenated input streams with constrained monotonic convolutional neural network (CNN) and unconstrained convolutional neural network (CNN) to produce the predictions along with their explanations in terms of similar images as well as complementary images. The system was designed for only binary classification.

4.2.5. Textual Justification

A model that can explain its decision in terms of sentences or phrases giving the reasoning can directly communicate with both expert and general users. A justification model that took inputs from the visual features of a classifier, as well as embeddings of the predictions, was used to generate a diagnostic sentence and visual heatmaps for breast mass classification [67]. A visual word constraint loss was applied in the training of the justification generator to produce justifications in the presence of only a limited number of medical reports. Such multimodal explanations can be used to obtain greater user confidence due to a similarity with the usual workflow and learning process.

4.2.6. Intrinsic Explainability

Intrinsic explainability refers to the ability of a model to explain its decisions in terms of human observable decision boundaries or features. These usually include relatively simpler models like regression, decision trees, and support vector machines (SVM) for a few dimensions where the decision boundaries can be observed. Recent studies to make deep learning model intrinsically explainable using different methods such as a hybrid with machine learning classifiers and visualizing the features in a segmentation space.

An example of the latter was presented in [68] using the latent space of the features of a variational autoencoder for classification and segmentation of the brain MRI of Alzheimer's patients. The classification was performed in a two-dimensional latent space using an multi layer perceptron (MLP). The segmentation was performed in a three-dimensional latent space in terms of the anatomical variability encoded in the discriminating features. This led to the visualization of the features of the classifier as global and local anatomical characteristics which were usually used for clinical decisions. A study for detection of autism pectrum disorder (ASD) from functional magnetic resonance imaging (fMRI) used a hybrid of deep learning and support vector machines (SVM) to perform explainable classification [69]. The support vector machines (SVM) was used as a classifier on the features of a deep learning model and the visualization of the decision boundary explained the model.

This subsection discussed a variety of non-attribution explainability methods but the list is not exhaustive as newer methods are published frequently due to high interest in the area. The design of these methods is more involved than the application of attribution based methods on the inputs of a trained model. Specific elements like concept vectors, expert-based rules, image retrieval methods need to be integrated often at a model training level. This added complexity can potentially provide more domain-specific explanations at the expense of higher design effort. Notably, a majority of these techniques are still a post-hoc step but for a specific architecture or domain. Moreover, we have limited our scope to medical imaging as that is the dominant approach for automated diagnosis because of the detailed information presented by the images. However, patient records also provide rich information for diagnosis and there were studies discussing their explainability. For example, in [70] a gated recurrent unit (GRU)-based recurrent neural network (RNN) for mortality prediction from diagnostic codes from electronic healthcare record (EHR) was presented. It used hierarchical attention in the network for interpretability and visualization of the results.

Table 2. Applications of explainability in medical imaging.

Method	Algorithm	Model	Application	Modality
Attribution	Gradient*I/P, GBP, LRP, occlusion [36]	3D CNN	Alzheimer's detection	Brain MRI
	GradCAM, GBP [37]	Custom CNN	Grading brain tumor	Brain MRI
	IG [38]	Inception-v4	DR grading	Fundus images
	EG [39]	Custom CNN	Lesion segmentation for AMD	Retinal OCT
	IG, SmoothGrad [41]	AlexNet	Estrogen receptor status	Breast MRI
	Saliency maps [42]	AlexNet	Breast mass classification	Breast MRI
	GradCAM, SHAP [49]	Inception	Melanoma detection	Skin images
	Activation maps [50]	Custom CNN	Lesion classification	Skin images
	DeepDreams [46]	Custom CNN	Segmentation of tumor from liver	CT imaging
	GSInquire, GBP, activation maps [47]	COVIDNet CNN	COVID-19 detection	X-ray images
Attention	Mapping between image to reports [56]	CNN & LSTM	Bladder cancer	Tissue images
	U-Net with shape attention stream [57]	U-net based	Cardiac volume estimation	Cardiac MRI
Concept vectors	TCAV [59]	Inception	DR detection	Fundus images
	TCAV with RCV [60]	ResNet101	Breast tumor detection	Breast lymph node images
	UBS [61]	SqueezeNet	Breast mass classification	Mammography images
Expert knowledge	Domain constraints [63]	U-net	Brain MLS estimation	Brain MRI
	Rule-based segmentation, perturbation [64]	VGG16	Lung nodule segmentation	Lung CT
Similar images	GMM and atlas [6]	3D CNN	MRI classification	3D MNIST, Brain MRI
	Triplet loss, kNN [65]	AlexNet based with shared weights	Melanoma	Dermoscopy images
	Monotonic constraints [66]	DNN with two streams	Melanoma detection	Dermoscopy images
Textual justification	LSTM, visual word constraint [67]	Breast mass classification	CNN	Mammography images
Intrinsic explainability	Deep Hierarchical Generative Models [68]	Auto-encoders	Classification and segmentation for Alzheimer's	Brain MRI
	SVM margin [69]	Hybrid of CNN & SVM	ASD detection	Brain fMRI

5. Discussion

There has been significant progress in explaining the decisions of deep learning models, especially those used for medical diagnosis. Understanding the features responsible for a certain decision is useful for the model designers to iron out reliability concerns for the end-users to gain trust and make better judgments. Almost all of these methods target local explainability, i.e., explaining the decisions for a single example. This then is extrapolated to a global level by averaging the highlighted features, especially in cases where the images have the same spatial orientation. However, emerging methods like concept vectors (Section 4.2.2) provide a more global view of the decisions for each class in terms of domain concepts.

It is important to analyze the features of a black-box which can make the right decision due to the wrong reason. It is a major issue that can affect performance when the system is deployed in the real world. Most of the methods, especially the attribution based are available as open-source implementations. However, some methods like GSInquire [48] which show higher performance on some metrics are proprietary. There is an increasing commercial interest in explainability, and specifically the attribution methods which can be leveraged for a variety of business use cases.

The explainability methods have two different but overlapping objectives for the two different user groups. Deep learning practitioners can use them to design better systems by analyzing the model features and understanding the interactions between the model and the data. The clinical end-users can be provided with the explanations as a reasoning for the model decision and hence build confidence and trust in the model decision and also help identify potentially questionable decisions. A recent study compared the understanding of explanations amongst data scientists [71]. In this study common issues like missing data and redundant features were introduced and the data scientists were provided explanations of the trained models in order to identify the problems. The study reported over trust on the models as they tried to justify the issues as meaningful features. This is contrary to lower trust and acceptance from end-users who are wary of the black-box nature. It is notable that the experienced data scientists were able to use them effectively for understanding model and data issues.

Studies analyzing the effect of explanations on the decisions of the clinical end-users show in general positive outcomes [38]. There are studies comparing explainability methods quantitatively [36,39] which are discussed previously. The quantitative analysis focuses on theoretical correctness and robustness while missing out on actual clinical usefulness. There is a pertinent need to perform end-user based qualitative comparison of explanations for medical imaging applications. This can help to identify the most relevant techniques for explaining decisions to the clinicians. Such studies can be performed using expert agreement where a panel of experts can be asked to rate the explanations. A similar approach was used for deep learning based methods in [72] and for clinical diagnosis in [73]. We are currently working on a quantitative and qualitative analysis of various XAI methods in the diagnosis of retinal disease. The explanations will have quantitative comparisons along with qualitative evaluation by expert clinicians rating the explanations. This would also help to evaluate the overlap between the clinical knowledge acquired through clinical training and experience and the model features acquired for the pattern recognition task for a given dataset.

Studies have extended existing explainability methods to better suit the challenges of the medical imaging domain. For example, [39] proposed Expressive gradients (EG), an extension of commonly used IG to cover the retinal lesions better while [60] extended concept vectors from [59] for continuous concepts like texture and shape. Such studies lead to the advancement of the explainability domain and provided customization without designing new methods from scratch. Despite all these advances, there is still a need to make the explainability methods more holistic and interwoven with uncertainty methods. Expert feedback must be incorporated into the design of such explainability methods to tailor the feedback for their needs. Initially, any clinical application of such explainable deep learning methods is likely to be a human-in-the-loop (HITL) hybrid keeping the clinical expert in the control of the process. It can be considered analogous to driving aids like adaptive cruise control or lane keep assistance in cars where the driver is still in control and responsible for the final decisions but with a reduced workload and an added safety net.

Another direction of work can be to use multiple modalities like medical images and patients' records together in the decision-making process and attribute the model decisions to each of them. This can simulate the diagnostic workflow of a clinician where both images and physical parameters of a patient are used to make a decision. This can potentially improve accuracy as well as explain the phenomena more comprehensively. To sum up, explainable diagnosis is making convincing strides but there is still some way to go to meet the expectations of end-users, regulators, and the general public.

Acronyms

AI	artificial intelligence
AMD	Age-related macular degeneration
ASD	autism pectrum disorder
CAD	Computer-aided diagnostics
CAM	Class activation maps
CNN	convolutional neural network
CNV	choroidal neovascularization
CT	computerized tomography
DME	diabetic macular edema
DNN	deep neural networks
DR	diabetic retinopathy
EG	Expressive gradients
EHR	electronic healthcare record
fMRI	functional magnetic resonance imaging
GBP	Guided backpropagation
GDPR	General Data Protection Regulation
GMM	Gaussian mixture model
GradCAM	Gradient weighted class activation mapping
GRU	gated recurrent unit
HITL	human-in-the-loop
IG	Integrated gradients
kNN	k nearest neighbors
LIFT	Deep Learning Important FeaTures
LRP	Layer wise relevance propagation
MLP	multi layer perceptron
MLS	midline shift
MRI	magnetic resonance imaging
OCT	optical coherence tomography
PCC	Pearson's correlation coefficient
RCV	Regression Concept Vectors
ReLU	rectified linear unit
RNN	recurrent neural network
SHAP	SHapley Additive exPlanations
SVM	support vector machines
TCAV	Testing Concept Activation Vectors
UBS	Uniform unit Ball surface Sampling

References

1. Jo, T.; Nho, K.; Saykin, A.J. Deep learning in Alzheimer's disease: Diagnostic classification and prognostic prediction using neuroimaging data. *Front. Aging Neurosci.* **2019**, *11*, 220. [CrossRef]
2. Hua, K.L.; Hsu, C.H.; Hidayati, S.C.; Cheng, W.H.; Chen, Y.J. Computer-aided classification of lung nodules on computed tomography images via deep learning technique. *OncoTargets Ther.* **2015**, *8*, 2015–2022.

3. Sengupta, S.; Singh, A.; Leopold, H.A.; Gulati, T.; Lakshminarayanan, V. Ophthalmic diagnosis using deep learning with fundus images–A critical review. *Artif. Intell. Med.* **2020**, *102*, 101758. [CrossRef] [PubMed]
4. Leopold, H.; Singh, A.; Sengupta, S.; Zelek, J.; Lakshminarayanan, V., Recent Advances in Deep Learning Applications for Retinal Diagnosis using OCT. In *State of the Art in Neural Networks*; El-Baz, A.S., Ed.; Elsevier: New York, NY, USA, 2020; in press.
5. Holzinger, A.; Biemann, C.; Pattichis, C.S.; Kell, D.B. What do we need to build explainable AI systems for the medical domain? *arXiv* **2017**, arXiv:1712.09923.
6. Stano, M.; Benesova, W.; Martak, L.S. Explainable 3D convolutional neural network using GMM encoding. In Proceedings of the Twelfth International Conference on Machine Vision, Amsterdam, The Netherlands, 16–18 November 2019; Volume 11433, p. 114331U.
7. Moccia, S.; Wirkert, S.J.; Kenngott, H.; Vemuri, A.S.; Apitz, M.; Mayer, B.; De Momi, E.; Mattos, L.S.; Maier-Hein, L. Uncertainty-aware organ classification for surgical data science applications in laparoscopy. *IEEE Trans. Biomed. Eng.* **2018**, *65*, 2649–2659. [CrossRef] [PubMed]
8. Adler, T.J.; Ardizzone, L.; Vemuri, A.; Ayala, L.; Gröhl, J.; Kirchner, T.; Wirkert, S.; Kruse, J.; Rother, C.; Köthe, U.; et al. Uncertainty-aware performance assessment of optical imaging modalities with invertible neural networks. *Int. J. Comput. Assist. Radiol. Surg.* **2019**, *14*, 997–1007. [CrossRef]
9. Meyes, R.; de Puiseau, C.W.; Posada-Moreno, A.; Meisen, T. Under the Hood of Neural Networks: Characterizing Learned Representations by Functional Neuron Populations and Network Ablations. *arXiv* **2020**, arXiv:2004.01254.
10. Arrieta, A.B.; Díaz-Rodríguez, N.; Del Ser, J.; Bennetot, A.; Tabik, S.; Barbado, A.; García, S.; Gil-López, S.; Molina, D.; Benjamins, R.; et al. Explainable Artificial Intelligence (XAI): Concepts, taxonomies, opportunities and challenges toward responsible AI. *Inf. Fusion* **2020**, *58*, 82–115. [CrossRef]
11. Stiglic, G.; Kocbek, P.; Fijacko, N.; Zitnik, M.; Verbert, K.; Cilar, L. Interpretability of machine learning based prediction models in healthcare. *arXiv* **2020**, arXiv:2002.08596.
12. Arya, V.; Bellamy, R.K.; Chen, P.Y.; Dhurandhar, A.; Hind, M.; Hoffman, S.C.; Houde, S.; Liao, Q.V.; Luss, R.; Mojsilović, A.; et al. One explanation does not fit all: A toolkit and taxonomy of ai explainability techniques. *arXiv* **2019**, arXiv:1909.03012.
13. Ying, Z.; Bourgeois, D.; You, J.; Zitnik, M.; Leskovec, J. Gnnexplainer: Generating explanations for graph neural networks. In Proceedings of the Advances in Neural Information Processing Systems 32, Vancouver, BC, Canada, 8–14 December 2019; Volume 32, pp. 9240–9251.
14. Wold, S.; Esbensen, K.; Geladi, P. Principal component analysis. *Chemom. Intell. Lab. Syst.* **1987**, *2*, 37–52. [CrossRef]
15. Maaten, L.V.D.; Hinton, G. Visualizing data using t-SNE. *J. Mach. Learn. Res.* **2008**, *9*, 2579–2605.
16. Safavian, S.R.; Landgrebe, D. A survey of decision tree classifier methodology. *IEEE Trans. Syst. Man Cybern.* **1991**, *21*, 660–674. [CrossRef]
17. Montavon, G.; Lapuschkin, S.; Binder, A.; Samek, W.; Müller, K.R. Explaining nonlinear classification decisions with deep taylor decomposition. *Pattern Recognit.* **2017**, *65*, 211–222. [CrossRef]
18. Ancona, M.; Ceolini, E.; Öztireli, C.; Gross, M. Towards better understanding of gradient-based attribution methods for deep neural networks. *arXiv* **2017**, arXiv:1711.06104.
19. Alber, M.; Lapuschkin, S.; Seegerer, P.; Hägele, M.; Schütt, K.T.; Montavon, G.; Samek, W.; Müller, K.R.; Dähne, S.; Kindermans, P.J. iNNvestigate neural networks. *J. Mach. Learn. Res.* **2019**, *20*, 1–8.
20. Zeiler, M.D.; Fergus, R. Visualizing and understanding convolutional networks. In Proceedings of the European Conference on Computer Vision, Zurich, Switzerland, 6–12 September 2014; Springer: Cham, Switzerland; pp. 818–833.
21. Goodfellow, I.J.; Shlens, J.; Szegedy, C. Explaining and harnessing adversarial examples. *arXiv* **2014**, arXiv:1412.6572.
22. Lipovetsky, S.; Conklin, M. Analysis of regression in game theory approach. *Appl. Stoch. Model. Bus. Ind.* **2001**, *17*, 319–330. [CrossRef]
23. Simonyan, K.; Vedaldi, A.; Zisserman, A. Deep inside convolutional networks: Visualising image classification models and saliency maps. *arXiv* **2013**, arXiv:1312.6034.
24. Springenberg, J.T.; Dosovitskiy, A.; Brox, T.; Riedmiller, M. Striving for simplicity: The all convolutional net. *arXiv* **2014**, arXiv:1412.6806.

25. Bach, S.; Binder, A.; Montavon, G.; Klauschen, F.; Müller, K.R.; Samek, W. On pixel-wise explanations for non-linear classifier decisions by layer-wise relevance propagation. *PLoS ONE* **2015**, *10*. [CrossRef] [PubMed]
26. Shrikumar, A.; Greenside, P.; Shcherbina, A.; Kundaje, A. Not just a black box: Learning important features through propagating activation differences. *arXiv* **2016**, arXiv:1605.01713.
27. Selvaraju, R.R.; Cogswell, M.; Das, A.; Vedantam, R.; Parikh, D.; Batra, D. Grad-cam: Visual explanations from deep networks via gradient-based localization. In Proceedings of the IEEE International Conference on Computer Vision, Venice, Italy, 22–29 October 2017; pp. 618–626. [CrossRef]
28. Sundararajan, M.; Taly, A.; Yan, Q. Axiomatic attribution for deep networks. In Proceedings of the 34th International Conference on Machine Learning, Sydney, Australia, 6–11 August 2017; Voume 70, pp. 3319–3328.
29. Kindermans, P.J.; Schütt, K.T.; Alber, M.; Müller, K.R.; Erhan, D.; Kim, B.; Dähne, S. Learning how to explain neural networks: Patternnet and patternattribution. *arXiv* **2017**, arXiv:1705.05598.
30. Shrikumar, A.; Greenside, P.; Kundaje, A. Learning important features through propagating activation differences. In Proceedings of the 34th International Conference on Machine Learning, Sydney, Australia, 6–11 August 2017; Voume 70, pp. 3145–3153.
31. Smilkov, D.; Thorat, N.; Kim, B.; Viégas, F.; Wattenberg, M. Smoothgrad: Removing noise by adding noise. *arXiv* **2017**, arXiv:1706.03825.
32. Chen, H.; Lundberg, S.; Lee, S.I. Explaining Models by Propagating Shapley Values of Local Components. *arXiv* **2019**, arXiv:1911.11888.
33. Yosinski, J.; Clune, J.; Bengio, Y.; Lipson, H. How transferable are features in deep neural networks? In Proceedings of the Advances in Neural Information Processing Systems, Montreal, QC, USA, 8–13 December 2014; pp. 3320–3328.
34. Singh, A.; Sengupta, S.; Lakshminarayanan, V. Glaucoma diagnosis using transfer learning methods. In *Proceedings of the Applications of Machine Learning*; International Society for Optics and Photonics (SPIE): Bellingham, WA, USA, 2019; Volume 11139, p. 111390U.
35. Deng, J.; Dong, W.; Socher, R.; Li, L.J.; Li, K.; Fei-Fei, L. Imagenet: A large-scale hierarchical image database. In Proceedings of the 2009 IEEE Conference on Computer Vision and Pattern Recognition, Miami, FL, USA, 20–25 June 2009; pp. 248–255.
36. Eitel, F.; Ritter, K.; Alzheimer's Disease Neuroimaging Initiative (ADNI). Testing the Robustness of Attribution Methods for Convolutional Neural Networks in MRI-Based Alzheimer's Disease Classification. In *Interpretability of Machine Intelligence in Medical Image Computing and Multimodal Learning for Clinical Decision Support, ML-CDS 2019, IMIMIC 2019*; Lecture Notes in Computer Science; Suzuki, K., et al., Eds.; Springer: Cham, Switzerland, 2019; Volume 11797. [CrossRef]
37. Pereira, S.; Meier, R.; Alves, V.; Reyes, M.; Silva, C.A. Automatic brain tumor grading from MRI data using convolutional neural networks and quality assessment. In *Understanding and Interpreting Machine Learning in Medical Image Computing Applications*; Springer: Cham, Switzerland, 2018; pp. 106–114.
38. Sayres, R.; Taly, A.; Rahimy, E.; Blumer, K.; Coz, D.; Hammel, N.; Krause, J.; Narayanaswamy, A.; Rastegar, Z.; Wu, D.; et al. Using a deep learning algorithm and integrated gradients explanation to assist grading for diabetic retinopathy. *Ophthalmology* **2019**, *126*, 552–564. [CrossRef]
39. Yang, H.L.; Kim, J.J.; Kim, J.H.; Kang, Y.K.; Park, D.H.; Park, H.S.; Kim, H.K.; Kim, M.S. Weakly supervised lesion localization for age-related macular degeneration detection using optical coherence tomography images. *PLoS ONE* **2019**, *14*, e0215076. [CrossRef]
40. Singh, A.; Sengupta, S.; Lakshminarayanan, V. Interpretation of deep learning using attributions: Application to ophthalmic diagnosis. In *Proceedings of the Applications of Machine Learning*; International Society for Optics and Photonics (SPIE): Bellingham, WA, USA, 2020; in press.
41. Papanastasopoulos, Z.; Samala, R.K.; Chan, H.P.; Hadjiiski, L.; Paramagul, C.; Helvie, M.A.; Neal, C.H. Explainable AI for medical imaging: Deep-learning CNN ensemble for classification of estrogen receptor status from breast MRI. In *Proceedings of the SPIE Medical Imaging 2020: Computer-Aided Diagnosis*; International Society for Optics and Photonics: Bellingham, WA, USA, 2020; Volume 11314, p. 113140Z.
42. Lévy, D.; Jain, A. Breast mass classification from mammograms using deep convolutional neural networks. *arXiv* **2016**, arXiv:1612.00542.

43. Szegedy, C.; Liu, W.; Jia, Y.; Sermanet, P.; Reed, S.; Anguelov, D.; Erhan, D.; Vanhoucke, V.; Rabinovich, A. Going deeper with convolutions. In Proceedings of the 2015 IEEE Conference on Computer Vision and Pattern Recognition (CVPR), Boston, MA, USA, 7–12 June 2015; pp. 1–9.
44. Krizhevsky, A.; Sutskever, I.; Hinton, G.E. Imagenet classification with deep convolutional neural networks. In Proceedings of the Advances in Neural Information Processing Systems, Lake Tahoe, NV, USA, 3–6 December 2012; pp. 1097–1105.
45. Mordvintsev, A.; Olah, C.; Tyka, M. Inceptionism: Going Deeper into Neural Networks. Google AI Blog. 2015. Available online: https://ai.googleblog.com/2015/06/inceptionism-going-deeper-into-neural.html (accessed on 23 May 2020)
46. Couteaux, V.; Nempont, O.; Pizaine, G.; Bloch, I. Towards Interpretability of Segmentation Networks by Analyzing DeepDreams. In *Interpretability of Machine Intelligence in Medical Image Computing and Multimodal Learning for Clinical Decision Support*; Springer: Cham, Switzerland, 2019; pp. 56–63.
47. Wang, L.; Wong, A. COVID-Net: A tailored deep convolutional neural network design for detection of COVID-19 cases from chest radiography images. *arXiv* **2020**, arXiv:2003.09871.
48. Lin, Z.Q.; Shafiee, M.J.; Bochkarev, S.; Jules, M.S.; Wang, X.Y.; Wong, A. Explaining with Impact: A Machine-centric Strategy to Quantify the Performance of Explainability Algorithms. *arXiv* **2019**, arXiv:1910.07387.
49. Young, K.; Booth, G.; Simpson, B.; Dutton, R.; Shrapnel, S. Deep neural network or dermatologist? In *Interpretability of Machine Intelligence in Medical Image Computing and Multimodal Learning for Clinical Decision Support*; Springer: Cham, Switzerland, 2019; pp. 48–55.
50. Van Molle, P.; De Strooper, M.; Verbelen, T.; Vankeirsbilck, B.; Simoens, P.; Dhoedt, B. Visualizing convolutional neural networks to improve decision support for skin lesion classification. In *Understanding and Interpreting Machine Learning in Medical Image Computing Applications*; Springer: Cham, Switzerland, 2018; pp. 115–123.
51. Wickstrøm, K.; Kampffmeyer, M.; Jenssen, R. Uncertainty and interpretability in convolutional neural networks for semantic segmentation of colorectal polyps. *Med Image Anal.* **2020**, *60*, 101619. [CrossRef] [PubMed]
52. Moccia, S.; De Momi, E.; Guarnaschelli, M.; Savazzi, M.; Laborai, A.; Guastini, L.; Peretti, G.; Mattos, L.S. Confident texture-based laryngeal tissue classification for early stage diagnosis support. *J. Med Imaging* **2017**, *4*, 034502. [CrossRef] [PubMed]
53. Lundberg, S.M.; Nair, B.; Vavilala, M.S.; Horibe, M.; Eisses, M.J.; Adams, T.; Liston, D.E.; Low, D.K.W.; Newman, S.F.; Kim, J.; et al. Explainable machine-learning predictions for the prevention of hypoxaemia during surgery. *Nat. Biomed. Eng.* **2018**, *2*, 749–760. [CrossRef]
54. Vaswani, A.; Shazeer, N.; Parmar, N.; Uszkoreit, J.; Jones, L.; Gomez, A.N.; Kaiser, Ł.; Polosukhin, I. Attention is all you need. In Proceedings of the Advances in Neural Information Processing Systems, Long Beach, CA, USA, 4–9 December 2017; pp. 5998–6008.
55. Bamba, U.; Pandey, D.; Lakshminarayanan, V. Classification of brain lesions from MRI images using a novel neural network. In *Multimodal Biomedical Imaging XV*; International Society for Optics and Photonics: Bellingham, WA, USA, 2020; Volume 11232, p. 112320K.
56. Zhang, Z.; Xie, Y.; Xing, F.; McGough, M.; Yang, L. Mdnet: A semantically and visually interpretable medical image diagnosis network. In Proceedings of the IEEE Conference on Computer Vision and Pattern Recognition, Honolulu, HI, USA, 21–26 July 2017; pp. 6428–6436.
57. Sun, J.; Darbeha, F.; Zaidi, M.; Wang, B. SAUNet: Shape Attentive U-Net for Interpretable Medical Image Segmentation. *arXiv* **2020**, arXiv:2001.07645.
58. Ronneberger, O.; Fischer, P.; Brox, T. U-net: Convolutional networks for biomedical image segmentation. In Proceedings of the International Conference on Medical Image Computing and Computer-Assisted Intervention, Munich, Germany, 5–9 October 2015; Springer: Cham, Switzerland; pp. 234–241.
59. Kim, B.; Wattenberg, M.; Gilmer, J.; Cai, C.; Wexler, J.; Viegas, F.; Sayres, R. Interpretability beyond feature attribution: Quantitative testing with concept activation vectors (tcav). *arXiv* **2017**, arXiv:1711.11279.
60. Graziani, M.; Andrearczyk, V.; Müller, H. Regression concept vectors for bidirectional explanations in histopathology. In *Understanding and Interpreting Machine Learning in Medical Image Computing Applications*; Springer: Cham, Switzerland, 2018; pp. 124–132.
61. Yeche, H.; Harrison, J.; Berthier, T. UBS: A Dimension-Agnostic Metric for Concept Vector Interpretability

Applied to Radiomics. In *Interpretability of Machine Intelligence in Medical Image Computing and Multimodal Learning for Clinical Decision Support*; Springer: Cham, Switzerland, 2019; pp. 12–20.

62. Iandola, F.N.; Han, S.; Moskewicz, M.W.; Ashraf, K.; Dally, W.J.; Keutzer, K. SqueezeNet: AlexNet-level accuracy with 50x fewer parameters and <0.5 MB model size. *arXiv* **2016**, arXiv:1602.07360.
63. Pisov, M.; Goncharov, M.; Kurochkina, N.; Morozov, S.; Gombolevsky, V.; Chernina, V.; Vladzymyrskyy, A.; Zamyatina, K.; Cheskova, A.; Pronin, I.; et al. Incorporating Task-Specific Structural Knowledge into CNNs for Brain Midline Shift Detection. In *Interpretability of Machine Intelligence in Medical Image Computing and Multimodal Learning for Clinical Decision Support*; Springer: Cham, Switzerland, 2019; pp. 30–38.
64. Zhu, P.; Ogino, M. Guideline-Based Additive Explanation for Computer-Aided Diagnosis of Lung Nodules. In *Interpretability of Machine Intelligence in Medical Image Computing and Multimodal Learning for Clinical Decision Support*; Springer: Cham, Switzerland, 2019; pp. 39–47.
65. Codella, N.C.; Lin, C.C.; Halpern, A.; Hind, M.; Feris, R.; Smith, J.R. Collaborative Human-AI (CHAI): Evidence-based interpretable melanoma classification in dermoscopic images. In *Understanding and Interpreting Machine Learning in Medical Image Computing Applications*; Springer: Cham, Switzerland, 2018; pp. 97–105.
66. Silva, W.; Fernandes, K.; Cardoso, M.J.; Cardoso, J.S. Towards complementary explanations using deep neural networks. In *Understanding and Interpreting Machine Learning in Medical Image Computing Applications*; Springer: Cham, Switzerland, 2018; pp. 133–140.
67. Lee, H.; Kim, S.T.; Ro, Y.M. Generation of Multimodal Justification Using Visual Word Constraint Model for Explainable Computer-Aided Diagnosis. In *Interpretability of Machine Intelligence in Medical Image Computing and Multimodal Learning for Clinical Decision Support*; Springer: Cham, Switzerland, 2019; pp. 21–29.
68. Biffi, C.; Cerrolaza, J.J.; Tarroni, G.; Bai, W.; De Marvao, A.; Oktay, O.; Ledig, C.; Le Folgoc, L.; Kamnitsas, K.; Doumou, G.; et al. Explainable Anatomical Shape Analysis through Deep Hierarchical Generative Models. *IEEE Trans. Med. Imaging* **2020**. [CrossRef]
69. Eslami, T.; Raiker, J.S.; Saeed, F. Explainable and Scalable Machine-Learning Algorithms for Detection of Autism Spectrum Disorder using fMRI Data. *arXiv* **2020**, arXiv:2003.01541.
70. Sha, Y.; Wang, M.D. Interpretable predictions of clinical outcomes with an attention-based recurrent neural network. In Proceedings of the 8th ACM International Conference on Bioinformatics, Computational Biology, and Health Informatics, Boston, MA, USA, 20–23 August 2017; pp. 233–240.
71. Kaur, H.; Nori, H.; Jenkins, S.; Caruana, R.; Wallach, H.; Wortman Vaughan, J. Interpreting Interpretability: Understanding Data Scientists' Use of Interpretability Tools for Machine Learning. In Proceedings of the CHI Conference on Human Factors in Computing Systems, Honolulu, HI, USA, 25–30 April 2020; pp. 1–14. [CrossRef]
72. Arbabshirani, M.R.; Fornwalt, B.K.; Mongelluzzo, G.J.; Suever, J.D.; Geise, B.D.; Patel, A.A.; Moore, G.J. Advanced machine learning in action: Identification of intracranial hemorrhage on computed tomography scans of the head with clinical workflow integration. *NPJ Digit. Med.* **2018**, *1*, 1–7. [CrossRef]
73. Almazroa, A.; Alodhayb, S.; Osman, E.; Ramadan, E.; Hummadi, M.; Dlaim, M.; Alkatee, M.; Raahemifar, K.; Lakshminarayanan, V. Agreement among ophthalmologists in marking the optic disc and optic cup in fundus images. *Int. Ophthalmol.* **2017**, *37*, 701–717. [CrossRef]

6

An Efficient Lightweight CNN and Ensemble Machine Learning Classification of Prostate Tissue using Multilevel Feature Analysis

Subrata Bhattacharjee [1], Cho-Hee Kim [2], Deekshitha Prakash [1], Hyeon-Gyun Park [1], Nam-Hoon Cho [3] and Heung-Kook Choi [1,*]

1 Department of Computer Engineering, u-AHRC, Inje University, Gimhae 50834, Korea; subrata_bhattacharjee@outlook.com (S.B.); deeskhithadp96@gmail.com (D.P.); gusrbs82@gmail.com (H.-G.P.)
2 Department of Digital Anti-Aging Healthcare, Inje University, Gimhae 50834, Korea; chgmlrla0917@naver.com
3 Department of Pathology, Yonsei University Hospital, Seoul 03722, Korea; cho1988@yumc.yonsei.ac.kr
* Correspondence: cschk@inje.ac.kr;

Abstract: Prostate carcinoma is caused when cells and glands in the prostate change their shape and size from normal to abnormal. Typically, the pathologist's goal is to classify the staining slides and differentiate normal from abnormal tissue. In the present study, we used a computational approach to classify images and features of benign and malignant tissues using artificial intelligence (AI) techniques. Here, we introduce two lightweight convolutional neural network (CNN) architectures and an ensemble machine learning (EML) method for image and feature classification, respectively. Moreover, the classification using pre-trained models and handcrafted features was carried out for comparative analysis. The binary classification was performed to classify between the two grade groups (benign vs. malignant) and quantile-quantile plots were used to show their predicted outcomes. Our proposed models for deep learning (DL) and machine learning (ML) classification achieved promising accuracies of 94.0% and 92.0%, respectively, based on non-handcrafted features extracted from CNN layers. Therefore, these models were able to predict nearly perfectly accurately using few trainable parameters or CNN layers, highlighting the importance of DL and ML techniques and suggesting that the computational analysis of microscopic anatomy will be essential to the future practice of pathology.

Keywords: prostate carcinoma; microscopic; convolutional neural network; machine learning; deep learning; handcrafted

---

1. Introduction

Image classification and analysis has become popular in recent years, especially for medical images. Cancer diagnosis and grading are often performed and evaluated using AI as these processes have become increasingly complex, because of growth in cancer incidence and the numbers of specific treatments. The analysis and classification of prostate cancer (PCa) are among the most challenging and difficult. PCa is the second most commonly diagnosed cancer among men in the USA and Europe, affecting approximately 25% of patients with cancer in the Western world [1]. PCa is a type of cancer that has always been an important challenge for pathologists and medical practitioners, with respect to detection, analysis, diagnosis, and treatment. Recently, researchers have analyzed PCa in young Korean men (<50 years of age), considering the pathological features of radical prostatectomy specimens and biochemical recurrence of PCa [2].

In the United States, thousands of people exhibit PCa. In 2017, there were approximately 161,360 new cases and 26,730 deaths, constituting 19% of all new cancer cases and 8% of all cancer deaths [3]. Therefore, it is important to detect PCa at an early stage to increase the survival rate. Currently, for the clinical diagnosis of PCa, methods that are performed in hospitals include a prostate-specific antigen test, digital rectal exam, trans-rectal ultrasound, and magnetic resonance imaging. Core needle biopsy examination is a common and useful technique, performed by insertion of a thin, hollow needle into the prostate gland to remove a tissue sample [4–6]. However, PCa diagnosis via microscopic biopsy images is challenging. Therefore, diagnostic accuracy may vary among pathologists.

Generally, in histopathology sections, pathologists categorize stained microscopy biopsy images into benign and malignant. To carry out PCa grading, pathologists use the Gleason grading system, which was originally based on the sum of the two Gleason scores for the most common so-called Gleason patterns (GPs). Many studies conclude that this is the recommended methodology for grading PCa [7]. The Gleason grading system defines five histological patterns from GP 1 (well differentiated) to GP 5 (poorly differentiated), with a focus on the shapes of atypical glands [8–11]. During the grossing study, the tumor affected in the prostate gland is extracted by the pathologist for examination under a microscope for cancerous cells [12,13]. In this cell culturing process, the tissues are stained with hematoxylin and eosin (H&E) compounds, yielding a combination of dark blue and bright pink colors, respectively [14–18]. In digital pathology, there are some protocols that every pathologist follows for preparing and staining the tissue slides. However, the acquisition systems and staining process vary from one pathologist to another. The generated tissue images with the variations in colour intensity and artifacts could impact the classification accuracy of the analysis [19,20].

DL and ML in AI have recently shown excellent performance in the classification of medical images. These techniques are used for computer vision tasks (e.g., segmentation, object detection, and image classification) and pattern recognition exploiting handcrafted features from a large-scale database, thus allowing new predictions from existing data [21–24]. DL is a class of ML algorithms, where multiple layers are used to extract higher-level features gradually from the raw input. ML is a branch of AI concentrated on application building that learns from data. ML algorithms are trained to learn features and patterns in huge amounts of data to make predictions based on new data. Both DL and ML have shown promising results in the field of medical imaging and have the potential to assist pathologists and radiologists with an accurate diagnosis; this may save time and minimize the costs of diagnosis [25–28]. For image classification, DL models are built to train, validate, and test thousands of images of different types for accurate prediction. These models consist of many layers through which a CNN transforms the images using functions such as convolution, kernel initialization, pooling, activation, padding, batch normalization, and stride.

The combination of image-feature engineering and ML classification has shown remarkable performance in terms of medical image analysis and classification. In contrast, CNN adaptively learns various image features to perform image transformation, focusing on features that are highly predictive for a specific learning objective. For instance, images of benign and malignant tissues could be presented to a network composed of convolutional layers with different numbers of filters that detect computational features and highlight the pixel pattern in each image. Based on these patterns, the network could use sigmoid and softmax classifiers to learn the extracted and important features, respectively. In DL, the "pipeline" of CNN's processing (i.e., from inputs to any output prediction) is opaque, performed automatically like a passage through a "black box" tunnel, where the user remains fully unaware of the process details. It is difficult to examine a CNN layer-by-layer. Therefore, each layer's visualization results and prediction mechanism are challenging to interpret.

The present paper proposes a pipeline for tissue image classification using DL and ML techniques. We developed two lightweight CNN (LWCNN) models for automatic detection of the GP in histological sections of PCa and extracted the non-handcrafted texture features from the CNN layers to classify these using an ensemble ML (EML) method. Color pre-processing was performed for enhancing images. To carry out a comparative analysis, the two types of hand-designed [29] features, such as the opposite color local binary patterns (OCLBP) [30] and improved OCLBP (IOCLBP) [30] were extracted and pre-trained models (VGG-16, ResNet-50, Inception-V3, and DenseNet-121) [31] were used for EML and DL classification, respectively. To avoid the complexity and build lightweight DL models, we used a few hidden layers and trainable parameters, and therefore, the models were named LWCNN.

The DL models were trained several times on the same histopathology dataset using different parameters and filters. For each round of training, we fine-tuned the hyperparameters, optimization function, and activation function to improve the model performance, including its accuracy. Binary classification is critical for PCa diagnosis because the goal of the pathologist is to identify whether each tumor is benign or malignant [32]. We generated a class activation map (CAM) using predicted images and created a heat map to visualize the method by which the LWCNN learned to recognize the pixel pattern (image texture) based on activation functions, thus interpreting the decision of the neural network. The CAM visualization results of the training and testing were difficult to interpret because CNNs are black-box models [33,34].

2. Related Work

A CNN was first used on medical images by Lo et al. [35,36]. Their model (LeNet) succeeded in a real-world application and could recognize hand-written digits [37]. Subsequent CNN-based methods showed the potential for automated image classification and prediction, especially after the introduction of AlexNet, a system that won the ImageNet challenge. In this era, the categorizing and auto-detection of cancer in the histological sections using machine assistance have shown excellent performance in the field of early detection of cancer.

Zheng et al. [38] developed a new CNN-based architecture for histopathological images, using the 3D multiparametric MRI data provided by PROSTATEx challenge. Data augmentation was performed through 3D rotation and slicing, to incorporate the 3D information of the lesion. They achieved the second-highest AUC (0.84) in the PROSTATEx challenge, which shows the great potential of deep learning for cancer imaging.

Han et al. [39] used breast cancer samples from the BreaKHis dataset to perform multi-classification using subordinate classes of breast cancer (ductal carcinoma, fibroadenoma, lobular carcinoma, adenosis, Phyllodes tumor, tubular adenoma, mucinous carcinoma, and papillary carcinoma). The author developed a new deep learning model and has achieved remarkable performance with an average accuracy of 93.2% on a large-scale dataset.

Kumar et al. [12] performed k-means segmentation to separate the background cells from the microscopy biopsy images. They extracted morphological and textural features from for automated detection and classification of cancer. They used different types of machine learning classifiers (random forest, Support vector machine, fuzzy k-nearest neighbor, and k-nearest neighbor) to classify connectivity, epithelial, muscular, and nervous tissues. Finally, the author obtained an average accuracy of 92.19% based on their proposed approach using a k-nearest neighbor classifier.

Abraham et al. [40] used multiparametric magnetic resonance images and presented a novel method for the grading of prostate cancer. They used VGG-16 CNN and an ordinal class classifier with J48 as the base classifier. The author used the PROSTATAx-2 2017 grand challenge dataset for their research work. Their method achieved a positive predictive value of 90.8%.

Yoo et al. [3] proposed an automated CNN-based pipeline for prostate cancer detection using diffusion-weighted magnetic resonance imaging (DWI) for each patient. They used a total of 427 patients as the dataset, out of these, 175 with PCa and 252 patients without PCa. The author used five CNNs based on the ResNet architecture and extracted first order statical features for classification. The analysis was carried out based on a slice- and patient-level. Finally, their proposed pipeline achieved the best result (AUC of 87%) using CNN1.

Turki [41] performed machine learning classification for cancer detection and used a data sample of colon, liver, thyroid cancer. They applied different ML algorithms, such as deep boost, AdaBoost, XgBoost, and support vector machines. The performance of the algorithms was evaluated using the area under the curve (AUC) and accuracy on real clinical data used classification.

Veta et al. [42] proposed different methods for the analysis of breast cancer histopathology images. They discussed different techniques for tissue image analysis and processing like tissue components segmentation, nuclei detection, tubules segmentation, mitotic detection, and computer-aided diagnosis. Before discussing the different image analysis algorithms, the author gave an overview of the tissue preparation, slide staining processes, and digitization of histological slides. In this paper, their approach is to perform clustering or supervised classification to acquire binary or probability maps for the different stains.

Moradi et al. [43] performed prostate cancer detection based on different image analysis techniques. The author used ultrasound, MRI, and histopathology images, and among these, ultrasound images were selected for cancer detection. For the classification of prostate cancer, feature extraction was carried out using the ultrasound echo radio-frequency (RF) signals, B-scan images, and Doppler images.

Alom et al. [44] proposed a deep CNN (DCNN) model for breast cancer classification. The model was developed based on the three powerful CNN architecture by combining the strength of the inception network (Inception-v4), the residual network (ResNet), and the recurrent convolutional neural network (RCNN). Thus, their proposed model was named as inception recurrent residual convolution neural network (IRRCNN). They used two publicly available datasets including BreakHis and Breast Cancer (BC) classification challenge 2015. The test results were compared against the existing state-of-art models for image-based, patch-based, image-level, and patient-level classification.

Wang et al. [45] proposed a novel method for the classification of colorectal cancer histopathological images. The author developed a novel bilinear convolutional neural network (BCNN) model that consists of two CNNs, and the outputs of the CNN layers are multiplied with the outer product at each spatial domain. Color deconvolution was performed to separate the tissue components (hematoxylin and eosin) for BCNN classification. Their proposed model performed better than the traditional CNN by classifying colorectal cancer images into eight different classes.

Bianconi et al. [20] compared the combination effect of six different colour pre-processing methods and 12 colour texture features on the patch-based classification of H&E stained images. They found that classification performance was poor using the generated colour descriptors. However, they achieved promising results using some pre-processing methods such as co-occurrence matrices, Gabor filters, and Local Binary Patterns.

Kather et al. [31] investigated the usefulness of image texture features, pre-trained convolutional networks against variants of local binary patterns for classifying different types of tissue sub-regions, namely stroma, epithelium, necrosis, and lymphocytes. They used seven different datasets of histological images for classifying the handcrafted and non-handcrafted features using standard classifiers (e.g., support vector machines) to obtain overall accuracy between 95% and 99%.

3. Tissue Staining and Data Collection

3.1. *Tissue Staining*

For the identification of cancerous cells, the prostate tissue was sectioned with a thickness of 4μm. The process of deparaffinization (i.e., removal of paraffin wax from slides prior to staining) is especially important after tissue sectioning because, otherwise, only poor staining may be achieved. However, in practice, each tissue section was deparaffinized and rehydrated in an appropriate manner and H&E staining was carried out successfully using an automated stainer (Autostainer XL, Leica). Hematoxylin and Eosin are positively and negatively charged, respectively. The nucleic acids in the nucleus are negatively charged components of basophilic cells; hematoxylin reacts with these components. Amino groups in proteins in the cytoplasm are positively charged components of acidophilic cells; eosin reacts with these components [46–48]. Figure 1 shows the visualization of the H&E stained biopsy image, which was analyzed using QuPath open-source software. The results of H&E staining are shown separately, with their respective chemical formulas.

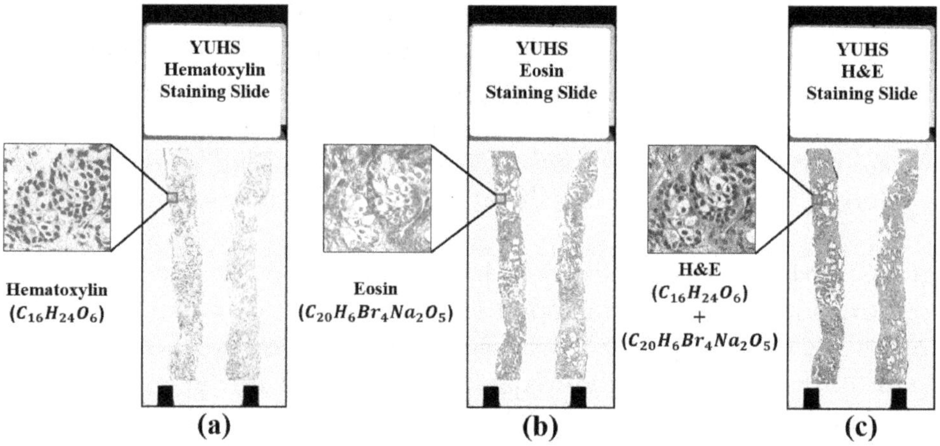

Figure 1. The visualization result of hematoxylin and eosin (H&E) staining slide. (**a**) Hematoxylin staining slide. (**b**) Eosin staining slide. (**c**) H&E staining slide obtained by combining (**a**,**b**). Note that the two slides (**a**,**b**) are highly dissimilar in texture, which is useful for analysis and classification.

3.2. Data Collection

The whole-slide H&E stained images of size 33,584 × 70,352 pixels were acquired from the pathology department of the Severance Hospital of Yonsei University. The slide images were further processed to generate multiple sizes (256 × 256, 512 × 512, and 1024 × 1024) of 2D patches by scanning at 40× optical magnification with 0.3NA objective using a digital camera (Olympus C-3000) which is attached to a microscope (Olympus BX-51). The extracted regions of interest (ROIs) were sent to the pathologist for prostate cancer (PCa) grading. Figure 2 shows an example of the cropped patches extracted from a whole-slide image. Regions containing background and adipose tissue were excluded. After the labeled patches were received, 6000 samples were selected, all with size 256 × 256 pixels (24 bit/pixel); the samples were divided equally into two classes: cancerous and non-cancerous. The tissue samples used in our research were extracted from 10 patients. These samples had an RGB color coding scheme (8 bits each for red, green, and blue).

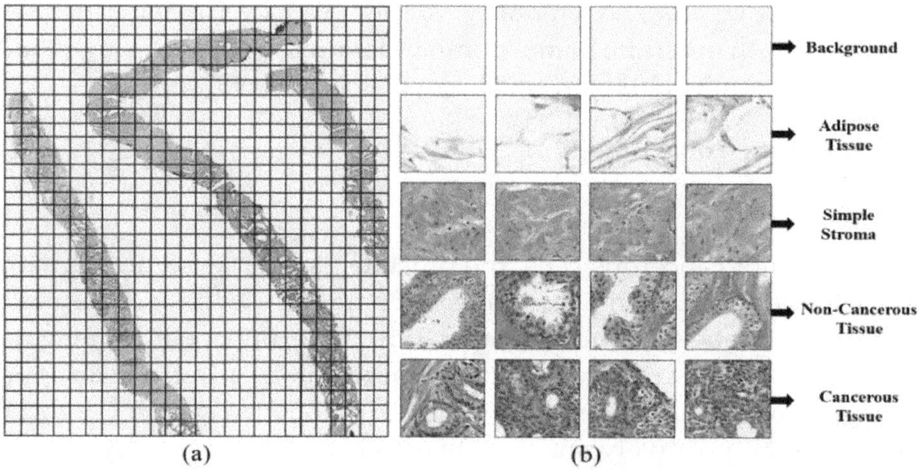

Figure 2. Data preparation of a sample histopathology slide from a prostatectomy. (**a**) An example of a whole-slide image where a sliding window method was applied to generate patch images. (**b**) The cropped patches obtained from (**a**) corresponded to the lowest and highest Gleason pattern, from well-differentiated to poorly differentiated, respectively. Among all patches in (**b**), the simple stroma, benign and malignant patches were selected for PCa analysis and classification.

4. Materials and Methods

4.1. Proposed Pipeline

Image and feature classification based on DL and ML methods showed some promising results in categorizing microscopic images of benign or malignant tissues. Our proposed pipeline for this paper is shown in Figure 3. Our analysis of a tissue image dataset was carried out in five phases, which include image pre-processing, analyze CNN models, feature analysis, model classification, and performance evaluation. In this study, we developed two LWCNN models (model 1 and model 2) and used state-of-art pre-trained models to carry out 2D image classification and perform a comparative analysis among the models. Also, EML classification was performed to classify the handcrafted (OCLBP and IOCLBP) and non-handcrafted (CNN-based) colour texture features extracted from tissue images.

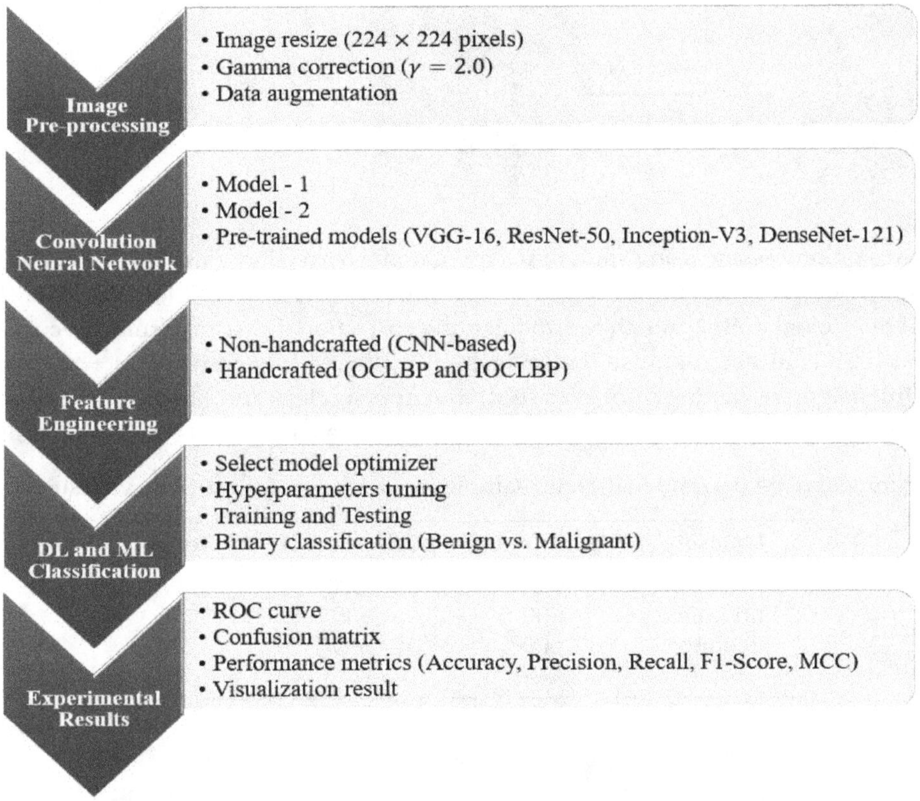

Figure 3. Proposed pipeline for image and feature classification based on a lightweight convolutional neural network (LWCNN) and ensemble machine learning (EML). LR: logistic regression, RF: random forest.

4.2. Image Preprocessing

In this phase, the preprocessing was carried out, whereby we resized the patches to 224 × 224 pixels for CNN training, and to adjust the contrast level of the image, power law (gamma) transformation [49,50] was applied to the resized images. The concept of gamma was used to encode and decode luminance values in image systems. Figure 4 illustrates the clarity of images before and after the application of this operation.

The dataset splitting was performed for training, validating, and testing the CNN models. The data samples were labeled with 0 (non-cancerous) and 1 (cancerous) for accurate classification and randomly assigned to one of three groups for training, validation, and testing, as shown in Table 1. The dataset used for DL and ML classification holds a total of 6000 samples. Out of these, 3600 were used for training, 1200 for validation, and 1200 for testing. Before the samples were fed to the network for classification, data augmentation was performed on the training set, which enabled analysis of model performance, reduction of overfitting problems, and improvement of generalization [51]. Therefore, to create some changes in the images, some transformations were applied using augmentation techniques, and these included rotation by 90°, transposition, random_brightening, and random_contrast, random_hue, and random_saturation, shown in Figure 5c,d. Keras and Tensorflow functions were used to execute data augmentation.

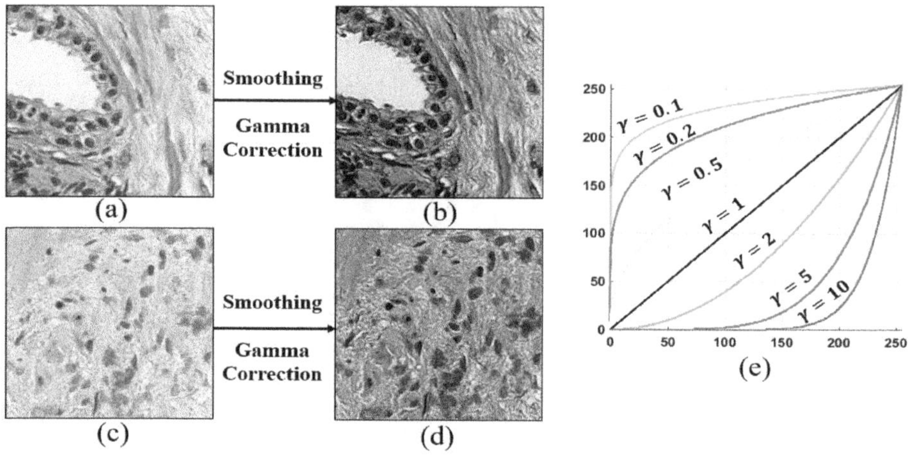

Figure 4. Image preprocessing using smoothing and gamma correction. (**a**,**c**) Original images of benign and malignant tissues, respectively. Here, the images are blurry and exhibit low contrast. (**b**,**d**) Images after removal of random noise, smoothing, and gamma correction. (**e**) Transformation curve for images with low and high contrast. Because the images in (**a**,**c**) have low contrast, $\gamma = 2$ was applied to adjust their intensities, obtaining images in (**b**,**d**) that appear clear and "fresh." Therefore, the tissue components were more visible after transformation, which was important for CNN classification.

Table 1. Assignment of benign and malignant samples into datasets for training, validation, and testing.

Dataset	Benign (0)	Malignant (1)	Total
Training	1800	1800	3600
Validation	600	600	1200
Testing	600	600	1200
Total	3000	3000	6000

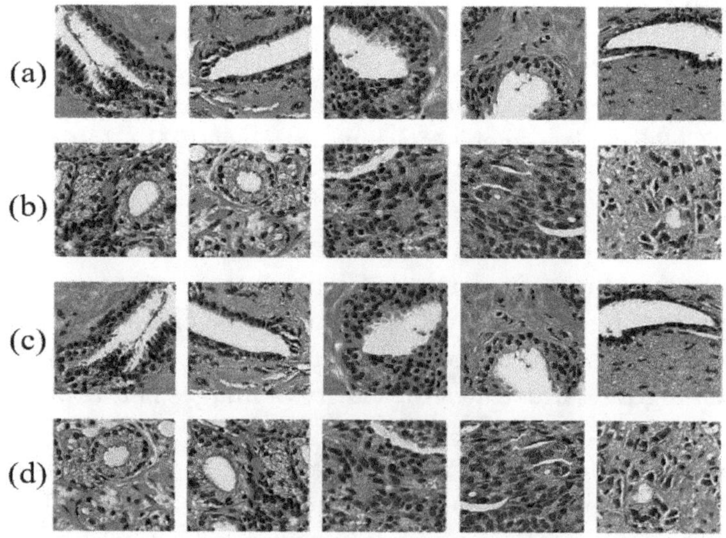

Figure 5. Randomly selected samples from the training dataset demonstrating data augmentation. (**a**,**b**) Images of benign and malignant tissues, respectively, before the transformation. (**c**,**d**) Transformed images from (**a**,**b**), respectively, after data augmentation.

4.3. Convolution Neural Network

To classify images of PCa, this paper introduces two LWCNN models to perform the classification of the GP and distinguish between two classes. Both model 1 and model 2 included CNN layers, such as those for input, convolution, rectified linear unit (ReLU), max pooling, dropout, flattening, GAP, and classification. Model 1 contained four convolutional blocks, with a depth of 10 layers, which interleaved two-dimensional (2D) convolutional layers (3 × 3 kernel, strides, and padding) with ReLU and batch normalization (BN) layers, followed by three max-pooling (2 × 2) and three dropout layers. To connect the neural network [52,53], a flattening layer and a sequence of three dense layers containing 1024, 1024, and 2 neurons were connected for feature classification and two probabilistic outputs. The sigmoid activation function [54,55] was used as a binary classifier. The numbers of filters in each block were 32, 64, 128, and 256. These filters acted as a sliding window over the entire image.

Model 2 contained three convolutional blocks, with a depth of seven layers, where the 2D convolutional, ReLU, and BN layers were identical to model 1 but were interleaved with two max-pooling (2 × 2) layers and one dropout layer. The numbers of convolutional filters in this model were 92, 192, and 384. A GAP layer was used instead of flattening, the classification section in this model also had three dense layers containing 64, 32, and 2 neurons. Here, a softmax [56,57] classifier was used to reduce binary loss. The input shape was set to 224 × 224 × 3 while building the model. The detailed design and specification of our lightweight CNN (LWCNN) models are shown in Figure 6 and Table 2, respectively. Model 2 was modified from model 1 based on multilevel feature analysis to improve classification accuracy and reduce validation loss, as shown in Figure 7.

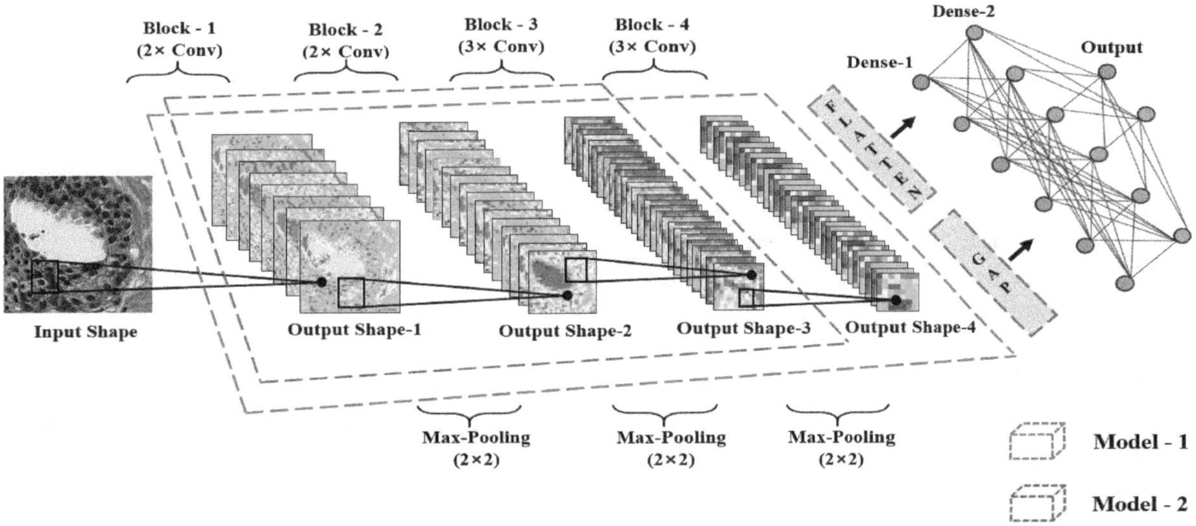

Figure 6. Structure of our lightweight convolutional neural networks for cancer image classification between two Gleason grade groups of prostate carcinoma. Spatial features are extracted from an image by convolving through one of the networks. Classification layers (flatten, global average pooling [GAP], dense-1, dense-2, and output) were used to find the required response based on features that were extracted by the convolutional neural network.

Table 2. Detailed information and specifications of lightweight convolutional neural network models. BN: batch normalization, GAP: global average pooling, ReLU: rectified linear unit.

	Layer Type	Filters	Output Shape	Kernel Size/Strides
	Model-1 Specification			
Input	Image	1	224 × 224 × 3	-
Block-1	2× convolutional + ReLU + BN	32	56 × 56 × 32	3 × 3/2
Block-2	2× convolutional + ReLU + BN	64	56 × 56 × 64	3 × 3/1

Table 2. *Cont.*

	Layer Type	Filters	Output Shape	Kernel Size/Strides
	Model-1 Specification			
-	Max pooling + dropout (0.25)	64	28 × 28 × 64	2 × 2/2
Block-3	3× convolutional + ReLU + BN	128	28 × 28 × 128	3 × 3/1
-	Max pooling + dropout (0.25)	128	14 × 14 × 128	2 × 2/2
Block-4	3× convolutional + ReLU + BN	256	14 × 14 × 256	3 × 3/1
-	Max pooling + dropout (0.25)	256	7 × 7 × 256	2 × 2/2
-	Flatten	-	12,544	-
-	Dense-1 + ReLU + BN	1024	1024	-
-	Dense-2 + ReLU + BN	1024	1024	-
-	Dropout (0.5)	1024	1024	-
Output	Sigmoid	2	2	-
	Model-2 specification			
Input	Image	1	224 × 224 × 3	-
Block-1	2× convolutional + ReLU + BN	92	56 × 56 × 92	5 × 5/2
Block-2	2× convolutional + ReLU + BN	192	56 × 56 × 192	3 × 3/1
-	Max pooling	192	28 × 28 × 192	2 × 2/2
Block-3	3× convolutional + ReLU + BN	384	28 × 28 × 384	3 × 3/1
-	Max pooling + dropout (0.25)	384	14 × 14 × 384	2 × 2/2
-	GAP	-	384	2 × 2/2
-	Dense-1 + ReLU + BN	64	64	-
-	Dense-2 + ReLU + BN	32	32	-
-	Dropout (0.5)	32	32	-
Output	Softmax	2	2	-

The multilevel feature maps were extracted after each convolutional block for pattern analysis and to understand the pixel distribution that the CNN detected, based on the number of convolution filters applied for edge detection and feature extraction. The convolution operation was performed by sliding the filter or kernel over the input image. Element-wise matrix multiplication was performed at each location in the image matrix and the output results were summed to generate the feature map. Max pooling was applied to reduce the input shape, prevent system memorization, and extract maximum information from each feature map. The feature maps from the first block held most of the information present in the image; that block acted as an edge detector. However, the feature map appeared more similar to an abstract representation and less similar to the original image, with advancement deeper into the network (see Figure 7). In block-3, the image pattern was somewhat visible, and by block-4, it became unrecognizable. This transformation occurred because deeper features encode high-level concepts, such as 2D information regarding the tissue (e.g., only spatial values of 0 or 1), while the CNN detects edges and shapes from low-level feature maps. Therefore, to improve the performance of the LWCNN, based on the observation that block-4 yielded unrecognizable images, model 2 was developed using three convolutional blocks, and selected as the model that this paper proposes.

To validate the performance of model 2 (LWCNN), we also included pre-trained CNN models (VGG-16, ResNet-50, Inceptio-V3, and DenseNet-121) for histopathology image classification. These models are very powerful and effective for extracting and classifying the deep CNN features. For each pre-trained network, the dense or classification block was configured according to the model specification. Sigmoid activation function was used for all the pre-trained models to perform binary classification.

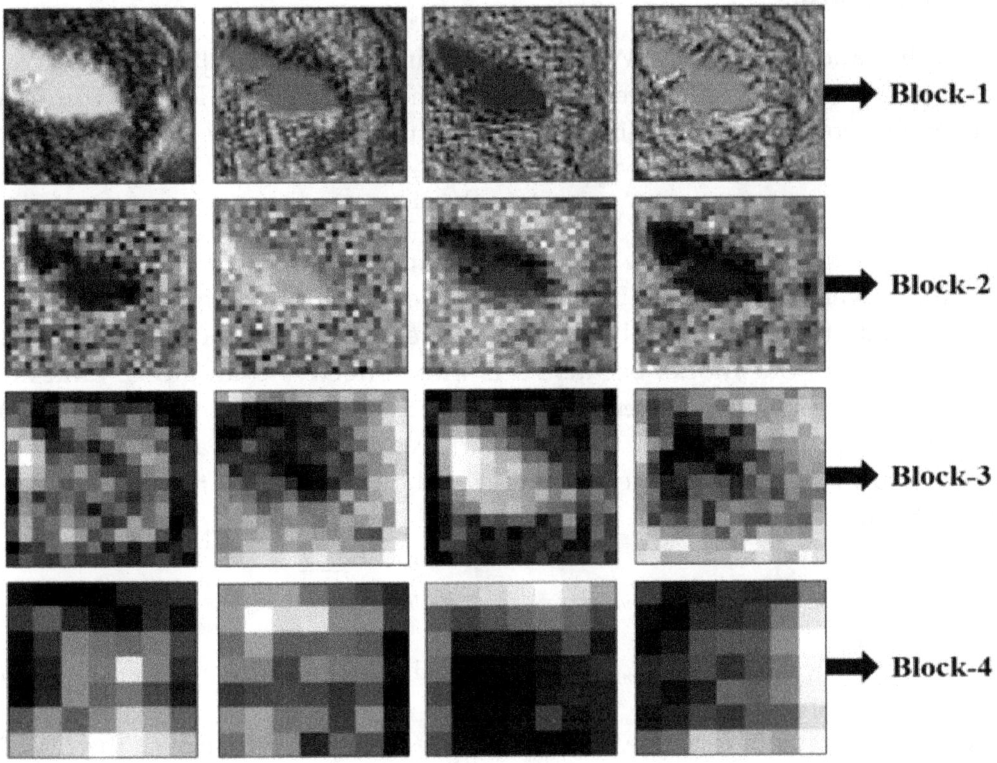

Figure 7. Multilevel feature map analysis for tissue image classification using a lightweight convolutional neural network. Visual analysis was performed by observing the pixel pattern in feature maps extracted from each block. Each block holds different information that is useful for convolutional neural network classification. Output shapes of feature maps from blocks 1–4 were: $56 \times 56 \times 92$, $28 \times 28 \times 192$, $14 \times 14 \times 384$, and $7 \times 7 \times 512$, respectively. Shown are four feature maps per block for the purpose of analysis, with 92, 192, 384, and 512 in each block, respectively. Analysis reveals that block-4 contains the maximum information regarding the image, but the resulting maps are less visually interpretable by people. With advancement deeper into the network, the feature maps become sparser, indicating that convolution filters detect fewer features. Therefore, block-4 was removed from model 2.

4.4. Feature Engineering

The extraction of texture features based on handcrafted and non-handcrafted was performed for ensemble machine learning (EML) classification. First, non-handcrafted or CNN-based features were extracted from the GAP layer of the proposed LWCNN (model 2). A different number of feature maps were generated from each CNN layer and the GAP mechanism was used to calculate the average value for each feature map. Second, a total of 20 handcrafted colour texture features were extracted using OCLBP and IOCLBP techniques. Out of these, 10 features were extracted using OCLBP, and 10 features using IOCLBP. The hand-designed feature analysis was performed for EML classification and compare with the non-handcrafted features classification results.

After we generate colour texture map, the LBP technique was applied to each colour channel (Red/Green/Blue) of OCLBP and IOCLBP separately. These state-of-art methods are the extensions of local binary patterns (LBP) and effective for colour image analysis. OCLBP and IOCLBP are the intra- and inter-channel descriptors with dissimilar local thresholding scheme (i.e., the peripheral pixels of OCLBP are thresholded at the central pixel value, and IOCLBP thresholding is based on the mean value) [30]. For each aforesaid state-of-art methods, the feature vector was obtained using general rotation-invariant operators (i.e., neighbor set of pixels p was placed on a circle of radius R) that can distinguish the spatial pattern and the contrast of local image texture. Therefore, the operators $p = 8$ and $R = 2$ were used to extract the colour features from the H&E stained tissue images.

4.5. DL and ML Classification

Prior to training and testing the LWCNN, pre-trained, and EML [58] models, we fine-tuned different types of parameters for better prediction and to minimize model loss. To compute the feature maps in each convolutional layer, a non-linear activation function (ReLU) was used, and the equation can be defined as:

$$A_{i,j,k} = \max\left(w_n^T I_{i,j} + b_n, 0\right) \tag{1}$$

where $A_{i,j,k}$ is the activation value of the nth feature map at the location (i, j), $I_{i,j}$ is the input patch, and w_n and b_n are the weight vector and bias term, respectively, of the nth filter.

BN was also used after each convolution layer to regularize the model, reducing the need for dropout. BN was used in our model because it is more effective than global data normalization. The latter normalization transforms the entire dataset so that it has a mean of zero and unit variance, while BN computes approximations of the mean and variance after each mini-batch. Therefore, BN enables the use of the ReLU activation function without saturating the model. Typically, BN is performed using the following equation:

$$\text{BN}\ (X_{normalize}) = (x_n - \mu_{mb}) / \sqrt{\sigma^2_{mb}} + c \tag{2}$$

where x_n is the d-dimensional input, μ_{mb} and σ^2_{mb} are the mean and variance, respectively, of the mini-batch, and c is a constant.

To optimize the weights of the network and analyze the performance of the LWCNN models, we performed a comparative analysis based on four different types of optimizers, namely stochastic gradient descent (SGD), Adadelta, Adam, and RMSprop. The results of comparative analysis are shown in the next section. The classification performance is measured using the cross-entropy loss, or log loss, whose output is a probability value between 0 and 1. To train our network, we used binary cross-entropy. The standard loss function for binary classification is given by:

$$Binary_{loss} = -\frac{1}{N}\sum_{i=1}^{N}[Y_i \times \log(M_w(X_i)) + (1 - Y_i) \times \log(1 - M_w(X_i))] \tag{3}$$

where N is the number of output class, X_i and Y_i are the input samples and target labels, respectively, and M_w is the model with network weight, w.

The hyperparameters were tuned while setting a minimum learning rate of 0.001 using the function known as ReduceLROnPlateau, a factor of 0.8 and patience of 10 were set; thus, if no improvement was observed in validation loss for 10 consecutive epochs, the learning rate was reduced by a factor of 0.8. The batch size was set to eight for training the model and regularization was applied by dropping out 25% and 50% of the weights in the convolution and dense blocks of LWCNN, respectively. The probabilistic output in the dense layer was computed using sigmoid and softmax classifiers.

In addition to CNN methods, traditional ML algorithms including logistic regression (LR) [59] and random forest (RF) [60] were used for features classification. In this paper, an ensemble voting method was proposed in which LR and RF classifiers were combined to create an EML model. This ensemble technique was used to classify the handcrafted and non-handcrafted features and compare the classification performance. The LWCNN, pre-trained, and EML models were tested using the unknown or unseen data samples. Typically, for ML classification, cross-validation was used by splitting the training data into k-fold (i.e., $k = 5$) to determine the model generalizability, and the result was computed by averaging the accuracies from each of the k trials. Prior to ML classification [61–63], the feature values for training and testing were normalized using the standard normal distribution function, which can be expressed as:

$$P_{i\_Normalised} = \frac{P_i - \mu}{\sigma} \tag{4}$$

where P_i is the ith pixel in an individual tissue image, and μ and σ are the mean and standard deviation of the dataset.

The DL and ML models were built with the Python 3 programming language using the Keras and Tensorflow libraries. Approximately 36 h were invested in fine-tuning the hyperparameters to achieve better accuracy. Figure 8 shows the entire process flow diagram for DL and ML classification. The hyperparameters that were used for DL and ML models are shown in Table 3.

The models were trained, validated, and tested on a PC with the following specifications: an Intel corei7 CPU (2.93 GHz), one NVIDIA GeForce RTX 2080 GPU, and 24 GB of RAM.

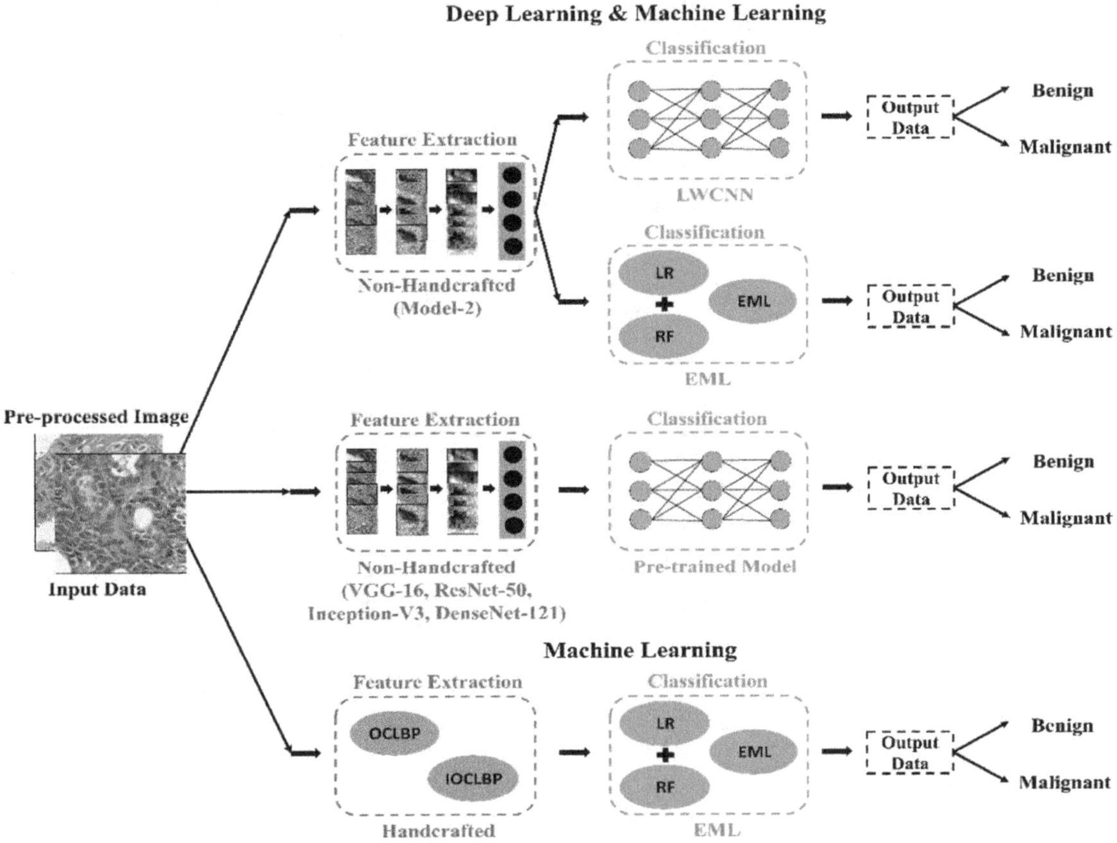

Figure 8. Flow diagram for DL and ML classification. Handcrafted and non-handcrafted colour texture descriptors were extracted for EML classification.

Table 3. Hyperparameters Tuning for DL and ML classifiers.

Models	Specification
Model-1, VGG-16, ResNet-50, Inception-V3, DenseNet-121	loss = binary_crossentropy; learning rate = start:1.0—auto reduce on plateau fraction: 0.8 after 10 consecutive non-declines of validation loss; classifier = sigmoid; epochs = 300
Model-2	loss = binary_crossentropy; learning rate = start:1.0—auto reduce on plateau fraction: 0.8 after 10 consecutive non-declines of validation loss; classifier = softmax; epochs = 300, kernel initializer = glorot_uniform
LR	C = 100, max_iter = 500, tol = 0.001, method = isotonic, penalty = l2
RF	n_estimators = 500, criterion = gini, max_depth = 9, min_samples_split = 5, min_samples_leaf = 4, method = isotonic

5. Experimental Results

This study mainly focuses on image classification based on AI. The proposed LWCNN (model 2) for tissue image classification and EML for feature classification produced reliable results, which met our requirements, at an acceptable speed. To develop DL models, a CNN approach was used as it is proven excellent performance in detecting specific regions for multiclass and binary classification. When splitting the dataset, a ratio of 8:2 was set for training and testing. Moreover, to validate the model after each epoch, the training set was further divided, such that 75% of the data was allocated for training and 25% was allocated for validation. Five-fold cross-validation was used during EML training. Algorithms used for preprocessing, data analysis, and classification were implemented in the MATLAB R2019a and PyCharm environments.

5.1. Performance Analysis

In this study, a binary classification approach was used to classify benign and malignant samples of prostate tissue. Two levels of classification were performed: DL (based on images) and ML (based on features). Table 4 shows the comparative analysis between the optimizers for model 1 and model 2, respectively. The developed LWCNN models were trained a couple of times by changing the optimizers during training.

Table 4. Comparison of the optimizers for tissue image classification.

	Model-1		Model-2	
Optimizers	**Test Loss (%)**	**Test Accuracy (%)**	**Test Loss (%)**	**Test Accuracy (%)**
SGD	0.51	85.7	0.25	93.3
RMSProp	1.00	85.5	0.62	89.3
Adam	0.45	84.4	0.28	91.1
Adadelta	0.54	89.1	0.25	94.0

From the above comparison table, we can analyze that the Adadelta performed the best and gave the best accuracies on test data for both the architectures. SGD and Adam performed close to Adadelta for model 2. On the other hand, RMSProp performed close to Adadelta for model 1. However, Adadelta (update version of Adam and Adagrad) is a more robust optimizer that restricts the window of accumulated past gradients to some fixed size w instead of accumulating all past square gradients. The comparison of these optimizers revealed that Aadelta is more stable and more rapid, hence, an overall improvement on SGD, RMSProp, and Adam. The behavior and performance of the optimizers were analyzed using the receiver operating characteristic (ROC) curve. It is a probabilistic curve that represents the diagnostic ability of a binary classifier system, including an indication of its effective threshold value. The area under the ROC curve (AUC) summarizes the extent to which a model can separate the two classes. Figure 9a,b show the ROC curve and corresponding AUC that depicts the effectiveness of different optimizers used for model 1 and model 2, respectively. For model 1, the AUCs were 0.95, 0.94, 0.96, and 0.93, and for model 2, 0.98, 0.97, 0.98, and 0.97 were obtained using Adadelta, RMSProp, SGD, and Adam, respectively.

Further, based on the optimum accuracy in Table 4, we carried out EML classification using the CNN extracted features from model 2, to analyze the efficiency of ML algorithms. Also, handcrafted features classification was performed to compare the performance with the non-handcrafted features classification results. Moreover, the EML model achieved promising results using the CNN-based features. Model 2 outperformed model 1 in overall accuracy, precision, recall, F1-score, and MCC, with values of 94.0%, 94.2%, 92.9%, 93.5%, and 87.0%, respectively. A confusion matrix (Figure 10) was generated based on the LWCNN model that yielded the optimum results, and thus most reliably distinguished malignant from benign tissue. Benign tissue was labeled as "0" and malignant was labeled as "1" to plot the confusion matrix for this binary classification. The four squares in the confusion matrix represent true positive, true negative, false positive, and false negative; their values were calculated using the test dataset based on the expected outcome and number of predictions of each class. Tables 5 and 6 show the overall comparative analysis for the DL and ML classification. The performance metrics used to evaluate the analysis results are accuracy, precision, recall, F1-score, and Matthews correlation coefficient (MCC).

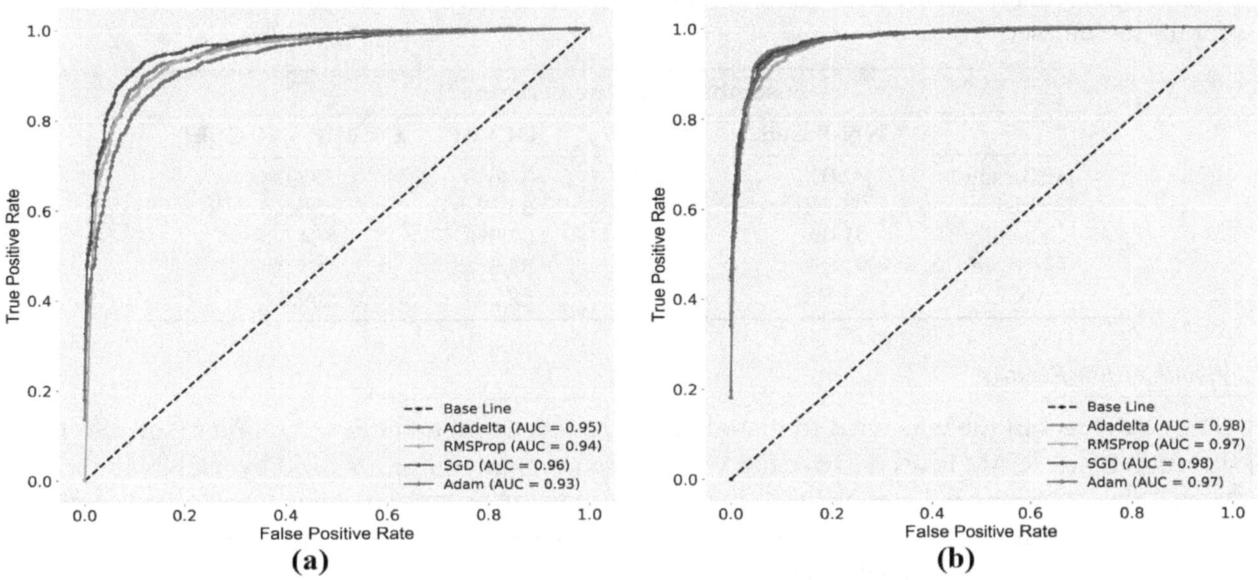

Figure 9. ROC curves for analyzing the behavior of different optimizers, generated by plotting predicted probability values (i.e., model's confidence scores). (**a**) Performance of model 1 based on sigmoid activation. (**b**) Performance of model 2 based on softmax activation function.

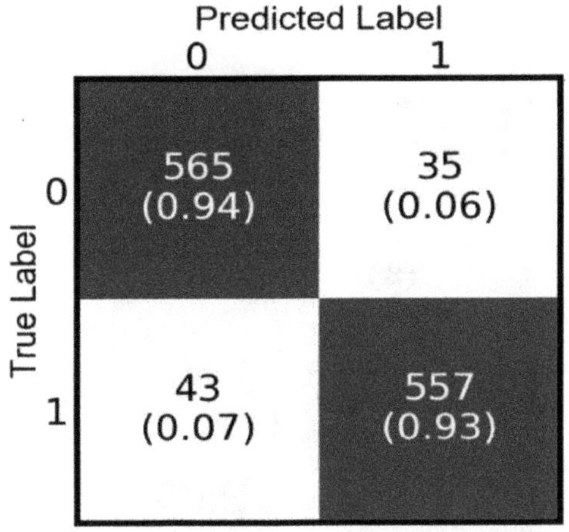

Figure 10. Confusion matrix of model 2, generated using the test dataset, showing results of binary classifications between benign (0) and malignant (1) tumors. Blue boxes at top-left and bottom-right represent true positive and true negative, respectively; white boxes at top-right and bottom-left represent false negative and false positive, respectively.

Table 5. Comparative analysis of lightweight and pre-trained CNN models based on non-handcrafted features. Metrics are for the test dataset.

	Deep Learning					
	Model-1	**Model-2**	**VGG-16**	**ResNet-50**	**Inception-V3**	**DenseNet-121**
Accuracy	89.1%	94.0%	92.0%	93.0%	94.6%	95.0%
Precision	89.2%	94.2%	92.2%	95.0%	96.5%	96.2%
Recall	89.1%	92.9%	91.9%	90.6%	93.2%	94.6%
F1-Score	89.0%	93.5%	92.0%	92.8%	94.8%	95.4%
MCC	78.3%	87.0%	84.0%	85.3%	89.5%	90.7%

Table 6. Comparative analysis of non-handcrafted and handcrafted features classification. Metrics are for the test dataset.

	Ensemble Machine Learning			
	CNN-Based	OCLBP	IOCLBP	OCLBP + IOCLBP
Accuracy	92.0%	69.3%	83.6%	85.0%
Precision	92.7%	66.0%	83.2%	85.5%
Recall	91.0%	70.6%	83.9%	84.5%
F1-Score	91.8%	68.2%	83.5%	85.0%
MCC	83.5%	38.6%	67.2%	69.8%

5.2. Visualization Results

The CAM technique was used to visualize the results from an activation layer (softmax) of the classification block. CAM is used to deduce which regions of an image are used by a CNN to recognize the precise class or group it contains [22,64]. Typically, it is difficult to visualize the results from hidden layers of a black box CNN model. More complexity is observed in feature maps with increasing depth in the network; thus, each image becomes increasingly abstract, encoding less information than the initial layers and appearing more blurred. Figure 11 shows the CAM results, indicating the method by which our DL network detected important regions; moreover, the network had learned a built-in mechanism to determine which regions merited attention. Therefore, this decision process was extremely useful in the classification network.

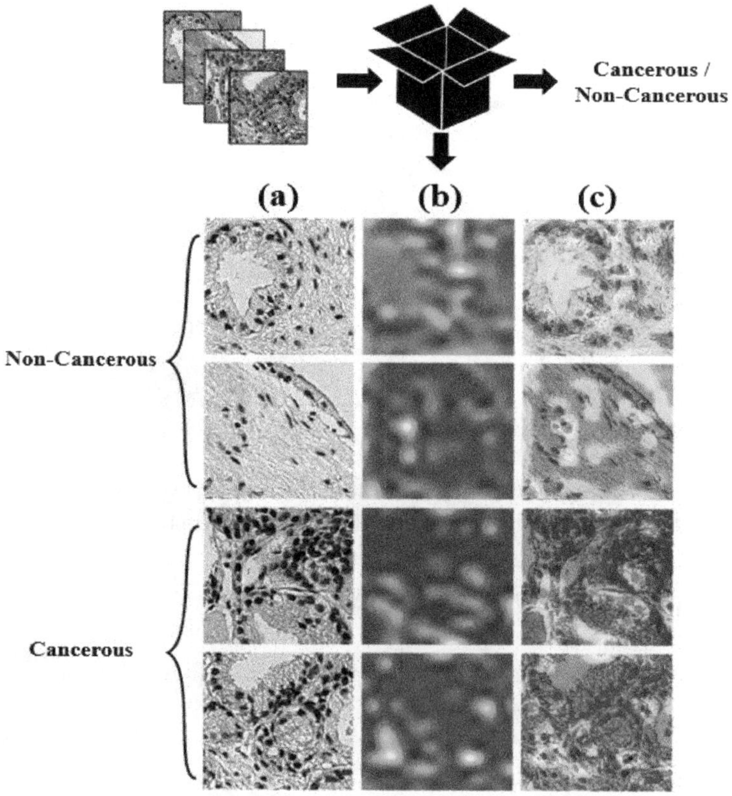

Figure 11. Class activation maps are extracted from one of the classification layers of our convolutional neural network. These show how images are classified and predicted by the neural network, although it is a black-box model. Top and bottom pairs of rows depict benign and malignant tissue images, respectively. (**a**) Input images with an RGB color scheme visualized as grayscale. (**b**) Activation map of classification block, showing detection of different regions in each tissue image. (**c**) Images overlaying (**a**,**b**), with spots indicating significant regions that the convolutional neural network used to identify a specific in that image.

Our CNN detected specific regions using the softmax classifier by incorporating spatially averaged information extracted by the GAP layer from the last convolution layer, which had an output shape of 14 × 14 × 384. The detected regions depicted in Figure 11c were generated by the application of a heat map to the CAM image in Figure 11b and overlaying that on the original image from Figure 11a. A heat map is highly effective for tissue image analysis; in this instance, it showed how the CNN detected each region of the image that is important for cancer classification. Doctors can use this information to better understand the classification (i.e., how the neural network predicted the presence of cancer in an image, based on the relevant regions). The visualization process was carried out using the test dataset, which was fed into the trained network of model 2.

In this study, supervised classification was performed for cancer grading, whereby our dataset was labeled with "0" and "1" to categorize benign and malignant tissue separately and independently. The probability distributions of data were similar in training and test sets, but the test dataset was independent of the training dataset. Therefore, after the model had been trained with several binary labeled cancer images, the unanalyzed dataset was fed to the network for accurate prediction between binary classes. Figure 12 shows examples of the binary classification results from our proposed model 2, with examples of images that were and were not predicted correctly. Notably, some images of benign were similar to malignant tissues and vice versa in terms of their nuclei distribution, intensity variation, and tissue texture. It was challenging for the model to correctly classify these images into the two groups.

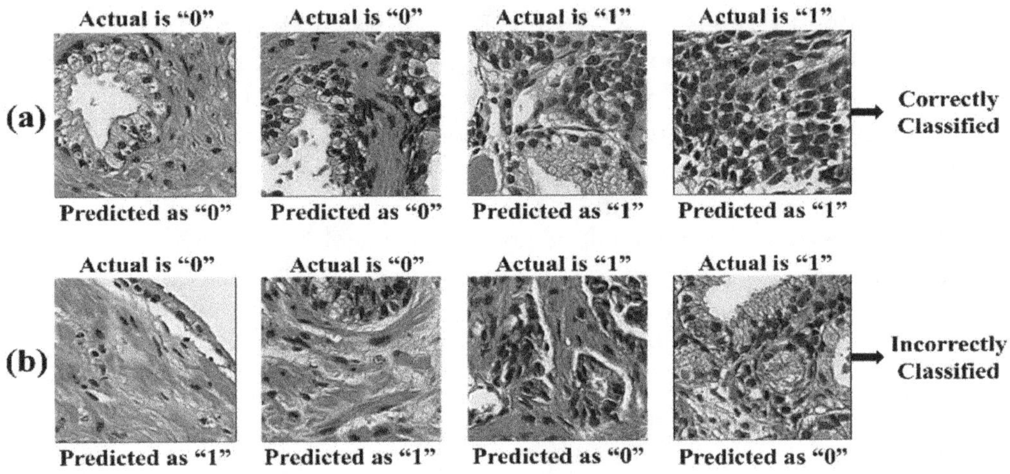

Figure 12. Cancer prediction using a binary labeled test dataset. Examples of images that were (**a**) correctly and (**b**) incorrectly classified, showing their actual and predicted labels.

6. Discussion

The main aim of this study was to develop LWCNN for benign and malignant tissue image classification based on multilevel feature map analysis and show the effectiveness of the model. Moreover, we developed an EML voting method for the classification of non-handcrafted (extracted from the GAP layer of model 2) and handcrafted (extracted using OCLBP and IOCLBP). Generally, in DL, the features are extracted automatically from raw data and further processed for classification using a neural network approach. However, for ML algorithms, features are extracted manually using different mathematical formulae; these are also regarded as handcrafted features. A CNN is suitable for complex detection tasks, such as analyses of scattered and finely drawn patterns in data. Of particular interest, in the malignant and benign classification task, model 2 was more effective than model 1.Indeed, model 1 performed below expectation, such that we modified it to improve performance, resulting in model 2. The modification comprised removal of the fourth convolutional block, flattening layer, and sigmoid activation function, as well as alterations of filter number and kernel size. Moreover, GAP replaced flattening after the third convolutional block, minimizing overfitting by reducing the total number of parameters in the model. The softmax activation function replaced the sigmoid activation function in the third dense layer. These modifications, based on the multilevel feature map analysis, improved the overall accuracy and localization ability of tissue image classification.

Furthermore, in this study, we have also compared our proposed CNN model with the well-known pre-trained models such as VGG-16, ResNet-50, Inception-V3, and DenseNet-121. Among these, DenseNet proved to give the highest accuracy of 95% followed by the Inception V3 with 94.6%. The pre-trained VGG-16 and ResNet-50 achieved 92% and 93%, respectively. Although DenseNet gained the highest accuracy among all the pre-trained models as well as our proposed model 2, it is not quite comparable with the motto of this paper. The ultimate goal of this paper was to develop a light-weighted CNN without a much-complicated structure with minimum possible convolutional layers and achieve better classification performance. Model 2 proved this hypothesis by achieving an overall accuracy of 94%. On the other hand, all the pre-trained models are well trained on a huge dataset (ImageNet) which includes 1000 classes. Therefore, it is evident that the classification of such models will be done accurately without much hassle. Nevertheless, the comparison of computational cost between the proposed LWCNN and other pre-trained models was performed to analyze the memory usage, trainable parameters, and learning (training and testing) time, shown in Table 7. First, according to the comparison Table 7, the number of trainable parameters used in the LWCNN model was reduced by more than 75% as compared to VGG-16, ResNet-50, and Inception-V3, and 2% as compared to DenseNet-121. Second, the memory usage of the proposed model was significantly less when compared to other models. Third, the time taken to train the proposed model was also drastically less. Among the pre-trained models, VGG-16 and ResNet-50 agree with the objective of this work. From Tables 5 and 7, it is evident that our LWCNN (model 2) is competitive and inexpensive, whereas, the state-of-art models were computationally expensive and achieved comparable results. Therefore, from this perspective, model 2 of our proposed work performed better than VGG-16 and ResNet-50 in terms of accuracy, besides employing a simple architecture.

Table 7. Comparing performance and computation cost of model-2 with other pre-trained models.

Models	Parameter (Trainable)	Model Memory Usage	Time to Solution (Minutes)	
			Train	Test
VGG-16	27,823,938	60.9 MB	570	<1
ResNet-50	23,538,690	148.4 MB	660	<1
Inception-V3	22,852,898	66.9 MB	600	<1
DenseNet-121	7,479,682	199.7 MB	700	<1
Model-2 (LWCNN)	5,386,638	44.7 MB	190	<1

Through fine-tuning of the hyperparameters, the CNN layers were determined to be optimal using the validation and test datasets. The modified, model 2 was adequate for the classification of benign and malignant tissue images. Our study examined the capability of the proposed LWCNN model to detect and forecast the histopathology images; a single activation map was extracted from each block (see Figure 13) to visualize the detection results using a heat map. Notably, we used an EML method for non-handcrafted and handcrafted features classification. However, the EML model was sufficiently powerful to classify the computational features extracted using the optimal LWCNN model, which predicted the samples of benign and malignant tissues almost perfectly accurately. Also, tissue samples that were classified and predicted using the softmax classifier are shown in quantile-quantile (Q–Q) plots of the prediction probability confidence for benign and malignant states in Figure 14a,b, respectively. These Q–Q plots allowed for the analysis of predictions. True and predicted probabilistic values were plotted according to true positive and true negative classifications of samples (see Figure 9), respectively.

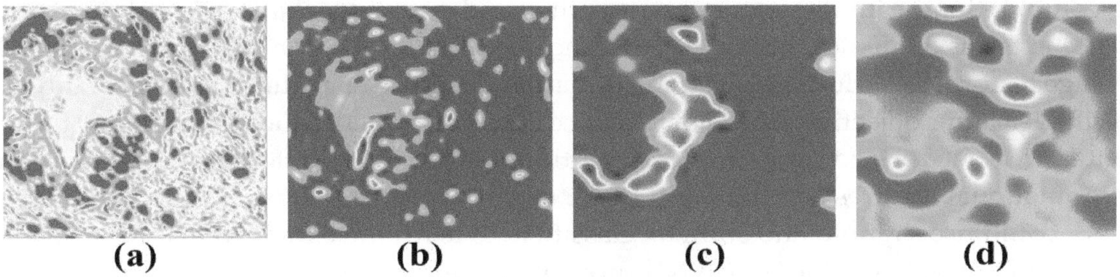

Figure 13. Visualizations of class activation maps generated from model 2, created using different numbers of filters. Outputs of (**a**) first convolutional, (**b**) second convolutional, (**c**) third convolutional, and (**d**) classification blocks. Colors indicate the most relevant regions for predicting the class of these histopathology images, as detected by the convolutional neural network.

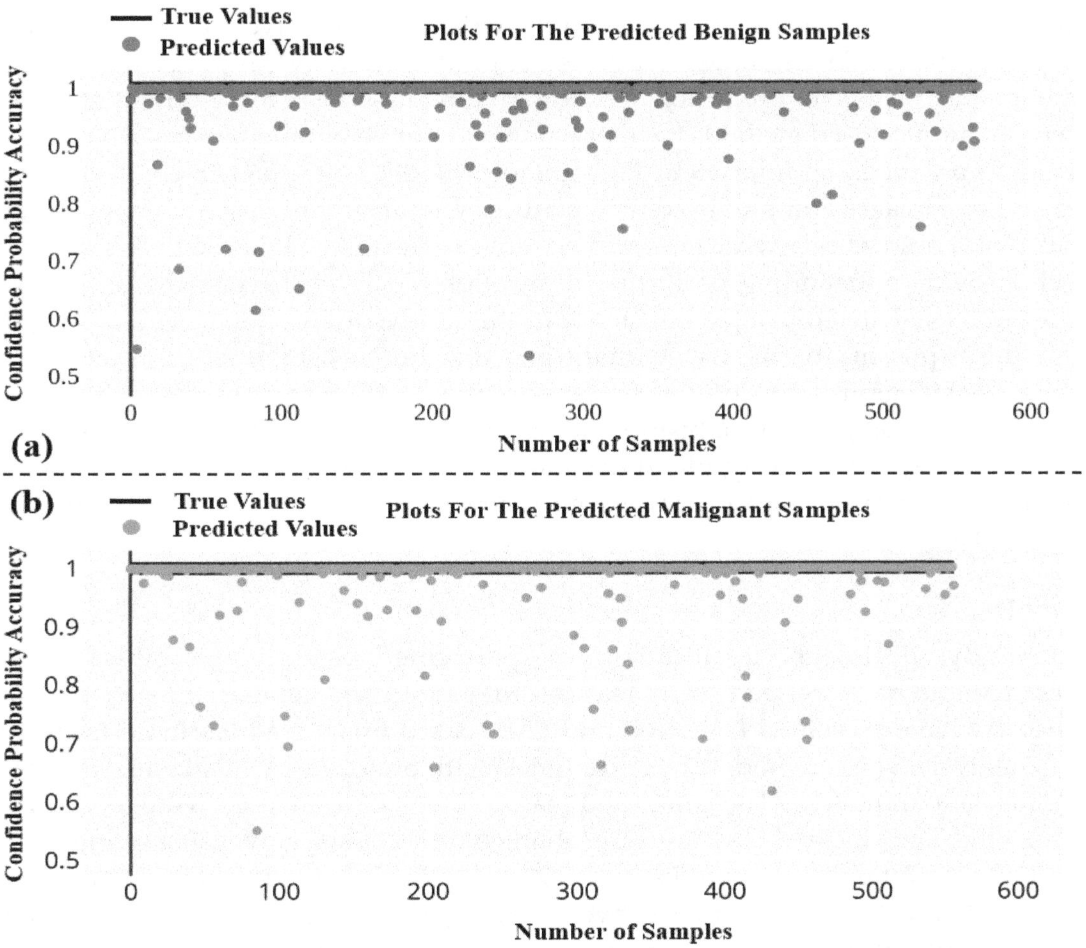

Figure 14. Quantile-quantile plot for true and predicted probabilistic values. (**a**) Samples that were benign and had true positive predictions. (**b**) Samples that were malignant and had true negative predictions.

In Q–Q plots, note that the black bar at the top parallel to the x-axis shows true probabilistic values; red (true positive) and blue (true negative) markers show the prediction confidence of each sample of a specific class. We used a softmax classifier, which normalizes the output of each unit to be between 0 and 1, ensuring that the probabilities always sum to 1. The number of samples used for each class was 600; the numbers correctly classified were 565 and 557 for true positive and true negative, respectively. A predicted probability value > 0.5 and <0.5 signifies an accurate classification and misclassification, respectively.

The combination of image-feature engineering and ML classification has shown remarkable performance in terms of medical image analysis and classification. In contrast, CNN adaptively learns various image features to perform image transformation, focusing on features that are highly predictive for a specific learning objective [65]. For instance, images of benign and malignant tissues could be presented to a network composed of convolutional layers with different numbers of filters that detect computational features and highlight the pixel pattern in each image. Based on these patterns, the network could use sigmoid and softmax classifiers to learn the extracted and important features, respectively. In DL, the "pipeline" of CNN's processing (i.e., from inputs to any output prediction) is opaque [66], performed automatically like a passage through a "black box" tunnel, where the user remains fully unaware of the process details. It is difficult to examine a CNN layer-by-layer. Therefore, each layer's visualization results and prediction mechanism are challenging to interpret.

Overall, all models performed well in tissue image classification, achieving comparable results. The EML method also worked well with CNN-extracted features, yielding comparable results. We conclude that, for image classification, models with very deep layers performed well by more accurately classifying the data samples. We aimed to build an LWCNN model with few feature-map layers and hyperparameters for prediction of cancer grading based on binary classification (i.e., benign vs. malignant). Our proposed methods have proven that lightweight models can achieve good results if the parameters are tuned appropriately. Furthermore, model 2 effectively recognized the histologic differences in tissue images and predicted their statuses with nearly perfect accuracy. The application of DL to histopathology is relatively new. However, it performs well and delivers accurate results. DL methods provide outstanding performance through black box layers; the outputs of each of these layers can be visualized using a heat map. In this study, our model provided insights into the histologic patterns present in each tissue image and can thus assist pathologists as a practical tool for analyzing tissue regions relevant to the worst prognosis. Heat map analyses suggested that the LWCNN can learn visual patterns of histopathological images containing different features relating to nuclear morphology, cell density, gland formation, and variations in the intensity of stroma and cytoplasm. Performance significantly improved when the first model was modified based on the feature map analysis.

7. Conclusions

In this study, 2D image classification was performed using PCa samples by leveraging non-handcrafted and handcrafted texture features to distinguish a malignant state of tissue from a benign state. We have presented LWCNN- and EML-based image and feature classification using feature map analysis. The DL models were designed with only a few CNN layers and trained with a small number of parameters. The computed feature maps of each layer were fed into these fully CNNs through the flattening and GAP layers, enabling binary classification using sigmoid and softmax classifiers. GAP and softmax were used for model 2, the optimal network in this paper. The GAP layer was used, instead of flattening, to minimize overfitting by reducing the total number of parameters in the model. This layer computes the mean value for each feature map, whereas flattening combined all feature maps extracted from the final convolution or pooling layers by changing the shape of the data from a 2D matrix of features into a one-dimensional array for passage to the fully CNN classifier. A comparative analysis was performed between the DL and EML classification results. Moreover, the computational cost was also compared among the models. The optimum LWCNN (i.e., model 2) and EML models (a combination of LR and RF classifiers) achieved nearly perfectly accurate results with significantly fewer trainable parameters. The proposed LWCNN model developed in the study achieved an overall accuracy of 94%, average precision of 94.2%, an average recall of 92.9%, an average f1-score of 93.5%, and MCC of 87%. On the other hand, using CNN-based features, the EML model achieved an overall accuracy of 92%, an average precision of 92.7%, an average recall of 91%, an average f1-score of 91.8%, and MCC of 83.5%.

To conclude, the analysis presented in this study is very encouraging. However, a model built for medical images may not work well for other types of images. There is a need to fine-tune the hyperparameters to control model overfitting and loss, thereby improving accuracy. The 2D LWCNN (model 2) developed in this study performed well, and therefore, the predicted true positive and true negative samples for benign and malignant, respectively, were plotted using Q-Q plots. The CAM technique was used to visualize the results of the block box CNN model. In the future, we will consider other methods and develop a more complex DL model and compare it with our optimal LWCNN model and other transfer learning models. Further, we will extend the research to multi-class classification (beyond binary) to simultaneously classify benign tissues, as well as grades 3–5.

Author Contributions: Funding acquisition, H.-K.C.; Methodology, S.B.; Resources, N.-H.C.; Supervision, H.-K.C.; Validation, H.-G.P.; Visualization, C.-H.K.; Writing—original draft, S.B.; Writing—review and editing, C.-H.K. and D.P. All authors have read and agreed to the published version of the manuscript.

References

1. Siegel, R.L.; Miller, K.D.; Jemal, A. Cancer statistics, 2015. *CA Cancer J. Clin.* **2015**, *65*, 5–29. [CrossRef]
2. Chung, M.S.; Shim, M.; Cho, J.S.; Bang, W.; Kim, S.I.; Cho, S.Y.; Rha, K.H.; Hong, S.J.; Hong, C.-H.; Lee, K.S.; et al. Pathological Characteristics of Prostate Cancer in Men Aged <50 Years Treated with Radical Prostatectomy: A Multi-Centre Study in Korea. *J. Korean Med. Sci.* **2019**, *34*, 78. [CrossRef]
3. Yoo, S.; Gujrathi, I.; Haider, M.A.; Khalvati, F. Prostate Cancer Detection using Deep Convolutional Neural Networks. *Sci. Rep.* **2019**, *9*, 19518. [CrossRef]
4. Humphrey, P.A. Diagnosis of adenocarcinoma in prostate needle biopsy tissue. *J. Clin. Pathol.* **2007**, *60*, 35–42. [CrossRef]
5. Van Der Kwast, T.H.; Lopes, C.; Santonja, C.; Pihl, C.-G.; Neetens, I.; Martikainen, P.; Di Lollo, S.; Bubendorf, L.; Hoedemaeker, R.F. Guidelines for processing and reporting of prostatic needle biopsies. *J. Clin. Pathol.* **2003**, *56*, 336–340. [CrossRef] [PubMed]
6. Kim, E.H.; Andriole, G.L. Improved biopsy efficiency with MR/ultrasound fusion-guided prostate biopsy. *J. Natl. Cancer Inst.* **2016**, *108*. [CrossRef] [PubMed]
7. Heidenreich, A.; Bastian, P.J.; Bellmunt, J.; Bolla, M.; Joniau, S.; Van Der Kwast, T.; Mason, M.; Matveev, V.; Wiegel, T.; Zattoni, F.; et al. EAU Guidelines on Prostate Cancer. Part 1: Screening, Diagnosis, and Local Treatment with Curative Intent—Update 2013. *Eur. Urol.* **2014**, *65*, 124–137. [CrossRef] [PubMed]
8. Humphrey, P.A. Gleason grading and prognostic factors in carcinoma of the prostate. *Mod. Pathol.* **2004**, *17*, 292–306. [CrossRef]
9. Nagpal, K.; Foote, D.; Liu, Y.; Chen, P.-H.C.; Wulczyn, E.; Tan, F.; Olson, N.; Smith, M.C.; Mohtashamian, A.; Wren, J.H.; et al. Development and validation of a deep learning algorithm for improving Gleason scoring of prostate cancer. *NPJ Digit. Med.* **2019**, *2*, 48. [CrossRef]
10. Alqahtani, S.; Wei, C.; Zhang, Y.; Szewczyk-Bieda, M.; Wilson, J.; Huang, Z.; Nabi, G. Prediction of prostate cancer Gleason score upgrading from biopsy to radical prostatectomy using pre-biopsy multiparametric MRI PIRADS scoring system. *Sci. Rep.* **2020**, *10*, 7722. [CrossRef]
11. Zhu, Y.; Freedland, S.J.; Ye, D. Prostate Cancer and Prostatic Diseases Best of Asia, 2019: Challenges and opportunities. *Prostate Cancer Prostatic Dis.* **2019**, *23*, 197–198. [CrossRef] [PubMed]
12. Kumar, R.; Srivastava, R.; Srivastava, S.K. Detection and Classification of Cancer from Microscopic Biopsy Images Using Clinically Significant and Biologically Interpretable Features. *J. Med. Eng.* **2015**, *2015*, 457906. [CrossRef] [PubMed]
13. Cahill, L.C.; Fujimoto, J.G.; Giacomelli, M.G.; Yoshitake, T.; Wu, Y.; Lin, D.I.; Ye, H.; Carrasco-Zevallos, O.M.; Wagner, A.A.; Rosen, S. Comparing histologic evaluation of prostate tissue using nonlinear microscopy and paraffin H&E: A pilot study. *Mod. Pathol.* **2019**, *32*, 1158–1167. [CrossRef]
14. Otali, D.; Fredenburgh, J.; Oelschlager, D.K.; Grizzle, W.E. A standard tissue as a control for histochemical and immunohistochemical staining. *Biotech. Histochem.* **2016**, *91*, 309–326. [CrossRef] [PubMed]
15. Alturkistani, H.A.; Tashkandi, F.M.; Mohammedsaleh, Z.M. Histological Stains: A Literature Review and Case Study. *Glob. J. Health Sci.* **2015**, *8*, 72. [CrossRef] [PubMed]

16. Zarella, M.D.; Yeoh, C.; Breen, D.E.; Garcia, F.U. An alternative reference space for H&E color normalization. *PLoS ONE* **2017**, *12*, 0174489.
17. Lahiani, A.; Klaiman, E.; Grimm, O. Enabling histopathological annotations on immunofluorescent images through virtualization of hematoxylin and eosin. *J. Pathol. Inform.* **2018**, *9*, 1. [CrossRef] [PubMed]
18. Gavrilovic, M.; Azar, J.C.; Lindblad, J.; Wählby, C.; Bengtsson, E.; Busch, C.; Carlbom, I.B. Blind Color Decomposition of Histological Images. *IEEE Trans. Med. Imaging* **2013**, *32*, 983–994. [CrossRef]
19. Bautista, P.A.; Yagi, Y. Staining Correction in Digital Pathology by Utilizing a Dye Amount Table. *J. Digit. Imaging* **2015**, *28*, 283–294. [CrossRef]
20. Bianconi, F.; Kather, J.N.; Reyes-Aldasoro, C.C. Evaluation of Colour Pre-Processing on Patch-Based Classification of H&E-Stained Images. In *Digital Pathology. ECDP*; Lecture Notes in Computer Science; Springer: Cham, Switzerland, 2019; Volume 11435, pp. 56–64. [CrossRef]
21. Diamant, A.; Chatterjee, A.; Vallières, M.; Shenouda, G.; Seuntjens, J. Deep learning in head & neck cancer outcome prediction. *Sci. Rep.* **2019**, *9*, 2764.
22. Yamashita, R.; Nishio, M.; Do, R.K.G.; Togashi, K. Convolutional neural networks: An overview and application in radiology. *Insights Imaging* **2018**, *9*, 611–629. [CrossRef] [PubMed]
23. Sahiner, B.; Pezeshk, A.; Hadjiiski, L.; Wang, X.; Drukker, K.; Cha, K.H.; Summers, R.M.; Giger, M.L. Deep learning in medical imaging and radiation therapy. *Med. Phys.* **2019**, *46*, e1–e36. [CrossRef] [PubMed]
24. Nanni, L.; Ghidoni, S.; Brahnam, S. Handcrafted vs. non-handcrafted features for computer vision classification. *Pattern Recognit.* **2017**, *71*, 158–172. [CrossRef]
25. Lundervold, A.S.; Lundervold, A. An overview of deep learning in medical imaging focusing on MRI. *Z. Med. Phys.* **2019**, *29*, 102–127. [CrossRef] [PubMed]
26. Lee, J.-G.; Jun, S.; Cho, Y.-W.; Lee, H.; Kim, G.B.; Seo, J.B.; Kim, N. Deep Learning in Medical Imaging: General Overview. *Korean J. Radiol.* **2017**, *18*, 570–584. [CrossRef] [PubMed]
27. Bi, W.L.; Hosny, A.; Schabath, M.B.; Giger, M.L.; Birkbak, N.J.; Mehrtash, A.; Allison, T.; Arnaout, O.; Abbosh, C.; Dunn, I.F.; et al. Artificial intelligence in cancer imaging: Clinical challenges and applications. *CA Cancer J. Clin.* **2019**, *69*, 127–157. [CrossRef]
28. Jha, S.; Topol, E.J. Adapting to Artificial Intelligence. *JAMA* **2016**, *316*, 2353–2354. [CrossRef] [PubMed]
29. Badejo, J.A.; Adetiba, E.; Akinrinmade, A.; Akanle, M.B. Medical Image Classification with Hand-Designed or Machine-Designed Texture Descriptors: A Performance Evaluation. In *Internatioanl Conference on Bioinformatics and Biomedical Engineering*; Springer: Cham, Switzerland, 2018; pp. 266–275. [CrossRef]
30. Bianconi, F.; Bello-Cerezo, R.; Napoletano, P. Improved opponent color local binary patterns: An effective local image descriptor for color texture classification. *J. Electron. Imaging* **2017**, *27*, 011002. [CrossRef]
31. Kather, J.N.; Bello-Cerezo, R.; Di Maria, F.; Van Pelt, G.W.; Mesker, W.E.; Halama, N.; Bianconi, F. Classification of Tissue Regions in Histopathological Images: Comparison Between Pre-Trained Convolutional Neural Networks and Local Binary Patterns Variants. In *Intelligent Systems Reference Library*; Springer: Cham, Switzerland, 2020; pp. 95–115. [CrossRef]
32. Khairunnahar, L.; Hasib, M.A.; Bin Rezanur, R.H.; Islam, M.R.; Hosain, K. Classification of malignant and benign tissue with logistic regression. *Inform. Med. Unlocked* **2019**, *16*, 100189. [CrossRef]
33. Guidotti, R.; Monreale, A.; Ruggieri, S.; Turini, F.; Giannotti, F.; Pedreschi, D. A Survey of Methods for Explaining Black Box Models. *ACM Comput. Surv.* **2019**, *51*, 93. [CrossRef]
34. Hayashi, Y. New unified insights on deep learning in radiological and pathological images: Beyond quantitative performances to qualitative interpretation. *Inform. Med. Unlocked* **2020**, *19*, 100329. [CrossRef]
35. Lo, S.-C.; Lou, S.-L.; Lin, J.-S.; Freedman, M.; Chien, M.; Mun, S. Artificial convolution neural network techniques and applications for lung nodule detection. *IEEE Trans. Med. Imaging* **1995**, *14*, 711–718. [CrossRef] [PubMed]
36. Lo, S.-C.B.; Chan, H.-P.; Lin, J.-S.; Li, H.; Freedman, M.T.; Mun, S.K. Artificial convolution neural network for medical image pattern recognition. *Neural Netw.* **1995**, *8*, 1201–1214. [CrossRef]
37. LeCun, Y.; Bottou, L.; Bengio, Y.; Haffner, P. Gradient-based learning applied to document recognition. *Proc. IEEE* **1998**, *86*, 2278–2324. [CrossRef]
38. Liu, S.; Zheng, H.; Feng, Y.; Li, W. Prostate cancer diagnosis using deep learning with 3D multiparametric MRI. In *Medical Imaging 2017: Computer-Aided Diagnosis*; SPIE 10134; International Society for Optics and Photonics: Orlando, FL, USA, 2017; p. 1013428.

39. Han, Z.; Wei, B.; Zheng, Y.; Yin, Y.; Li, K.; Li, S. Breast Cancer Multi-classification from Histopathological Images with Structured Deep Learning Model. *Sci. Rep.* **2017**, *7*, 4172. [CrossRef]
40. Abraham, B.; Nair, M.S. Automated grading of prostate cancer using convolutional neural network and ordinal class classifier. *Inform. Med. Unlocked* **2019**, *17*, 100256. [CrossRef]
41. Truki, T. An Empirical Study of Machine Learning Algorithms for Cancer Identification. In Proceedings of the 2018 IEEE 15th International Conference on Networking, Sensing and Control (ICNSC), Zhuhai, China, 27–29 March 2018; pp. 1–5.
42. Veta, M.M.; Pluim, J.P.W.; Van Diest, P.J.; Viergever, M.A. Breast Cancer Histopathology Image Analysis: A Review. *IEEE Trans. Biomed. Eng.* **2014**, *61*, 1400–1411. [CrossRef]
43. Moradi, M.; Mousavi, P.; Abolmaesumi, P. Computer-Aided Diagnosis of Prostate Cancer with Emphasis on Ultrasound-Based Approaches: A Review. *Ultrasound Med. Biol.* **2007**, *33*, 1010–1028. [CrossRef]
44. Alom, Z.; Yakopcic, C.; Nasrin, M.S.; Taha, T.M.; Asari, V.K. Breast Cancer Classification from Histopathological Images with Inception Recurrent Residual Convolutional Neural Network. *J. Digit. Imaging* **2019**, *32*, 605–617. [CrossRef]
45. Wang, C.; Shi, J.; Zhang, Q.; Ying, S. Histopathological image classification with bilinear convolutional neural networks. In Proceedings of the 2017 39th Annual International Conference of the IEEE Engineering in Medicine and Biology Society (EMBC), Seogwipo, Korea, 15–16 July 2017; Volume 2017, pp. 4050–4053.
46. Smith, S.A.; Newman, S.J.; Coleman, M.P.; Alex, C. Characterization of the histologic appearance of normal gill tissue using special staining techniques. *J. Vet. Diagn. Investig.* **2018**, *30*, 688–698. [CrossRef]
47. Vodyanoy, V.; Pustovyy, O.; Globa, L.; Sorokulova, I. Primo-Vascular System as Presented by Bong Han Kim. *Evid. Based Complement. Altern. Med.* **2015**, *2015*, 361974. [CrossRef] [PubMed]
48. Larson, K.; Ho, H.H.; Anumolu, P.L.; Chen, M.T. Hematoxylin and Eosin Tissue Stain in Mohs Micrographic Surgery: A Review. *Dermatol. Surg.* **2011**, *37*, 1089–1099. [CrossRef] [PubMed]
49. Huang, S.-C.; Cheng, F.-C.; Chiu, Y.-S. Efficient Contrast Enhancement Using Adaptive Gamma Correction With Weighting Distribution. *IEEE Trans. Image Process.* **2012**, *22*, 1032–1041. [CrossRef] [PubMed]
50. Rahman, S.; Rahman, M.; Abdullah-Al-Wadud, M.; Al-Quaderi, G.D.; Shoyaib, M. An adaptive gamma correction for image enhancement. *EURASIP J. Image Video Process.* **2016**, *2016*, 35. [CrossRef]
51. Shorten, C.; Khoshgoftaar, T.M. A survey on Image Data Augmentation for Deep Learning. *J. Big Data* **2019**, *6*, 60. [CrossRef]
52. Lecun, Y.; Bengio, Y.; Hinton, G. Deep learning. *Nature* **2015**, *521*, 436–444. [CrossRef]
53. Kieffer, B.; Babaie, M.; Kalra, S.; Tizhoosh, H.R. Convolutional neural networks for histopathology image classification: Training vs. Using pre-trained networks. In Proceedings of the 2017 Seventh International Conference on Image Processing Theory, Tools and Applications (IPTA), Montreal, QC, Canada, 28 November–1 December 2017; pp. 1–6.
54. Mourgias-Alexandris, G.; Tsakyridis, A.; Passalis, N.; Tefas, A.; Vyrsokinos, K.; Pleros, N. An all-optical neuron with sigmoid activation function. *Opt. Express* **2019**, *27*, 9620–9630. [CrossRef]
55. Elfwing, S.; Uchibe, E.; Doya, K. Sigmoid-weighted linear units for neural network function approximation in reinforcement learning. *Neural Netw.* **2018**, *107*, 3–11. [CrossRef]
56. Kouretas, I.; Paliouras, V. Simplified Hardware Implementation of the Softmax Activation Function. In Proceedings of the 2019 8th International Conference on Modern Circuits and Systems Technologies (MOCAST), Thessaloniki, Greece, 13–15 May 2019; pp. 1–4.
57. Zhu, Q.; He, Z.; Zhang, T.; Cui, W. Improving Classification Performance of Softmax Loss Function Based on Scalable Batch-Normalization. *Appl. Sci.* **2020**, *10*, 2950. [CrossRef]
58. Dietterich, T.G. Ensemble Methods in Machine Learning. In *International Workshop on Multiple Classifier System*; Springer: Berlin, Heidelberg, 2000; pp. 1–15. [CrossRef]
59. Dikaios, N.; Alkalbani, J.; Sidhu, H.S.; Fujiwara, T.; Abd-Alazeez, M.; Kirkham, A.; Allen, C.; Ahmed, H.; Emberton, M.; Freeman, A.; et al. Logistic regression model for diagnosis of transition zone prostate cancer on multi-parametric MRI. *Eur. Radiol.* **2015**, *25*, 523–532. [CrossRef]
60. Nguyen, C.; Wang, Y.; Nguyen, H.N. Random forest classifier combined with feature selection for breast cancer diagnosis and prognostic. *J. Biomed. Sci. Eng.* **2013**, *6*, 551–560. [CrossRef]
61. Cruz, J.A.; Wishart, D.S. Applications of Machine Learning in Cancer Prediction and Prognosis. *Cancer Inform.* **2006**, *2*, 59–77. [CrossRef]

62. Tang, T.T.; Zawaski, J.A.; Francis, K.N.; Qutub, A.A.; Gaber, M.W. Image-based Classification of Tumor Type and Growth Rate using Machine Learning: A preclinical study. *Sci. Rep.* **2019**, *9*, 12529. [CrossRef] [PubMed]
63. Madabhushi, A.; Lee, G. Image analysis and machine learning in digital pathology: Challenges and opportunities. *Med. Image Anal.* **2016**, *33*, 170–175. [CrossRef] [PubMed]
64. Yang, W.; Huang, H.; Zhang, Z.; Chen, X.; Huang, K.; Zhang, S. Towards Rich Feature Discovery With Class Activation Maps Augmentation for Person Re-Identification. In Proceedings of the 2019 IEEE/CVF Conference on Computer Vision and Pattern Recognition (CVPR), Long Beach, CA, USA, 15–20 June 2019; pp. 1389–1398.
65. Hou, X.; Gong, Y.; Liu, B.; Sun, K.; Liu, J.; Xu, B.; Duan, J.; Qiu, G. Learning Based Image Transformation Using Convolutional Neural Networks. *IEEE Access* **2018**, *6*, 49779–49792. [CrossRef]
66. Chai, X.; Gu, H.; Li, F.; Duan, H.; Hu, X.; Lin, K. Deep learning for irregularly and regularly missing data reconstruction. *Sci. Rep.* **2020**, *10*, 3302. [CrossRef]

Morphological Estimation of Cellularity on Neo-Adjuvant Treated Breast Cancer Histological Images

Mauricio Alberto Ortega-Ruiz [1,2,*], Cefa Karabağ [2], Victor García Garduño [3] and Constantino Carlos Reyes-Aldasoro [4,*]

1 Universidad del Valle de México, Departamento de Ingeniería, Campus Coyoacán, Ciudad de México 04910, Mexico
2 Department of Electrical & Electronic Engineering, School of Mathematics, Computer Science and Engineering, City, University of London, London EC1V 0HB, UK; cefa.karabag.1@city.ac.uk
3 Departamento de Ingeniería en Telecomunicaciones, Facultad de Ingeniería, Universidad Nacional Autónoma de México, Av. Universidad 3000, Ciudad Universitaria, Coyoacán, Ciudad de México 04510, Mexico; france@marconi.fi-b.unam.mx
4 giCentre, Department of Computer Science, School of Mathematics, Computer Science and Engineering, City, University of London, London EC1V 0HB, UK
* Correspondence: mauricio.ortega@city.ac.uk (M.A.O.-R.); reyes@city.ac.uk (C.C.R.-A.)

Abstract: This paper describes a methodology that extracts key morphological features from histological breast cancer images in order to automatically assess Tumour Cellularity (TC) in Neo-Adjuvant treatment (NAT) patients. The response to NAT gives information on therapy efficacy and it is measured by the residual cancer burden index, which is composed of two metrics: TC and the assessment of lymph nodes. The data consist of whole slide images (WSIs) of breast tissue stained with Hematoxylin and Eosin (H&E) released in the 2019 SPIE Breast Challenge. The methodology proposed is based on traditional computer vision methods (K-means, watershed segmentation, Otsu's binarisation, and morphological operations), implementing colour separation, segmentation, and feature extraction. Correlation between morphological features and the residual TC after a NAT treatment was examined. Linear regression and statistical methods were used and twenty-two key morphological parameters from the nuclei, epithelial region, and the full image were extracted. Subsequently, an automated TC assessment that was based on Machine Learning (ML) algorithms was implemented and trained with only selected key parameters. The methodology was validated with the score assigned by two pathologists through the intra-class correlation coefficient (ICC). The selection of key morphological parameters improved the results reported over other ML methodologies and it was very close to deep learning methodologies. These results are encouraging, as a traditionally-trained ML algorithm can be useful when limited training data are available preventing the use of deep learning approaches.

Keywords: neo-adjuvant treatment; digital pathology; tumour cellularity; machine learning

1. Introduction

Digital pathology has recently become a major player in Cancer research, disease detection, classification, and even in outcome prognosis [1–4]. Perhaps the most common imaging technique is Hematoxylin and Eosin (H&E), where H stains nuclei blue and E stains cytoplasm pink [5]. Additionally, other immunohistochemistry methods (IHC) that use antibodies to stain antigens or proteins in the tissue are more specific and they can complement H&E [6]. For instance, the cluster of differentiation 31 (CD31), which is commonly found on endothelial cells, is used as an indication of the growth of blood vessels in tumours, or angiogenesis [7–9]. CD34 is found on hematopoietic cells, mesenchymal stem cells, and it is required in certain processes, like infiltration of eosinophils into the colon [10], or the dendritic cell trafficking and pathology in pneumonitis [11], Ki67 is normally associated with cell proliferation and it can be used as a prognostic factor for gliomas [12], breast cancer [13], and colorectal adenocarcinomas [14]. Computer-assisted diagnosis (CAD) [2] is based on the quantitative analysis to grade the level of the disease, but, recently, other clinical-pathological relationships with the data have been explored [15,16]. For example, a better understanding of mechanisms of the disease evolution process [1] and even prognosis information [3].

Breast Cancer is a common disease both in terms of incidence and deaths, with approximately 252,710 new cases and 40,610 deaths in 2017 in the United States alone [17]. In 2018, 30% of new cases Cancer among females cases in the US were breast cancer, which placed it the second place in mortality [18]. Numerous imaging analysis methods are employed in order to study these cancers [19]. Common treatments for breast cancer are surgery, radiation, chemotherapy, or targeted therapy. Breast cancer neo-adjuvant treatment (NAT) is a therapy for advanced cases that provides useful information for breast-conserving surgery [20]. NAT provides prognostic and survival information [21] as well as a rate of local recurrence [22]. The efficacy of NAT is determined by means of the pathological complete response (pCR) and this can be assessed by the Residual Cancer Burden (RCB) [23]. RCB is supported by two metrics: residual Tumour Cellularity (TC) within the Tumour Bed (TB) and the assessment of lymph nodes. RCB is scored in a continuous value, but it is further categorised in four classes RCB-0 to RCB-III. Subsequently, TC, which is defined as the fraction of malignant cells within the image patch, is a key parameter for RCB computation [24,25]. Currently, TC is manually assessed by an eye-balling routine estimating the proportion of TB and this procedure is time-consuming and requires an experienced pathologist.

Neo-adjuvant treatment (NAT) chemotherapy refers to a treatment that is administrated before Cancer surgery [26–28]. The first successful results of NAT chemotherapy were demonstrated in the 1980s [29,30]. Some of the benefits of NAT are: tumour size reduction, better prognostics, and, even in some cases, surgery can be avoided [31]. In addition, patients with large tumours could be eligible for breast-conserving or a less tumour size surgery extraction.

TC assessment problem was first addressed by a hand engineering approach based on nuclei segmentation and feature extraction. In the first step, nuclei segmentation needs to be implemented [1]. This is a challenging task and some common techniques are based on active contours [32], watersheds [33], or graph cuts [34], which are either designed for nuclei [33] or lymphocytes segmentation. [32] Based on the segmentation application, speed, accuracy, or automation level might be required [34]. In the present study, automated segmentation is performed and, as it has been reported in some tissue classification studies, accuracy nuclei segmentation does not guarantee better outcome assessment between benign and malignant tissue [2]. When processing a high number of image files, speed constraint is preferable. After segmentation, many features can be extracted, for instance, cell shape, size, and texture [33–35], and also, features from regional and the global image can provide valuable information [36]. These parameters can be used for diagnostic purposes to classify tissue malignancy [36–39] and also for grade disease level assignment. Ref. [33] For instance, a study conducted by Dong and co-authors [40] categorised intraductal lesions in breast cancer by an adequate feature extraction and machine learning (ML) classification.

ML algorithms are trained to learn from the parameters extracted [15]. Some supervised algorithms are Support Vector Machines [41], Boosted Trees [42], and K-Nearest Neighbours [43]. Besides diagnosis, different new clinicopathological relationships with features have been discovered, for example, [16] revealed the relation between stroma morphology and prognosis of breast cancer patients and [44] studied quantification and distribution of tumour-infiltrating lymphocytes (TILs) as prognostic and predictive biomarker.These type of digital pathology methodologies can also useful for TC assessment. A full hand-engineering method for this task was proposed by Peikari [45]. This methodology was based on the extraction of a vector with 125 parameters [45].

Separate to traditional ML techniques, another approach to estimate TC is by Deep Learning (DL) techniques. In the last decade, there has been increased interest in DL methods. One of the main architectures or models is based on the use of neural networks, and a particular case is a Convolutional Neural Network (CNN) [46]. The main advantage of DL techniques is that they do not require the extraction of features manually or by training, as the network learns a series of parameters and weights by itself. However, to achieve this, the network requires a relatively large number of training images with labels, and the number of training data can impact on the performance. In many histopathology applications, labelled training data are still limited as compared to other imaging applications, such as everyday images, like cats and dogs. With the spread use of whole slide digital scanners [47], numerous histopathology images have become available for research purposes. Some have been released to the research community in general in the form of challenges (e.g., https://grand-challenge.org/challenges/) in order to encourage research groups globally to work together, gather annotations, provide training, and testing data sets and benchmark algorithms. The present work follows the 2019 SPIE-AAPM-NCI BreastPathQ: Cancer Cellularity Challenge with the specific objective of "development of quantitative biomarkers for the determination of cancer cellularity from whole slide images (WSI) of breast cancer hematoxylin and eosin (H&E) stained pathological slides" (https://breastpathq.grand-challenge.org/) and addresses the development of quantitative biomarkers for the challenge.

CNNs have been used for different Histopathology tasks, like segmentation [48,49], detection of a specific image properties [50] , and image grade classification [38,51]. Breast cancer tumour cellularity has also been addressed by deep techniques. For instance, Ziang Pei [52] implemented a direct method based on deep and transfer learning approach with the advantage of avoiding cell segmentation. Akbar [20] presented a traditional hand-engineering approach and a deep neural network.

The methodology in this study is based on a hand-engineering approach similar to the one that was described by [45] based on a 125 parameter vector size, but we selected 22 parameters after a correlation analysis of extracted features with TC. Additionally, the methodology described here is similar to Dong et al. parameters from nuclei; we also include parameters from the neighbourhood of the nuclei and from the full image patch. The study by Fondon [36] also analysed regions around the nuclei; however, our study includes morphology parameters from whole breast ducts region. Thus, the main contributions of this paper in the methodology are the segmentation algorithm that is based on the enhancement of the nuclei region, and an algorithm for breast ducts detection and the parameter derivation and selection and its correlation to tumour cellularity. In the results, the correlation analysis of the morphological parameters with cellularity revealed that stroma concentration has the strongest correlation with TC, which is in agreement with the results that were presented by [16]. Finally, the results were validated with the ICC and compared with similar studies [20,45] indicating an increase in ICC. The methodology described only requires a reduced set of training parameters. Therefore, the methodology described in this paper improves previous results and it may be useful in cases when large training data sets, which are normally required for deep learning approaches, are not available.

2. Materials and Methods

2.1. Materials

The data set used in this work consists of 2579 patches of tissue stained with H&E, which were extracted from 64 different patients under Neo-adjuvant Treatment. The size of each patch is 512 × 512 pixels. As a reference, a breast tissue is formed of a connective tissue, named stroma, as seen in pink. Lymphocytes can be seen as dark blue round objects and fat zones as white areas. It also contains ducts,which are responsible for carrying milk, and sometimes arteries, which can be seen as regular clusters of darker blue nuclei grouped into the region (Figure 1).

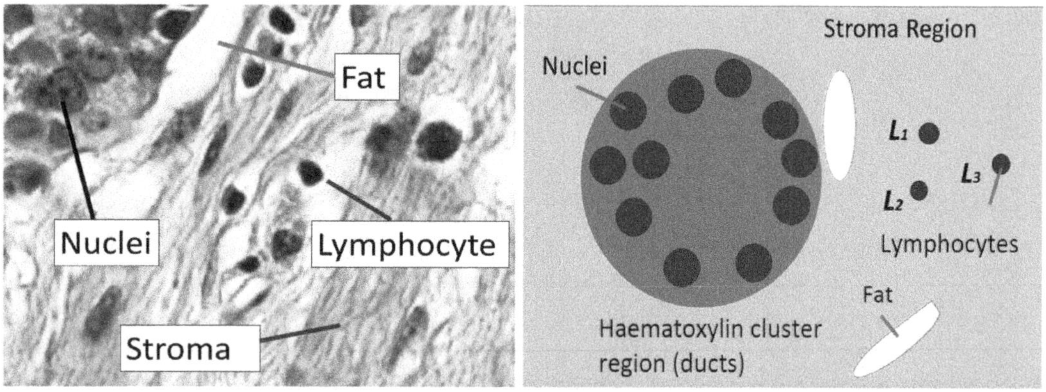

(a) (b)

Figure 1. (**a**) Stroma region which shows several clusters, regions of fat as well as some lymphocytes. (**b**) Graphical description of the elements that are analysed in this work. Within a stroma, the connective tissue shown in pink region, ducts appear as clusters stained with haematoxylin and contain several nuclei. Outside these ducts, regions of fat appear white and lymphocytes appear purple.

The residual cellularity of each patch was evaluated by 2 pathologists and this assessment was considered to be the ground truth (GT) for this study. The data was released as part of the challenge 2019 and it was collected at the Sunnybrook Health Sciences Centre, Toronto. It comprises a set of whole slide images (WSIs) that have been stained with H&E [45] from 64 patients with residual invasive breast cancer on re-section specimens following NAT therapy. The specimens were handled according to routine clinical protocols and WSIs were scanned at 20× magnification (0.5 μm/pixel).

The images were divided into a training and validation set of images. The cellularity value distribution for the whole data-set is uneven, i.e., most of the patches correspond to cellularity zero and fewer patches were available for higher cellularity. The training images were selected uniformly distributed from cellularity zero to one in order to have an even amount of benign and malignant nuclei. First, 212 images with selected cellularity values from 0 to 1 were processed and 4533 nuclei cells from those selected images were extracted and its corresponding features computed and used as a training set. The remaining 2367 patches were used for validation. Figure 2 shows the selected patches with different levels of cellularity. A third set of test data of 1119 images was available for the challenge contest. These three sets were used in this work.

2.2. Methodology

The proposed methodology consists of a sequence of traditional image processing routines, computer vision, and machine learning algorithms that automatically process the full validation set. A large amount of morphological parameters can be extracted and stored orderly in an output table file. A master control routine is responsible for selecting one by one the corresponding image patch to be processed. There are two operational modes. A manualmode useful to train machine learning algorithms. In this mode, nuclei from the selected image with a known classification assignment are fed to the algorithm and output features are saved in an output data file. Subsequently, an automated mode processes the full validation set and gives a TC estimation. This mode is able to process thousands of patch images. Figure 3 presents this process in a diagram.

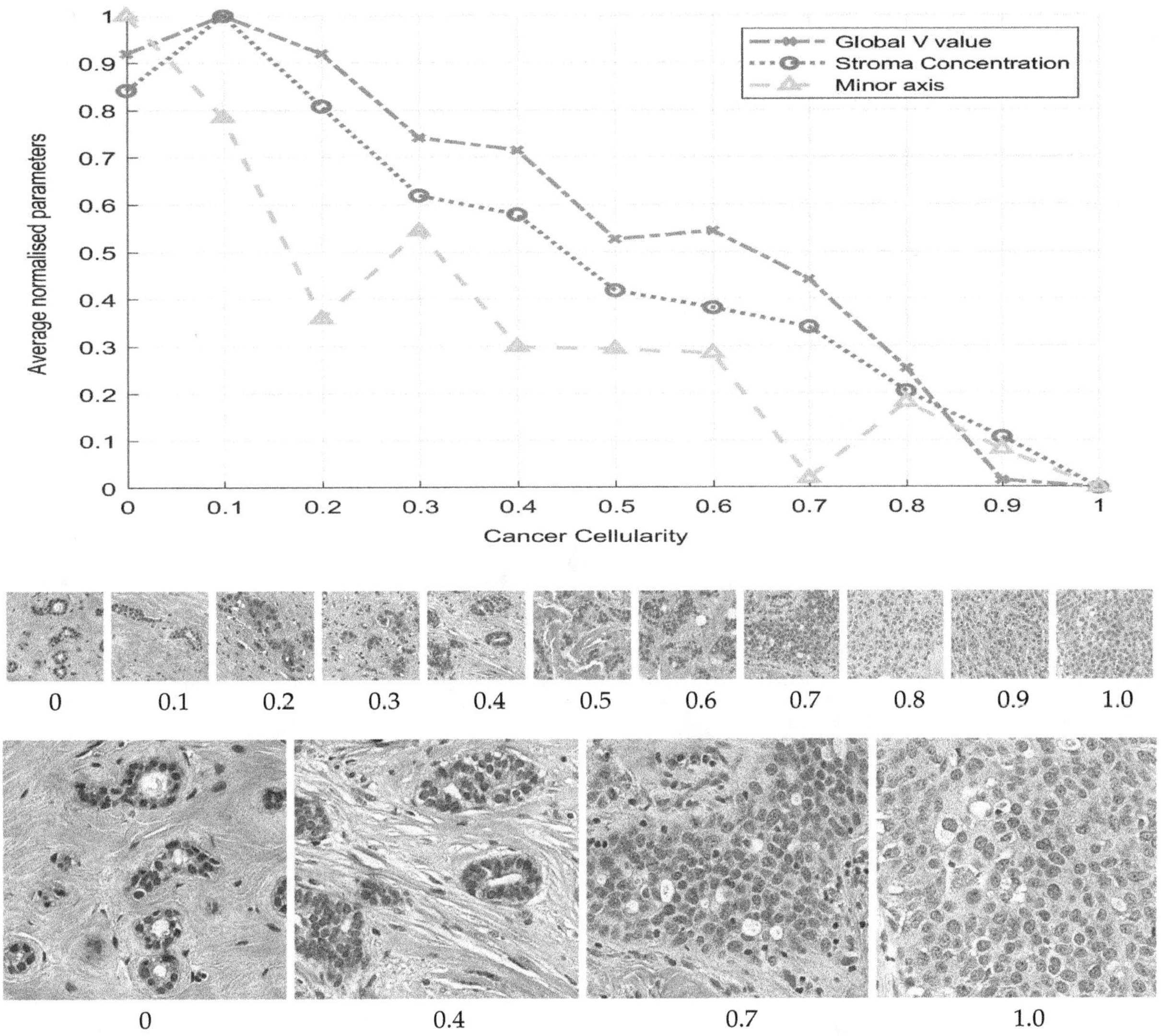

Figure 2. Graphical display of three selected morphological parameters against the cellularity: Global stroma filtered region (o), minor axis (△) and Value concentration in region (x). Cellularity was manually ranked by a pathologist and the parameters automatically extracted. The plots represent average parameter value normalised with maximum value to be compared in the same graph. The graph indicates an inverse relationship between respective parameter and cellularity. Thumbnails show images with cellularity values from zero to one and magnified versions of cases with values 0, 0.4, 0.7, and 1, where the prevalence of cancerous cells can be clearly observed.

The methodology was implemented in Matlab® (The Mathworks™, Natick, MA, USA) 2019b version, with functions from the digital image processing, statistical, and machine learning toolboxes. Additionally, QuPath [53], an open source software for digital pathology image analysis, was used to validate the segmentation results obtained by the methodology. Three regions of interest were selected from each image patch, and more than 150 morphological parameters were extracted at inner segmented cell region, neighbourhood around segmented cell, and the full image patch.

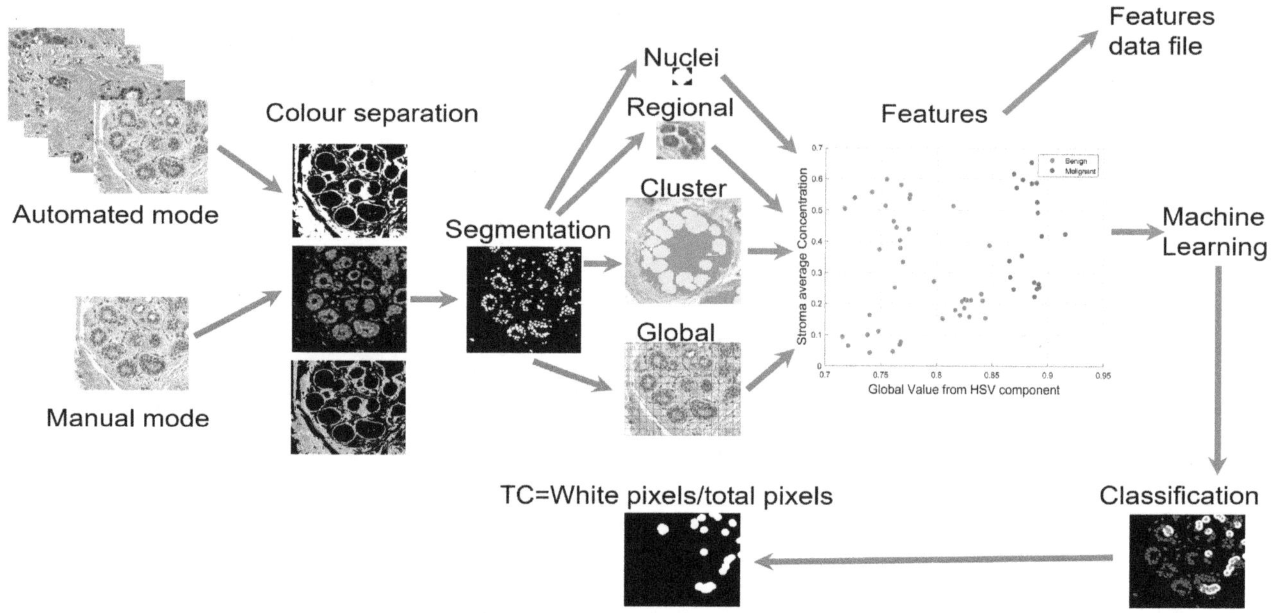

Figure 3. Graphical illustration of the pipeline of the methodology. Under two operational modes images are processed to extract features at nuclei, regional, cluster, and global image regions either to classify and assign Cellularity or to extract same features in order to an archive output.

2.3. Segmentation of Nuclei

At the nuclei region, cells from the image patch are segmented by colour separation and binarisation. The image is converted to HSV colour space and, by K-means clustering [54], three main colour images are extracted, say Ip for pink, Ib for blue, and Iba for the remaining background component image. A special procedure enhances Ib and weakens background region is calculated as:

$$In = K_1(Io. * Im) + K_2 Io + \gamma(Im, 0.1) \quad (1)$$

where Io is the RGB image converted to gray levels and Im is gray image after a median filter of size 3×3 was applied. γ is the gamma correction Im of parameter 0.1 represented as $\gamma(Im,\ 0.1)$. This value was selected as low to start from a lighter background. K_1 and K_2 are constants that control enhancement of nuclei and weaken background intensity, respectively, and they were experimentally adjusted. First, both of the constants were fixed to 0.5 and, as K_1 is increased and K_2 is reduced, the nuclei region is enhanced. The enhanced image In is binarised by Otsu's algorithm [55] combined with watershed [56] separation of touching nuclei. This segmentation procedure is seen in Figure 4 for three TC cases. A validation analysis of this procedure was done by means of Jaccard Index [57], as shown in (e). The reference images were obtained by a manual segmentation while using the QuPath platform. The results indicate an average Jaccard index of 0.73 after comparing cases of low, medium, and high TC. Although this result might be improved, Peikari and co-authors [45] suggest that cell segmentation accuracy does not have a significant effect in TC assessment.

2.4. Extraction of Morphological Parameters

Using the binary image, a set of morphological parameters has been obtained: area, perimeter, roundness, eccentricity, centroid X, centroid Y, major axis, minor axis, and orientation angle. Additionally, a sub region inside the segmented cell body was determined in order to compute the texture and mean HSV values of the nuclei cell body.

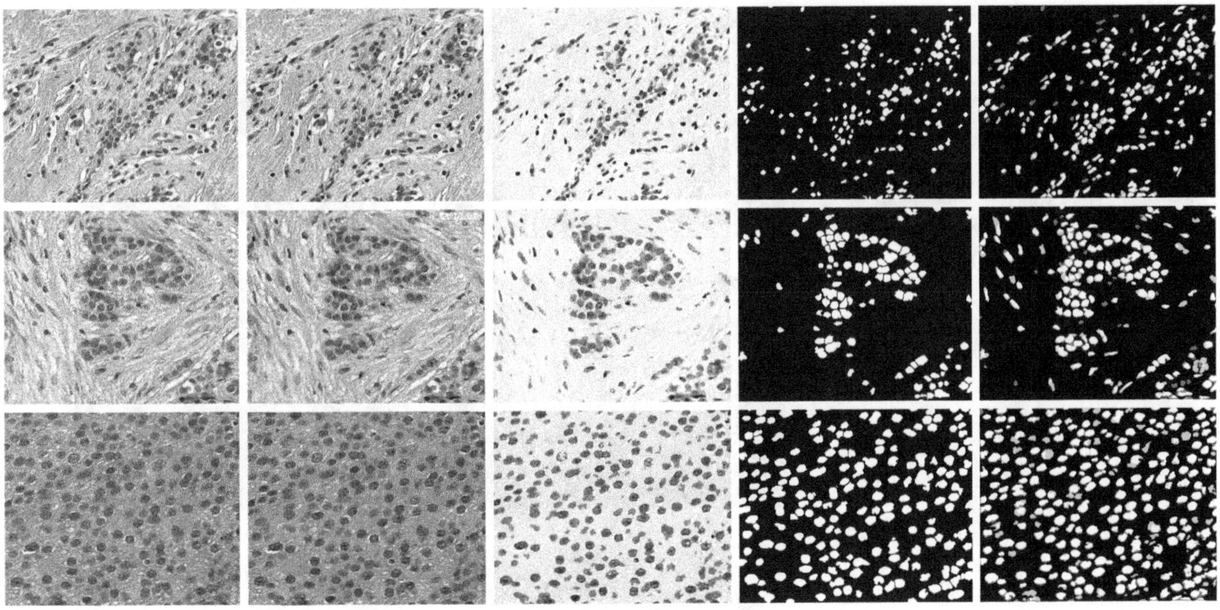

Figure 4. Enhancement of nuclei area. First row corresponds to a Tumour Cellularity (TC) value of zero, second row is an example of TC= 0.5 and third row is TC= 1. Images in column (**a**) are the original image, (**b**) gray level images, (**c**) enhanced images, notice that the nuclei region is darker whilst background becomes lighter, (**d**) Binary image obtained with an adaptive threshold value estimated directly from strongest correlated parameter, and (**e**) validation of nuclei segmentation by Jaccard index. Reference image was manually segmented by using QuPath Platform.

The parameters were extracted from different window sizes surrounding the segmented cell: $30 \times 30, 60 \times 60, 90 \times 90$, and 120×120 pixels. The statistical analysis indicated that the best correlation was obtained from the smallest window size. The parameters estimated are the four bins histogram from HSV image and also the regional concentration R of Ip, Iba, and Ib from its binary image, determined by the ratio of total white pixels T_W by total pixels T_P inside window neighbourhood region, $R = T_W/T_P$. Figure 5 shows a sample patch image, with its corresponding pink, blue, binary, and concentration image components. Brown areas indicate low concentration and white and yellow areas are high concentration. Breast normal tissue images present ducts and sometimes arteries, which are clearly seen as regular clusters of darker blue nuclei grouped into the region, see Figure 6. These are detected based on set theory: let U be the full image, D be the cluster or duct, $D \subseteq U \neq \emptyset$. Subsequently, D regions are obtained by subtracting background image Iba from original image U. The following morphological parameters can be extracted from these regions: total cluster area, roundness, number of cells inside cluster, and distance from cells centroid to cluster centroid.

Concentration parameters from the complete full image patch were computed using original RGB image and transformed to HSV. Additionally, a pink colour filter was implemented by means of the Matlab® colour thresholder, which extracts stroma region from the image and computes its mean value. A summary of the full set of features extracted is presented in Table 1; notice that regional parameters are computed at the different window sizes.

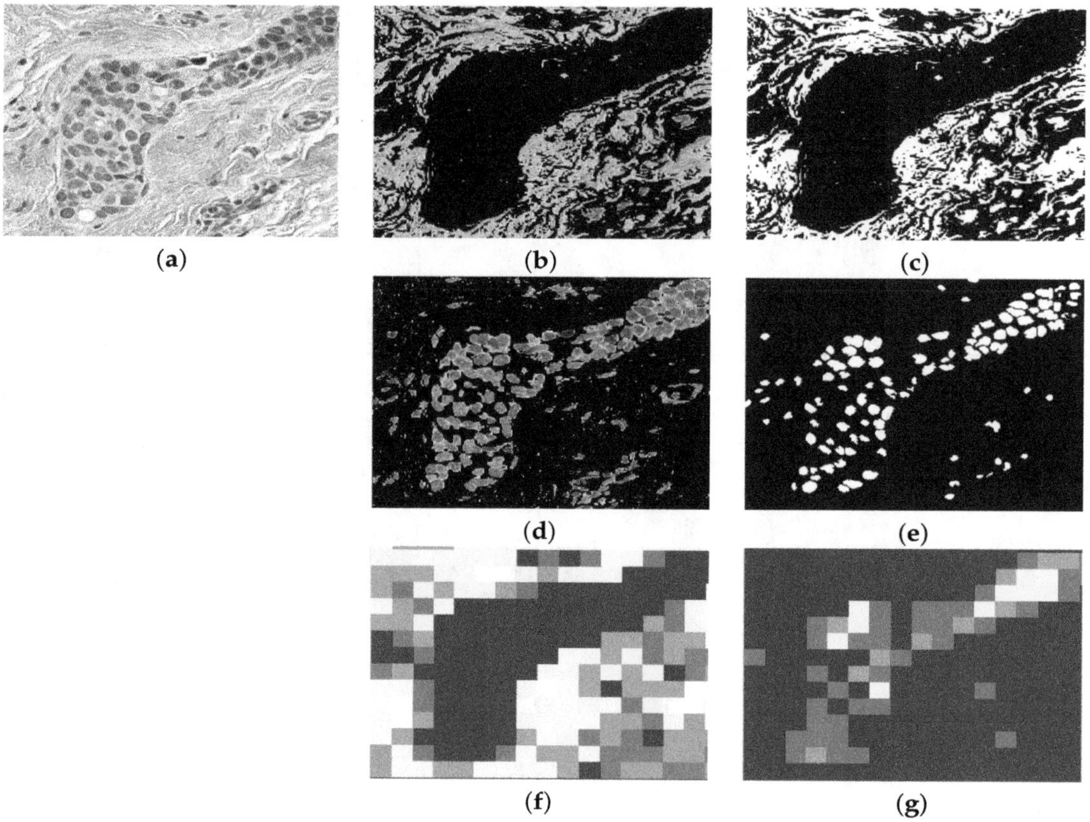

Figure 5. Regional analysis of the data. (**a**) Original image. (**b**) Ip, stroma region image obtained from colour separation. (**c**) Binarised Ip image. (**d**) Ib nuclei image obtained from colour separation. (**e**) Binarised Ib image. (**f**) Regional image concentration of Ip in which brown colour indicates the lowest and white is the highest region concentration. (**g**) Regional density concentration of Ib. This example was processed at 30×30 pixels window.

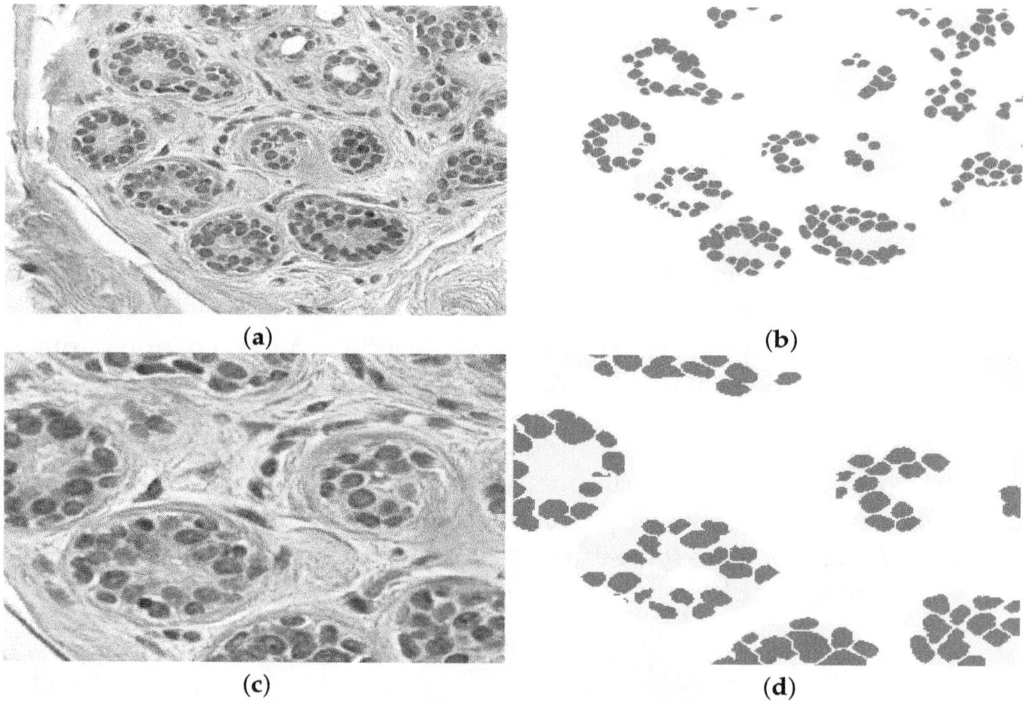

Figure 6. (**a**) The original patch with clear breast ducts. (**b**) Clusters detected by the methodology, every duct or cluster is in yellow and cells inside are in red. Background is labelled in white. (**c**,**d**) Magnified regions of (**a**,**b**).

Table 1. Summary of extracted features. Features at regional level are computed at four different window sizes. Features from the full image represent average values.

Nuclei	**Area**	**Eccentricity**	**Roundness**	**Centroid x, y**
	Perimeter	Orientation	Major Axis	Minor Axis
	Mean Texture Contrast 1	Mean Texture Contrast 2	Mean Texture Homogenity 1	Mean Texture Homogenity 2
	Mean H value inside nuclei	Mean V value inside nuclei	Mean S value inside nuclei	
Regional Concentrations	Stroma Ip	Background Iba	Nuclei Ib	Epithelial tissue from Ib
	Mean H in window	Mean S in window 2	Mean V in window	
	Mean intensity Histogram H 1	Mean intensity Histogram H 2	Mean intensity Histogram H 3	Mean intensity Histogram H 4
	Mean intensity Histogram S 1	Mean intensity Histogram S 2	Mean intensity Histogram S 3	Mean intensity Histogram S 4
	Mean intensity Histogram V 1	Mean intensity Histogram V 2	Mean intensity Histogram V 3	Mean intensity Histogram V 4
Clusters (ducts)	Cluster area	Cluster roundness	Cells inside cluster	Distance to centroid
Global Image Concentrations	Stroma Ip	Background Iba	Nuclei Ib	
	H value	V Value	S Value	

2.5. Correlation Analysis of Morphological Parameters to TC

The full training set was processed to determine all of the morphological parameters at the three region of interest and those corresponding to Cellularity values equal to $(0, 0.1, 0.2, \ldots, 1.0)$ were selected, and their mean, standard deviation, maximum, and minimum values were computed. Subsequently, a linear regression and lasso analysis were determined from both analyses. Parameters of coefficient above 0.80 from linear regression and in concordance with lasso selected parameters after redundant removal yield 22 parameters that have the strongest correlation with TC. The plot in in Figure 2 illustrates three parameters with the strongest correlation with TC.

First, the morphological parameters related to segmented nuclei are: eccentricity, roundness, major axis, minor axis, and perimeter. Subsequently, parameters computed at neighbourhood region are: nuclei density concentration, Hue, Value, and Saturation histograms of the regional HSV colour map image. Finally, parameters that are computed from the full image are: HSV average values from HSV components, nuclei concentration, basement concentration, and stroma average concentration determined at output of the pink colour filter. Some of these parameters are graphically displayed in Figure 7.

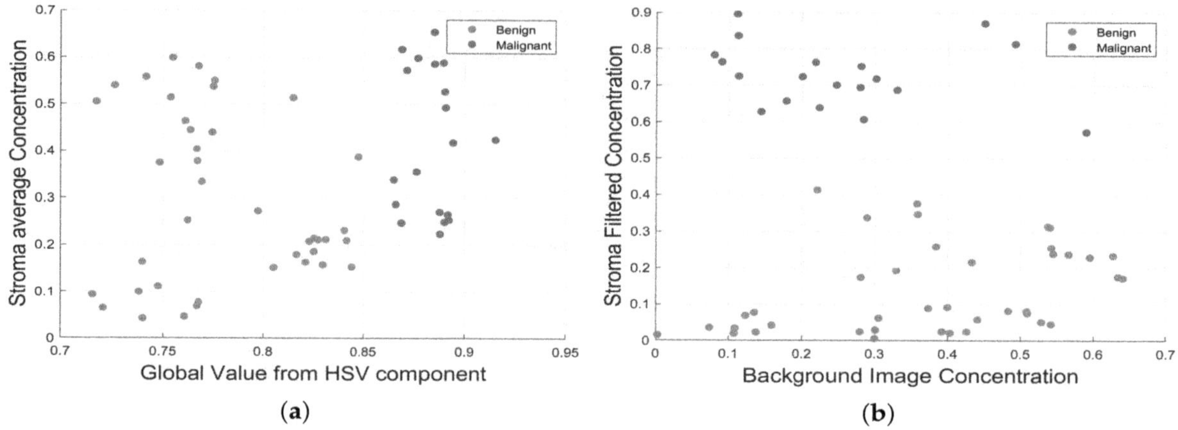

Figure 7. Morphological relationship between the four strongest correlated parameters. (**a**) Global value from HSV component and Stroma average Concentration. (**b**) Background Image Concentration and Stroma Filtered Concentration. In both cases, the benign and malignant cells are highlighted with different colours, which indicate a clear separation.

2.6. *Training of Machine Learning Algorithms*

Machine learning algorithms were trained with the parameter vector of size 22 determined by the statistical correlation analysis. From the training set, 4533 segmented cells were processed and its corresponding extracted parameters were used to generate a prediction function that classifies nuclei cells between malignant and normal cells. Three algorithms were tested: Support Vector Machines, Nearest K-Network, and AdaBoost. The accuracy of training process for every selected method with the training data showed values up to 0.99 due to a high correlation selected features used for training. TPR achieved are 0.97 for SVM, 0.95 for AdaBoost, and 0.97 for KNN (Figure 8). Support Vector Machines (SVM) is a training algorithm for optimal margin classifier [41], and it is based on a determination of a decision function of pattern vectors x of dimension n classifying in either A or B, in our case benign or malignant cells. The input is a set of p examples of x_i, i.e., the 22 strongest correlated features extracted. K-Nearest Neighbour method [42] was also selected, because it is one of the most well known algorithms within clustering and data classification, in our case between benign and malignant classes. AdaBoost [43] is a decision tree type learning algorithm that starts from observations of a certain item that is represented by branches and goes to conclusions about item target value or leaves. It has a best performance on binary classification problems.

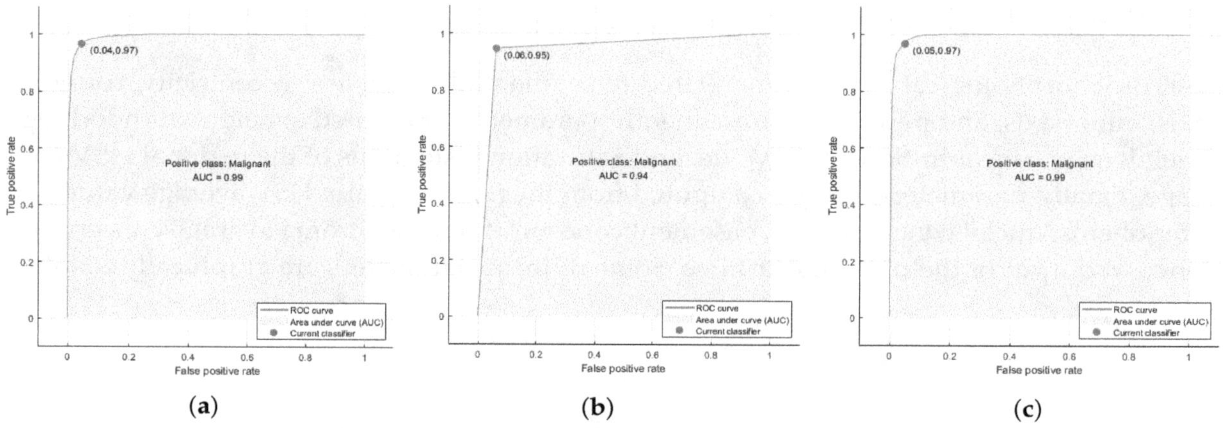

Figure 8. (**a**) Receiver operating characteristic (ROC) curves obtained during training phase for the three selected algorithms. (**a**) Support Vector Machines (SVM), (**b**) AdaBoost , and (**c**) K-Nearest Neighbour (KNN). The higher accuracy value achieved is obtained only with the training set that is highly correlated with Tumour Cellularity (TC).

2.7. Assessment of Tumour Cellularity

The methodology to estimate TC is illustrated in Figure 9, with three representative images with increasing TC from top to bottom in each row. In Figure 9a the nuclei are segmented and their corresponding parameters are extracted. Subsequently, the prediction function classifies every cell in either benign (green) or malignant (red), as illustrated in Figure 9b. Next, an estimation of full cell cytoplasm is done by morphological dilation drawn as the white circles around malignant cells (Figure 9c). The full cellularity that is detected region is shown in Figure 9d. TC is computed as the ratio of the area that is covered by cellularity (white in the figure) over the total area (white and black in figure).

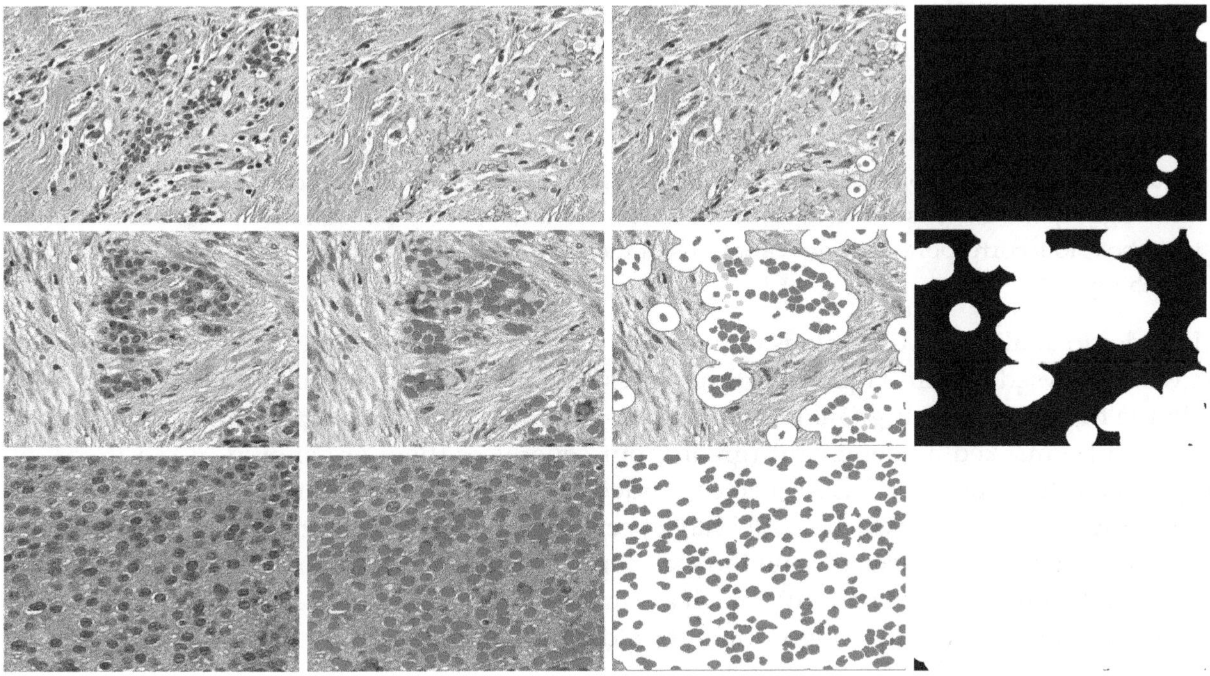

(a) (b) (c) (d)

Figure 9. Visual description of the method. Three TC cases are presented in each row: 0, 0.5 and 1. (**a**) The original image, the image is segmented and key parameters are computed, then a classification predictor estimates either malignant or benign cells, shown in red and green, respectively in (**b**). A dilation of segmented malignant nuclei estimates full cytoplasm of every detected malignant cell (**c**) and TB region is shown in white in (**d**). The cellularity metrics calculated by the proposed methodology are: $TC = 0.0113$, $TC = 0.5181$ and $TC = 0.9936$.

3. Results

An automated estimation of TC was computed from two test data sets. Three prediction functions that were trained by machine learning algorithms were determined to be used with the automated processing software of breast cancer images that classifies cells and computes TC. The method was tested with a training set of 2579 images that were already classified by a pathologist with a TC value. Additionally, it was tested with the 1119 images for submission of SPIE Breast Challenge, with an unknown TC value. Figure 10 shows the statistical behaviour of the method's result for the training set as boxplots.

Dispersion plot indicates the method for approximating to the pathologist classification assignment. The results have a better approximation at higher cellularity values ($TC > 0.70$) and performs well with KNN algorithm. Additionally, around the middle region ($0.4 < TC < 0.6$) has a good approximation with AdaBoost. At low cellularity values ($TC < 0.3$), three methods present deviation, with its higher at cellularity zero, which correspond to images with only benign nuclei cells. According to Minimum Square Error (MSE), SVM performs better overall in the cellularity region.

This result can be validated by a visual inspection of boxplots of Figure 10 in the three cases there is a positive correlation between the actual cellularity (horizontal) and the estimated cellularity (vertical). However, SVM shows less dispersion, especially in the lower values of cellularity as compared with the other two techniques.

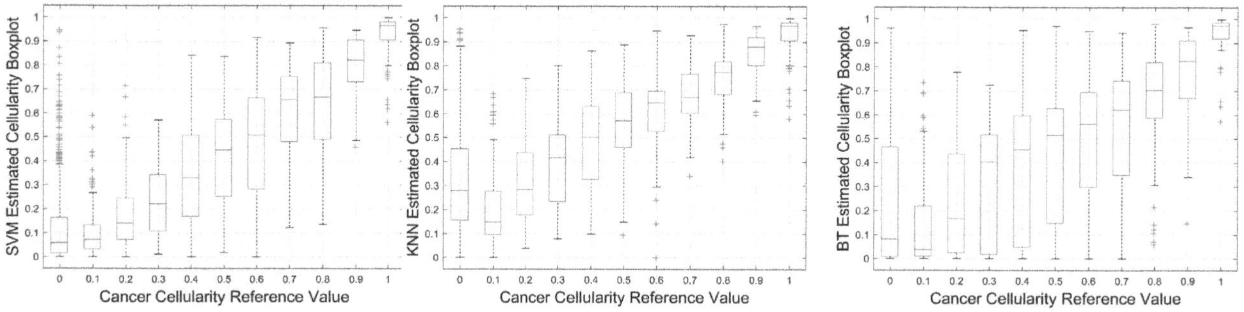

(a) (b)

Figure 10. Results of implementation on Training Data. Boxplots for the Cancer Cellularity Reference Value against: (**a**) SVM estimation, (**b**) KNN estimation and (**c**) BT Estimation. It should be noted that large boxplots correspond to large variations of the estimations and as such, SVM shows the lowest variability

In order to analyse the limitations of the algorithm, the TC assessment outcomes with the highest errors were analysed. Figure 11 presents three cases where the TC was incorrectly calculated. All three cases in the figure are of benignant tissue with no cellularity; this means that most of the segmented cells should be marked as benignant (green), but several of them are shown in red (b–d), which corresponds to false-positive cases. The expanded area around the cell (e) yields a high TC value instead of the correct value which should have been zero. We assume that this problem is because of the limited amount of cells used to train the algorithm. This problem also explains some of the outliers on the boxplots presented in Figure 10, which are mainly observed at low cellularity. Additionally, this suggests that other classification algorithms should be evaluated.

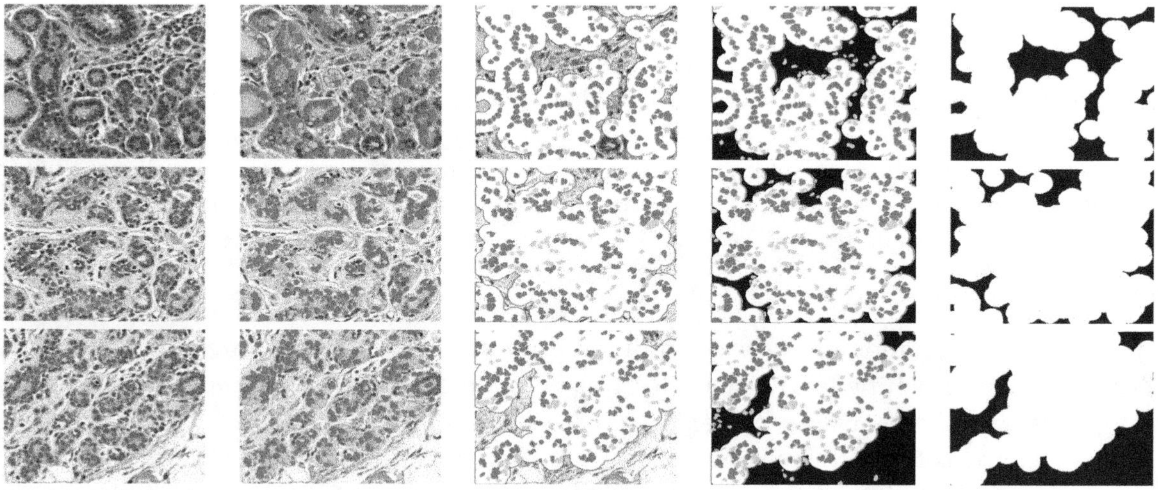

(a) (b) (c) (d) (e)

Figure 11. Three cases where the TC was incorrectly calculated. Each row corresponds to a patch with incorrect TC. Column (**a**) illustrates the original image, and columns (**b–e**) show the step by step process to assess cellularity. (**b**) Corresponds to the segmented image and classified into benign (green) and malignant (red). Columns (**c**,**d**) show expanded region of malignant cells. Column (**e**) corresponds to cancer cell region in white, used to compute TC. Three worst cases correspond to a TC of zero; this means there would not be any malignant cell and TC image must be completely black. Several cells were miss classified which yields to a TC wrong assessment. Estimated TC values are: 0.75, 0.81, and 0.75, instead of zero.

Statistical analysis of the training set revealed 22 key parameters that have a strong correlation to TC. The Stroma concentration (r = −0.9786), global Value of HSV component (r = −0.9728), regional histogram bins (r = −0.9659), and minor axis (r = 0.8939) from nuclei morphology were the strongest parameters, as shown in Figure 2.

This result revealed that the stroma region has a significant relation to TC, which is in agreement with the results of the hand engineering method by [45] that was trained by a 125-dimensional feature vector reported a 0.75 ICC (first column of Table 2). Lower and upper-bounds are shown in square brackets. Our methodology is also a hand engineering, but trained with only 22 key morphological parameters (second column of Table 2), indicates a 0.78 ICC. This result outperformed those that were obtained by the method of Peikari. The results based on Deep Learning techniques like a combined hand engineering Deep Neural Network reported by Akbar [20] is slightly above the proposed methodology (third column of Table 2). Finally, the methodology proposed was used to process the test set and the results were submitted to the challenge contest. The prediction probability result obtained from contest was $P_k = 0.76$.

Table 2. Comparison of the Intra-class Correlation Coefficients (ICC) of the proposed methodology against a Hand Engineering Methodology (Peikari [45]) and a combined deep learning and hand engineering methodology (Akbar [20]). Lower and upper bounds are shown in square brackets. Notice the closeness of the results of the proposed methodology against the Deep Learning approach.

	Hand Engineering (Peikari)	**Key Parameters (Our methodology)**	**Combined Deep Network (Akbar)**
ICC	0.75	0.78	0.79
[L,U]	[0.71, 0.79]	[0.75, 0.80]	[0.76, 0.81]

4. Discussion

A computer methodology that automatically processes H&E histopathology digital images based in the extraction of main morphological parameters at a cell, regional, and global level is presented in this paper. The methodology processed a training set of breast cancer images under NAT treatment and the results indicate 22 key morphological parameters are strongly correlated with cellularity. Interesting results were revealed from the correlation analysis of the morphological parameters. The strongest related parameter was stroma density, in agreement with Beck et al. [16], which is, the histology of stroma correlates with prognostic in breast cancer. Three different machine learning algorithms for cell classification were evaluated and compared in order to determine tumour regions. The best result was obtained with Support Vector Machines (SVM) algorithm. The relevance of this paper is a selection of a key parameters to train the algorithms, which results in a better performance of similar techniques; however, the reported deep learning algorithms outperform this result, which is a motivation to explore these techniques in the future.

Author Contributions: Conceptualisation, M.A.O.-R. and C.C.R.-A.; methodology, M.A.O.-R. and C.C.R.-A.; software, M.A.O.-R.; validation, M.A.O.-R., V.G.G. and C.C.R.-A.; formal analysis, M.A.O.-R. and C.C.R.-A.; investigation, M.A.O.-R. and C.C.R.-A.; resources, M.A.O.-R. and C.C.R.-A.; data curation, M.A.O.-R. and C.C.R.-A.; writing—original draft preparation, M.A.O.-R., C.K. and C.C.R.-A.; writing—review and editing, M.A.O.-R., C.K., V.G.G. and C.C.R.-A.; visualisation, M.A.O.-R. and C.C.R.-A.; supervision, V.G.G. and C.C.R.-A. All authors have read and agreed to the published version of the manuscript.

Acknowledgments: The authors would like to thank Sunnybrook Health Sciences Centre, Toronto, for the breast cancer NAT images. We also would like to thank Kenny H. Chan for validating our test results which were submitted to SPIE Breast Challenge contest.

Abbreviations

The following abbreviations are used in this manuscript:

TC	Tumour Cellularity
NAT	Neo-Adjuvant treatment
WSIs	Whole slide images
H&E	Hematoxylin and Eosin
ICC	Intraclass correlation coefficient
ML	Machine Learning
IHC	Immunohistochemistry
CAD	Computer-assisted diagnosis
RCB	Residual Cancer Burden
pCR	Pathological complete response
TB	Tumour Bed
GT	Ground Truth
HSV	Hue, Saturation, Value
RGB	Red, Green, Blue
SVM	Support Vector Machines

References

1. Irshad, H.; Veillard, A.; Roux, L.; Racoceanu, D. Methods for nuclei detection, segmentation, and classification in digital histopathology: A review-current status and future potential. *IEEE Rev. Biomed. Eng.* **2013**, *7*, 97–114. [CrossRef] [PubMed]
2. Gurcan, M.N.; Boucheron, L.E.; Can, A.; Madabhushi, A.; Rajpoot, N.M.; Yener, B. Histopathological Image Analysis: A Review. *IEEE Rev. Biomed. Eng.* **2009**, *2*, 147–171. [CrossRef] [PubMed]
3. Madabhushi, A.; Lee, G. Image analysis and machine learning in digital pathology: Challenges and opportunities. *Med. Image Anal.* **2016**, *33*, 170–175. [CrossRef] [PubMed]
4. Kather, J.N.; Krisam, J.; Charoentong, P.; Luedde, T.; Herpel, E.; Weis, C.A.; Gaiser, T.; Marx, A.; Valous, N.A.; Ferber, D.; et al. Predicting survival from colorectal cancer histology slides using deep learning: A retrospective multicenter study. *PLoS Med.* **2019**, *16*, e1002730. [CrossRef] [PubMed]
5. Chan, J.K.C. The Wonderful Colors of the Hematoxylin–Eosin Stain in Diagnostic Surgical Pathology. *Int. J. Surg. Pathol.* **2014**, *22*, 12–32. [CrossRef] [PubMed]
6. Di Cataldo, S.; Ficarra, E.; Macii, E. Computer-aided techniques for chromogenic immunohistochemistry: Status and directions. *Comput. Biol. Med.* **2012**, *42*, 1012–1025. [CrossRef]
7. Okamura, S.; Osaki, T.; Nishimura, K.; Ohsaki, H.; Shintani, M.; Matsuoka, H.; Maeda, K.; Shiogama, K.; Itoh, T.; Kamoshida, S. Thymidine kinase-1/CD31 double immunostaining for identifying activated tumor vessels. *Biotech. Histochem. Off. Publ. Biol. Stain Comm.* **2019**, *94*, 60–64. [CrossRef]
8. Mohamed, S.Y.; Mohammed, H.L.; Ibrahim, H.M.; Mohamed, E.M.; Salah, M. Role of VEGF, CD105, and CD31 in the Prognosis of Colorectal Cancer Cases. *J. Gastrointest. Cancer* **2019**, *50*, 23–34. [CrossRef]
9. Reyes-Aldasoro, C.C.; Williams, L.J.; Akerman, S.; Kanthou, C.; Tozer, G.M. An automatic algorithm for the segmentation and morphological analysis of microvessels in immunostained histological tumour sections. *J. Microsc.* **2011**, *242*, 262–278. [CrossRef]
10. Maltby, S.; Wohlfarth, C.; Gold, M.; Zbytnuik, L.; Hughes, M.R.; McNagny, K.M. CD34 is required for infiltration of eosinophils into the colon and pathology associated with DSS-induced ulcerative colitis. *Am. J. Pathol.* **2010**, *177*, 1244–1254. [CrossRef]
11. Blanchet, M.R.; Bennett, J.L.; Gold, M.J.; Levantini, E.; Tenen, D.G.; Girard, M.; Cormier, Y.; McNagny, K.M. CD34 is required for dendritic cell trafficking and pathology in murine hypersensitivity pneumonitis. *Am. J. Respir. Crit. Care Med.* **2011**, *184*, 687–698. [CrossRef] [PubMed]
12. Chen, W.J.; He, D.S.; Tang, R.X.; Ren, F.H.; Chen, G. Ki-67 is a valuable prognostic factor in gliomas: Evidence from a systematic review and meta-analysis. *Asian Pac. J. Cancer Prev.* **2015**, *16*, 411–420. [CrossRef] [PubMed]

13. Ishibashi, N.; Nishimaki, H.; Maebayashi, T.; Hata, M.; Adachi, K.; Sakurai, K.; Masuda, S.; Okada, M. Changes in the Ki-67 labeling index between primary breast cancer and metachronous metastatic axillary lymph node: A retrospective observational study. *Thorac. Cancer* **2019**, *10*, 96–102. [CrossRef] [PubMed]
14. Sen, A.; Mitra, S.; Das, R.N.; Dasgupta, S.; Saha, K.; Chatterjee, U.; Mukherjee, K.; Datta, C.; Chattopadhyay, B.K. Expression of CDX-2 and Ki-67 in different grades of colorectal adenocarcinomas. *Indian J. Pathol. Microbiol.* **2015**, *58*, 158–162. [CrossRef]
15. Komura, D.; Ishikawa, S. Machine learning methods for histopathological image analysis. *Comput. Struct. Biotechnol. J.* **2018**, *16*, 34–42. [CrossRef]
16. Beck, A.H.; Sangoi, A.R.; Leung, S.; Marinelli, R.J.; Nielsen, T.O.; van de Vijver, M.J.; West, R.B.; van de Rijn, M.; Koller, D. Systematic analysis of breast cancer morphology uncovers stromal features associated with survival. *Sci. Transl. Med.* **2011**, *3*, 108ra113. [CrossRef]
17. DeSantis, C.E.; Ma, J.; Goding Sauer, A.; Newman, L.A.; Jemal, A. Breast cancer statistics, 2017, racial disparity in mortality by state. *CA A Cancer J. Clin.* **2017**, *67*, 439–448. [CrossRef]
18. Siegel, R.L.; Miller, K.D.; Jemal, A. Cancer statistics, 2019. *CA A Cancer J. Clin.* **2019**, *69*, 7–34. [CrossRef]
19. Veta, M.; Pluim, J.P.W.; Diest, P.J.V.; Viergever, M.A. Breast Cancer Histopathology Image Analysis: A Review. *IEEE Trans. Biomed. Eng.* **2014**, *61*, 1400–1411. [CrossRef]
20. Akbar, S.; Peikari, M.; Salama, S.; Panah, A.Y.; Nofech-Mozes, S.; Martel, A.L. Automated and manual quantification of tumour cellularity in digital slides for tumour burden assessment. *Sci. Rep.* **2019**, *9*, 1–9. [CrossRef]
21. Nahleh, Z.; Sivasubramaniam, D.; Dhaliwal, S.; Sundarajan, V.; Komrokji, R. Residual cancer burden in locally advanced breast cancer: A superior tool. *Curr. Oncol.* **2008**, *15*, 271–278. [CrossRef] [PubMed]
22. Kaufmann, M.; Hortobagyi, G.N.; Goldhirsch, A.; Scholl, S.; Makris, A.; Valagussa, P.; Blohmer, J.U.; Eiermann, W.; Jackesz, R.; Jonat, W.; et al. Recommendations from an international expert panel on the use of neoadjuvant (primary) systemic treatment of operable breast cancer: An update. *J. Clin. Oncol. Off. J. Am. Soc. Clin. Oncol.* **2006**, *24*, 1940–1949. [CrossRef] [PubMed]
23. Symmans, W.F.; Peintinger, F.; Hatzis, C.; Rajan, R.; Kuerer, H.; Valero, V.; Assad, L.; Poniecka, A.; Hennessy, B.; Green, M.; et al. Measurement of residual breast cancer burden to predict survival after neoadjuvant chemotherapy. *J. Clin. Oncol. Off. J. Am. Soc. Clin. Oncol.* **2007**, *25*, 4414–4422. [CrossRef]
24. Kumar, S.; Badhe, B.A.; Krishnan, K.; Sagili, H. Study of tumour cellularity in locally advanced breast carcinoma on neo-adjuvant chemotherapy. *J. Clin. Diagn. Res.* **2014**, *8*, FC09. [PubMed]
25. Peintinger, F.; Kuerer, H.M.; McGuire, S.E.; Bassett, R.; Pusztai, L.; Symmans, W.F. Residual specimen cellularity after neoadjuvant chemotherapy for breast cancer. *Br. J. Surg.* **2008**, *95*, 433–437. [CrossRef]
26. Okines, A.F. T-DM1 in the Neo-Adjuvant Treatment of HER2-Positive Breast Cancer: Impact of the KRISTINE (TRIO-021) Trial. *Rev. Recent Clin. Trials* **2017**, *12*, 216–222. [CrossRef]
27. van Zeijl, M.C.T.; van den Eertwegh, A.J.; Haanen, J.B.; Wouters, M.W.J.M. (Neo)adjuvant systemic therapy for melanoma. *Eur. J. Surg. Oncol. J. Eur. Soc. Surg. Oncol. Br. Assoc. Surg. Oncol.* **2017**, *43*, 534–543. [CrossRef]
28. Tann, U.W. Neo-adjuvant hormonal therapy of prostate cancer. *Urol. Res.* **1997**, *25*, S57–S62. [CrossRef]
29. Bourut, C.; Chenu, E.; Mathé, G. Can neo-adjuvant chemotherapy prevent residual tumors? *Bull. Soc. Sci. Medicales Grand-Duche Luxemb.* **1989**, *126*, 59–63.
30. Stolwijk, C.; Wagener, D.J.; Van den Broek, P.; Levendag, P.C.; Kazem, I.; Bruaset, I.; De Mulder, P.H. Randomized neo-adjuvant chemotherapy trial for advanced head and neck cancer. *Neth. J. Med.* **1985**, *28*, 347–351.
31. Rastogi, P.; Wickerham, D.L.; Geyer, C.E.; Mamounas, E.P.; Julian, T.B.; Wolmark, N. Milestone clinical trials of the National Surgical Adjuvant Breast and Bowel Project (NSABP). *Chin. Clin. Oncol.* **2017**, *6*, 7. [CrossRef]
32. Fatakdawala, H.; Xu, J.; Basavanhally, A.; Bhanot, G.; Ganesan, S.; Feldman, M.; Tomaszewski, J.E.; Madabhushi, A. Expectation–Maximization-Driven Geodesic Active Contour With Overlap Resolution (EMaGACOR): Application to Lymphocyte Segmentation on Breast Cancer Histopathology. *IEEE Trans. Biomed. Eng.* **2010**, *57*, 1676–1689. [CrossRef] [PubMed]
33. Veta, M.; van Diest, P.J.; Kornegoor, R.; Huisman, A.; Viergever, M.A.; Pluim, J.P.W. Automatic Nuclei Segmentation in H&E Stained Breast Cancer Histopathology Images. *PLoS ONE* **2013**, *8*, e70221. [CrossRef]
34. Al-Kofahi, Y.; Lassoued, W.; Lee, W.; Roysam, B. Improved Automatic Detection and Segmentation of Cell Nuclei in Histopathology Images. *IEEE Trans. Biomed. Eng.* **2010**, *57*, 841–852. [CrossRef] [PubMed]

35. Yamada, M.; Saito, A.; Yamamoto, Y.; Cosatto, E.; Kurata, A.; Nagao, T.; Tateishi, A.; Kuroda, M. Quantitative nucleic features are effective for discrimination of intraductal proliferative lesions of the breast. *J. Pathol. Inform.* **2016**, *7*. [CrossRef]
36. Fondón, I.; Sarmiento, A.; García, A.I.; Silvestre, M.; Eloy, C.; Polónia, A.; Aguiar, P. Automatic classification of tissue malignancy for breast carcinoma diagnosis. *Comput. Biol. Med.* **2018**, *96*, 41–51. [CrossRef]
37. De Lima, S.M.L.; da Silva-Filho, A.G.; dos Santos, W.P. Detection and classification of masses in mammographic images in a multi-kernel approach. *Comput. Methods Programs Biomed.* **2016**, *134*, 11–29. [CrossRef]
38. Araújo, T.; Aresta, G.; Castro, E.; Rouco, J.; Aguiar, P.; Eloy, C.; Polónia, A.; Campilho, A. Classification of breast cancer histology images using Convolutional Neural Networks. *PLoS ONE* **2017**, *12*, e0177544. doi:10.1371/journal.pone.0177544. [CrossRef]
39. Niu, Q.; Jiang, X.; Li, Q.; Zheng, Z.; Du, H.; Wu, S.; Zhang, X. Texture features and pharmacokinetic parameters in differentiating benign and malignant breast lesions by dynamic contrast enhanced magnetic resonance imaging. *Oncol. Lett.* **2018**, *16*, 4607–4613. [CrossRef]
40. Dong, F.; Irshad, H.; Oh, E.Y.; Lerwill, M.F.; Brachtel, E.F.; Jones, N.C.; Knoblauch, N.W.; Montaser-Kouhsari, L.; Johnson, N.B.; Rao, L.K.F.; et al. Computational Pathology to Discriminate Benign from Malignant Intraductal Proliferations of the Breast. *PLoS ONE* **2014**, *9*, e114885. [CrossRef]
41. Boser, B.E.; Guyon, I.M.; Vapnik, V.N. A Training Algorithm for Optimal Margin Classifiers. In Proceedings of the 5th Annual ACM Workshop on Computational Learning Theory, Pittsburgh, PA, USA, 27–29 July 1992; ACM Press New York, NY, USA, 1992; pp. 144–152.
42. Cover, T.; Hart, P. Nearest neighbor pattern classification. *IEEE Trans. Inf. Theory* **1967**, *13*, 21–27. [CrossRef]
43. Schapire, R.E.; Singer, Y. Improved boosting algorithms using confidence-rated predictions. *Mach. Learn.* **1999**, *37*, 297–336. [CrossRef]
44. Romagnoli, G.; Wiedermann, M.; Hübner, F.; Wenners, A.; Mathiak, M.; Röcken, C.; Maass, N.; Klapper, W.; Alkatout, I. Morphological Evaluation of Tumor-Infiltrating Lymphocytes (TILs) to Investigate Invasive Breast Cancer Immunogenicity, Reveal Lymphocytic Networks and Help Relapse Prediction: A Retrospective Study. *Int. J. Mol. Sci.* **2017**, *18*, 1936. [CrossRef] [PubMed]
45. Peikari, M.; Salama, S.; Nofech-Mozes, S.; Martel, A.L. Automatic cellularity assessment from post-treated breast surgical specimens. *Cytom. Part A J. Int. Soc. Anal. Cytol.* **2017**, *91*, 1078–1087. [CrossRef] [PubMed]
46. Soffer, S.; Ben-Cohen, A.; Shimon, O.; Amitai, M.M.; Greenspan, H.; Klang, E. Convolutional Neural Networks for Radiologic Images: A Radiologist's Guide. *Radiology* **2019**, *290*, 590–606. [CrossRef] [PubMed]
47. Kumar, N.; Gupta, R.; Gupta, S. Whole Slide Imaging (WSI) in Pathology: Current Perspectives and Future Directions. *J. Digit. Imaging* **2020**. [CrossRef]
48. Sirinukunwattana, K.; Raza, S.E.A.; Tsang, Y.W.; Snead, D.R.J.; Cree, I.A.; Rajpoot, N.M. Locality Sensitive Deep Learning for Detection and Classification of Nuclei in Routine Colon Cancer Histology Images. *IEEE Trans. Med. Imaging* **2016**, *35*, 1196–1206. [CrossRef]
49. Huang, L.; Xia, W.; Zhang, B.; Qiu, B.; Gao, X. MSFCN-multiple supervised fully convolutional networks for the osteosarcoma segmentation of CT images. *Comput. Methods Programs Biomed.* **2017**, *143*, 67–74. [CrossRef]
50. Arjmand, A.; Angelis, C.T.; Christou, V.; Tzallas, A.T.; Tsipouras, M.G.; Glavas, E.; Forlano, R.; Manousou, P.; Giannakeas, N. Training of Deep Convolutional Neural Networks to Identify Critical Liver Alterations in Histopathology Image Samples. *Appl. Sci.* **2020**, *10*, 42. [CrossRef]
51. Xu, J.; Luo, X.; Wang, G.; Gilmore, H.; Madabhushi, A. A Deep Convolutional Neural Network for segmenting and classifying epithelial and stromal regions in histopathological images. *Neurocomputing* **2016**, *191*, 214–223. [CrossRef]
52. Pei, Z.; Cao, S.; Lu, L.; Chen, W. Direct Cellularity Estimation on Breast Cancer Histopathology Images Using Transfer Learning. *Comput. Math. Methods Med.* **2019**, *2019*, 3041250. [CrossRef]
53. Bankhead, P.; Loughrey, M.B.; Fernández, J.A.; Dombrowski, Y.; McArt, D.G.; Dunne, P.D.; McQuaid, S.; Gray, R.T.; Murray, L.J.; Coleman, H.G.; et al. QuPath: Open source software for digital pathology image analysis. *Sci. Rep.* **2017**, *7*, 16878. [CrossRef]
54. Arthur, D.; Vassilvitskii, S. K-means++: The advantages of careful seeding. In Proceedings of the 18th Annual ACM-SIAM Symposium on Discrete Algorithms, New Orleans, LA, USA, 7–9 January 2007; pp. 1027–1035.
55. Otsu, N. A Threshold Selection Method from Gray-Level Histograms. *IEEE Trans. Syst. Man Cybern.* **1979**, *9*, 62–66. [CrossRef]

56. Yang, X.; Li, H.; Zhou, X. Nuclei Segmentation Using Marker-Controlled Watershed, Tracking Using Mean-Shift, and Kalman Filter in Time-Lapse Microscopy. *IEEE Trans. Circuits Syst. I* **2006**, *53*, 2405–2414. [CrossRef]
57. Jaccard, P. Étude comparative de la distribution florale dans une portion des Alpes et des Jura. *Bull. Soc. Vaudoise Sci. Nat.* **1901**, *37*, 547–579.

8

A Survey of Deep Learning for Lung Disease Detection on Medical Images: State-of-the-Art, Taxonomy, Issues and Future Directions

Stefanus Tao Hwa Kieu [1], Abdullah Bade [1], Mohd Hanafi Ahmad Hijazi [2,*] and Hoshang Kolivand [3]

[1] Faculty of Science and Natural Resources, Universiti Malaysia Sabah, Kota Kinabalu 88400, Sabah, Malaysia; stefanuskieu@gmail.com (S.T.H.K.); abb@ums.edu.my (A.B.)
[2] Faculty of Computing and Informatics, Universiti Malaysia Sabah, Kota Kinabalu 88400, Sabah, Malaysia
[3] School of Computer Science and Mathematics, Liverpool John Moores University, Liverpool L3 3AF, UK; H.Kolivand@ljmu.ac.uk
* Correspondence: hanafi@ums.edu.my

Abstract: The recent developments of deep learning support the identification and classification of lung diseases in medical images. Hence, numerous work on the detection of lung disease using deep learning can be found in the literature. This paper presents a survey of deep learning for lung disease detection in medical images. There has only been one survey paper published in the last five years regarding deep learning directed at lung diseases detection. However, their survey is lacking in the presentation of taxonomy and analysis of the trend of recent work. The objectives of this paper are to present a taxonomy of the state-of-the-art deep learning based lung disease detection systems, visualise the trends of recent work on the domain and identify the remaining issues and potential future directions in this domain. Ninety-eight articles published from 2016 to 2020 were considered in this survey. The taxonomy consists of seven attributes that are common in the surveyed articles: image types, features, data augmentation, types of deep learning algorithms, transfer learning, the ensemble of classifiers and types of lung diseases. The presented taxonomy could be used by other researchers to plan their research contributions and activities. The potential future direction suggested could further improve the efficiency and increase the number of deep learning aided lung disease detection applications.

Keywords: deep learning; lung disease detection; taxonomy; medical images

---

1. Introduction

Lung diseases, also known as respiratory diseases, are diseases of the airways and the other structures of the lungs [1]. Examples of lung disease are pneumonia, tuberculosis and Coronavirus Disease 2019 (COVID-19). According to Forum of International Respiratory Societies [2], about 334 million people suffer from asthma, and, each year, tuberculosis kills 1.4 million people, 1.6 million people die from lung cancer, while pneumonia also kills millions of people. The COVID-19 pandemic impacted the whole world [3], infecting millions of people and burdening healthcare systems [4]. It is clear that lung diseases are one of the leading causes of death and disability in this world. Early detection plays a key role in increasing the chances of recovery and improve long-term survival rates [5,6]. Traditionally, lung disease can be detected via skin test, blood test, sputum sample test [7], chest X-ray examination and computed tomography (CT) scan examination [8]. Recently, deep learning has shown great potential when applied on medical images for disease detection, including lung disease.

Deep learning is a subfield of machine learning relating to algorithms inspired by the function and structure of the brain. Recent developments in machine learning, particularly deep learning, support the identification, quantification and classification of patterns in medical images [9]. These developments were made possible due to the ability of deep learning to learned features merely from data, instead of hand-designed features based on domain-specific knowledge. Deep learning is quickly becoming state of the art, leading to improved performance in numerous medical applications. Consequently, these advancements assist clinicians in detecting and classifying certain medical conditions efficiently [10].

Numerous works on the detection of lung disease using deep learning can be found in the literature. To the best of our knowledge, however, only one survey paper has been published in the last five years to analyse the state-of-the-art work on this topic [11]. In that paper, the history of deep learning and its applications in pulmonary imaging are presented. Major applications of deep learning techniques on several lung diseases, namely pulmonary nodule diseases, pulmonary embolism, pneumonia, and interstitial lung disease, are also described. In addition, the analysis of several common deep learning network structures used in medical image processing is presented. However, their survey is lacking in the presentation of taxonomy and analysis of the trend of recent work. A taxonomy shows relationships between previous work and categorises them based on the identified attributes that could improve reader understanding of the topic. Analysis of trend, on the other hand, provides an overview of the research direction of the topic of interest identified from the previous work. In this paper, a taxonomy of deep learning applications on lung diseases and a trend analysis on the topic are presented. The remaining issues and possible future direction are also described.

The aims of this paper are as follows: (1) produce a taxonomy of the state-of-the-art deep learning based lung disease detection systems; (2) visualise the trends of recent work on the domain; and (3) identify the remaining issues and describes potential future directions in this domain. This paper is organised as follows. Section 2 presents the methodology of conducting this survey. Section 3 describes the general processes of using deep learning to detect lung disease in medical images. Section 4 presents the taxonomy, with detailed explanations of each subtopic within the taxonomy. The analysis of trend, research gap and future directions of lung disease detection using deep learning are presented in Section 5. Section 6 describes the limitation of the survey. Section 7 concludes this paper.

2. Methodology

In this section, the methodology used to conduct the survey of recent lung disease detection using deep learning is described. Figure 1 shows the flowchart of the methodology used.

First, a suitable database, as a main source of reference, of articles was identified. The Scopus database was selected as it is one of the largest databases of scientific peer-reviewed articles. However, several significant articles, indexed by Google Scholar but not Scopus, are also included based on the number of citations that they have received. Some preprint articles on COVID-19 are also included as the disease has just recently emerged. To ensure that this survey only covers the state-of-the-art works, only articles published recently (2016–2020) are considered. However, several older but significant articles are included too. To search for all possible deep learning aided lung disease detection articles, relevant keywords were used to search for the articles. The keywords used were "deep learning", "detection", "classification", "CNN", "lung disease", "Tuberculosis", "pneumonia", "lung cancer", "COVID-19" and "Coronavirus". Studies were limited to articles written in English only. At the end of this phase, we identified 366 articles.

Second, to select only the relevant works, screening was performed. During the screening, only the title and abstract were assessed. The main selection criteria were this survey is only interested in work, whereby deep learning algorithms were applied to detect the relevant diseases. Articles considered not relevant were excluded. Based on the screening performed, only 98 articles were shortlisted.

Last, for all the articles screened, the eligibility inspection was conducted. Similar criteria, as in the screening phase, were used, whereby the full-text inspection of the articles was performed instead. All 98 screened articles passed this phase and were included in this survey. Out of the eligible articles, 90 were published in 2018 and onwards. This signifies that lung disease detection using deep learning is still a very active field. Figure 1 shows the numbers of studies identified, screened, assessed for eligibility and included in this survey.

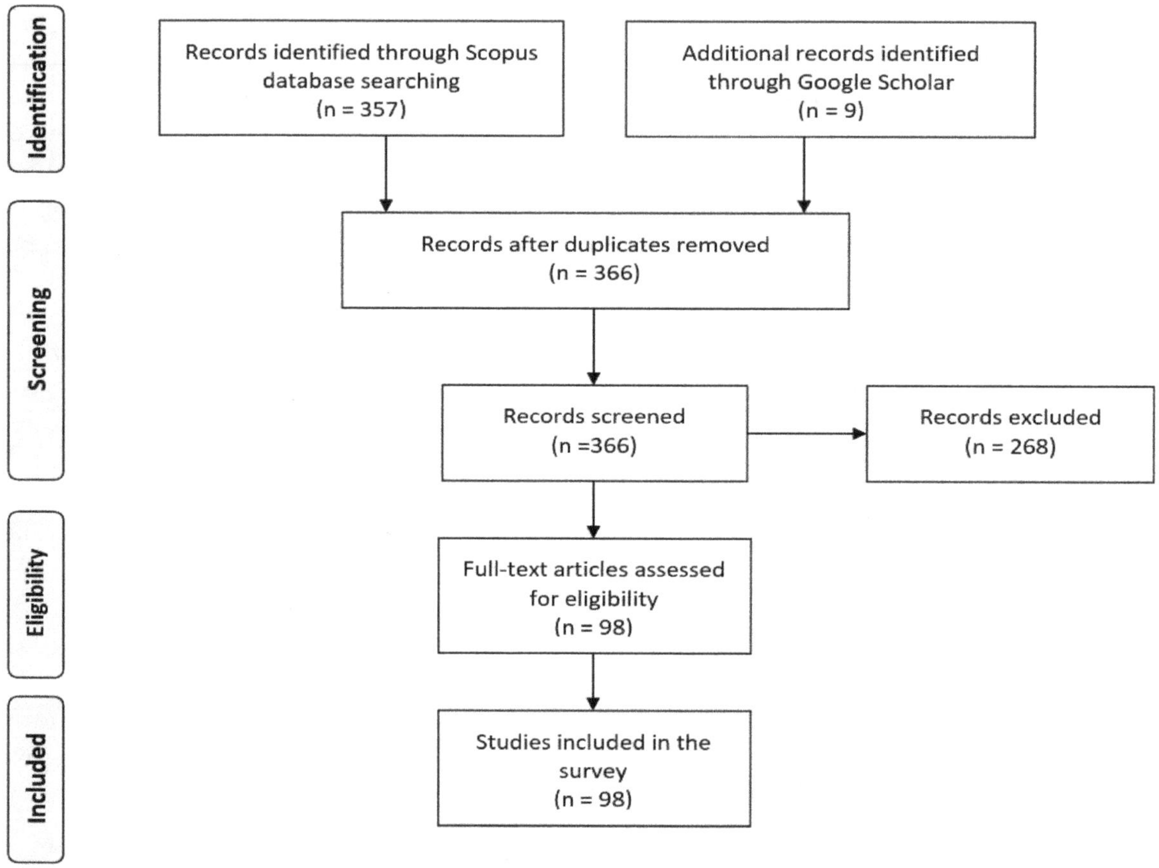

Figure 1. Flow diagram of the methodology used to conduct this survey.

3. The Basic Process to Apply Deep Learning for Lung Disease Detection

In this section, the process of how deep learning is applied to identify lung diseases from medical images is described. There are mainly three steps: image preprocessing, training and classification. Lung disease detection generally deals with classifying an image into healthy lungs or disease-infected lungs. The lung disease classifier, sometimes known as a model, is obtained via training. Training is the process in which a neural network learns to recognise a class of images. Using deep learning, it is possible to train a model that can classify images into their respective class labels. Therefore, to apply deep learning for lung disease detection, the first step is to gather images of lungs with the disease to be classified. The second step is to train the neural network until it is able to recognise the diseases. The final step is to classify new images. Here, new images unseen by the model before are shown to the model, and the model predicts the class of those images. The overview of the process is illustrated in Figure 2.

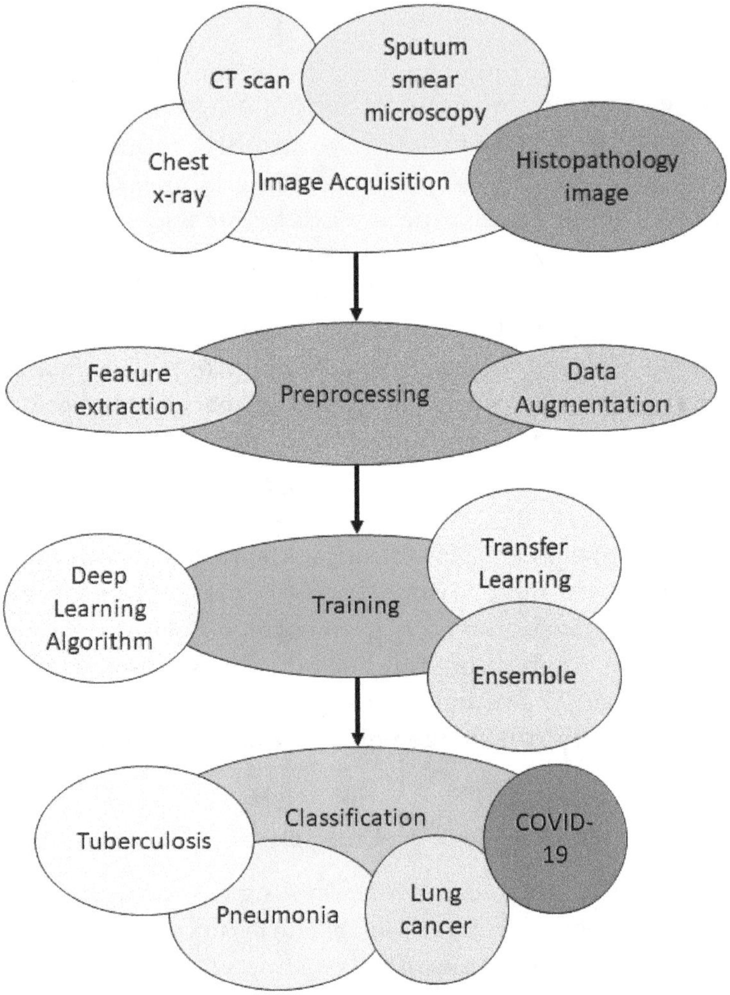

Figure 2. Overview of using deep learning for lung disease detection.

3.1. Image Acquisition Phase

The first step is to acquire images. To produce a classification model, the computer needs to learn by example. The computer needs to view many images to recognise an object. Other types of data, such as time series data and voice data, can also be used to train deep learning models. In the context of the work surveyed in this paper, the relevant data required to detect lung disease will be images. Images that could be used include chest X-ray, CT scan, sputum smear microscopy and histopathology image. The output of this step is images that will later be used to train the model.

3.2. Preprocessing Phase

The second step is preprocessing. Here, the image could be enhanced or modified to improve image quality. Contrast Limited Adaptive Histogram Equalisation (CLAHE) could be performed to increase the contrast of the images [12]. Image modification such as lung segmentation [13] and bone elimination [14] could be used to identify the region of interest (ROI), whereby the detection of the lung disease can then be performed on the ROI. Edge detection could also be used to provide an alternate data representation [15]. Data augmentation could be applied to the images to increase the amount of available data. Feature extraction could also be conducted so that the deep learning model could identify important features to identify a certain object or class. The output of this step is a set of images whereby the quality of the images is enhanced, or unwanted objects have been removed. The output of this step is images that were enhanced or modified that will later be used in training.

3.3. Training Phase

In the third step, namely training, three aspects could be considered. These aspects are the selection of deep learning algorithm, usage of transfer learning and usage of an ensemble. There are numerous deep learning algorithm, for example deep belief network (DBN), multilayer perceptron neural network (MPNN), recurrent neural network (RNN) and the aforementioned CNN. Different algorithms have different learning styles. Different types of data work better with certain algorithms. CNN works particularly well with images. Deep learning algorithm should be chosen based on the nature of the data at hand. Transfer learning refers to the transfer of knowledge from one model to another. Ensemble refers to the usage of more than one model during classification. Transfer learning and ensemble are techniques used to reduce training time, improve classification accuracy and reduce overfitting [16]. Further details concerning these two aspects could be found in Sections 4.5 and 4.6, respectively. The output of this step is models generated from the data learned.

3.4. Classification Phase

In the fourth and final step, which is classification, the trained model will predict which class an image belongs to. For example, if a model was trained to differentiate X-ray images of healthy lungs and tuberculosis-infected lungs, it should be able to correctly classify new images (images that are never seen by the model before) into healthy lungs or tuberculosis-infected lungs. The model will give a probability score for the image. The probability score represents how likely an image belongs to a certain class. At the end of this step, the image will be classified based on the probability score given to it by the model.

4. The Taxonomy of State-Of-The-Art Work on Lung Disease Detection Using Deep Learning

In this section, a taxonomy of the recent work on lung disease detection using deep learning is presented, which is the first contribution of this paper. The taxonomy is built to summarise and provide a clearer picture of the key concepts and focus of the existing work. Seven attributes were identified for inclusion in the taxonomy. These attributes were chosen as they were imminent and can be found in all the articles being surveyed. The seven attributes included in the taxonomy are image types, features, data augmentation, types of deep learning algorithms, transfer learning, the ensemble of classifiers and types of lung diseases. Sections 4.1–4.7 describe each attribute in detail, whereby the review of relevant works is provided. Section 4.8 describes the datasets used by the works surveyed. Figure 3 shows the taxonomy of state-of-the-art lung disease detection using deep learning.

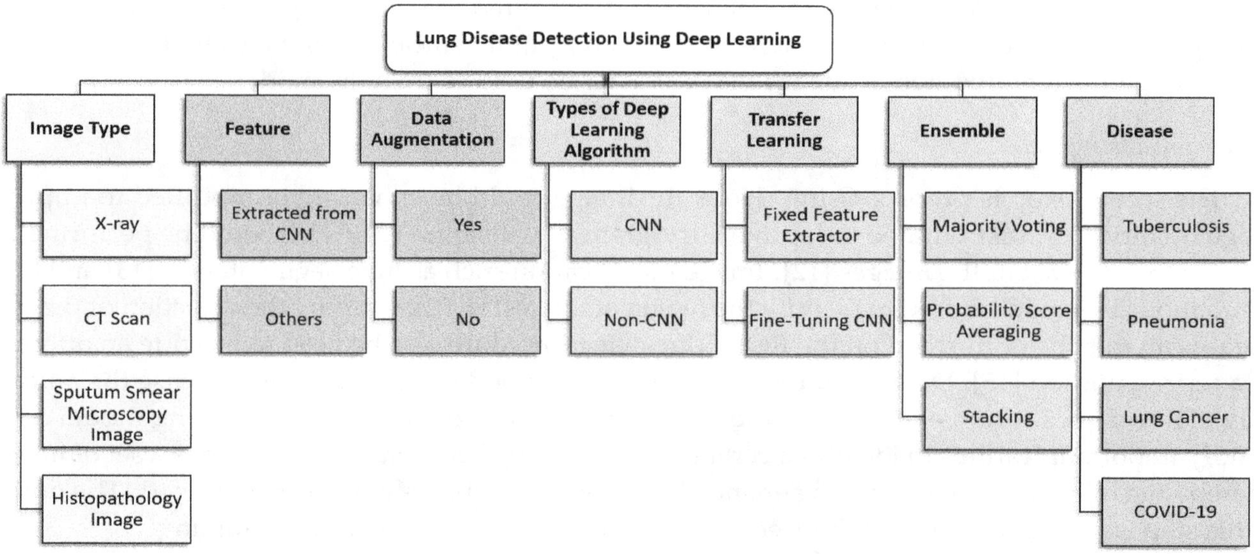

Figure 3. Taxonomy of lung disease detection using deep learning.

4.1. Image Type

In the papers surveyed, four types of images were used to train the model: chest X-ray, CT scans, sputum smear microscopy images and histopathology images. These images are described in detail in Sections 4.1.1–4.1.4. It should be noted that there are other imaging techniques exist such as positron emission tomography (PET) and magnetic resonance imaging (MRI) scans. Both PET and MRI scans could also be used to diagnose health conditions and evaluate the effectiveness of ongoing treatment. However, none of the papers surveyed used PET or MRI scans.

4.1.1. Chest X-rays

An X-ray is a diagnostic test that helps clinicians identify and treat medical problems [17]. The most widely performed medical X-ray procedure is a chest X-ray, and a chest X-ray produces images of the blood vessels, lungs, airways, heart and spine and chest bones. Traditionally, medical X-ray images were exposed to photographic films, which require processing before they can be viewed. To overcome this problem, digital X-rays are used [18]. Figure 4 shows several examples of chest X-ray with different lung conditions taken from various datasets.

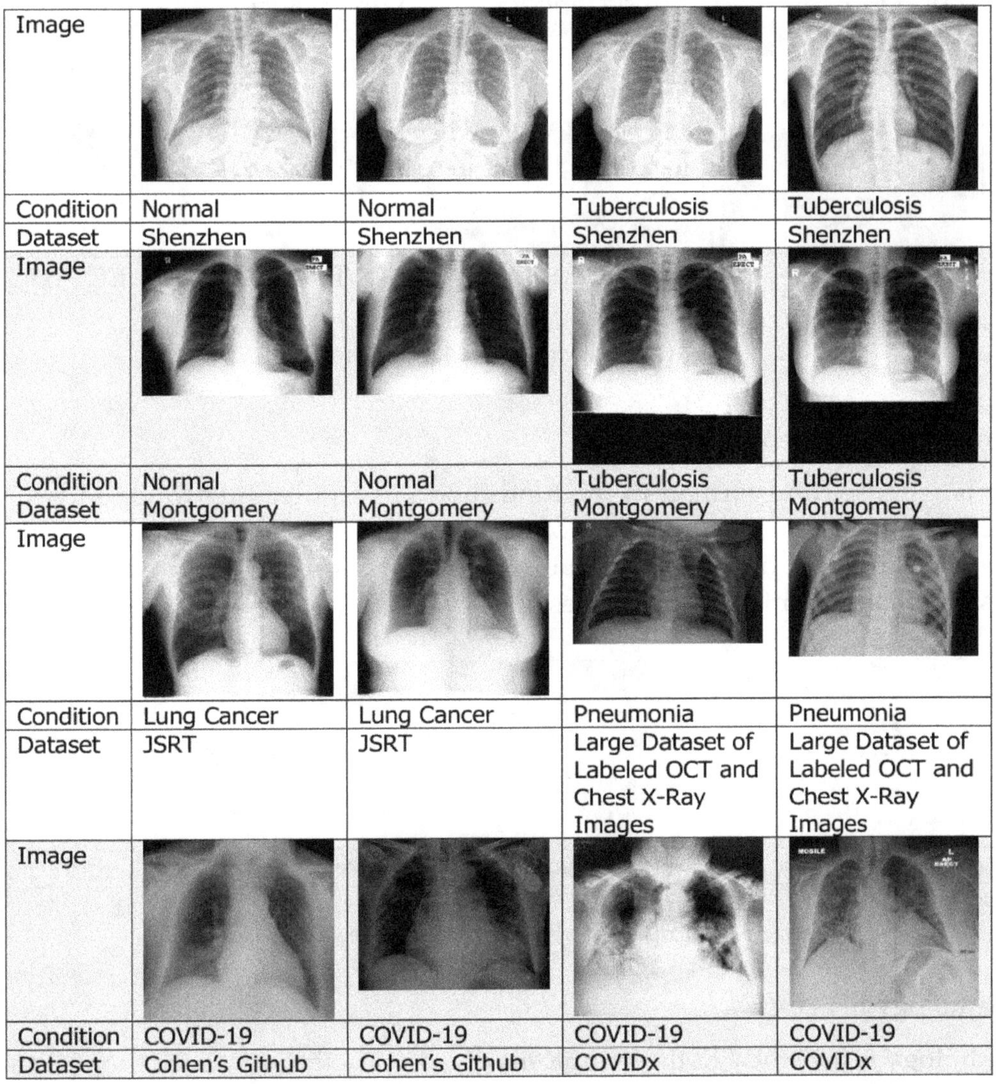
Image
Condition | Normal | Normal | Tuberculosis | Tuberculosis
Dataset | Shenzhen | Shenzhen | Shenzhen | Shenzhen
Image
Condition | Normal | Normal | Tuberculosis | Tuberculosis
Dataset | Montgomery | Montgomery | Montgomery | Montgomery
Image
Condition | Lung Cancer | Lung Cancer | Pneumonia | Pneumonia
Dataset | JSRT | JSRT | Large Dataset of Labeled OCT and Chest X-Ray Images | Large Dataset of Labeled OCT and Chest X-Ray Images
Image
Condition | COVID-19 | COVID-19 | COVID-19 | COVID-19
Dataset | Cohen's Github | Cohen's Github | COVIDx | COVIDx

Figure 4. Examples of chest X-ray images.

Among the papers surveyed, the majority of them used chest X-rays. For example, X-rays were used for tuberculosis detection [19], pneumonia detection [20], lung cancer detection [14] and COVID-19 detection [21].

4.1.2. CT Scans

A CT scan is a form of radiography that uses computer processing to create sectional images at various planes of depth from images taken around the patient's body from different angles [22]. The image slices can be shown individually, or they can be stacked to produce a 3D image of the patient, showing the tissues, organs, skeleton and any abnormalities present [23]. CT scan images deliver more detailed information than X-rays. Figure 5 shows examples of CT scan images taken from numerous datasets. CT scans have been used to detect lung disease in numerous work found in the literature, for example for tuberculosis detection [24], lung cancer detection [25] and COVID-19 detection [26].

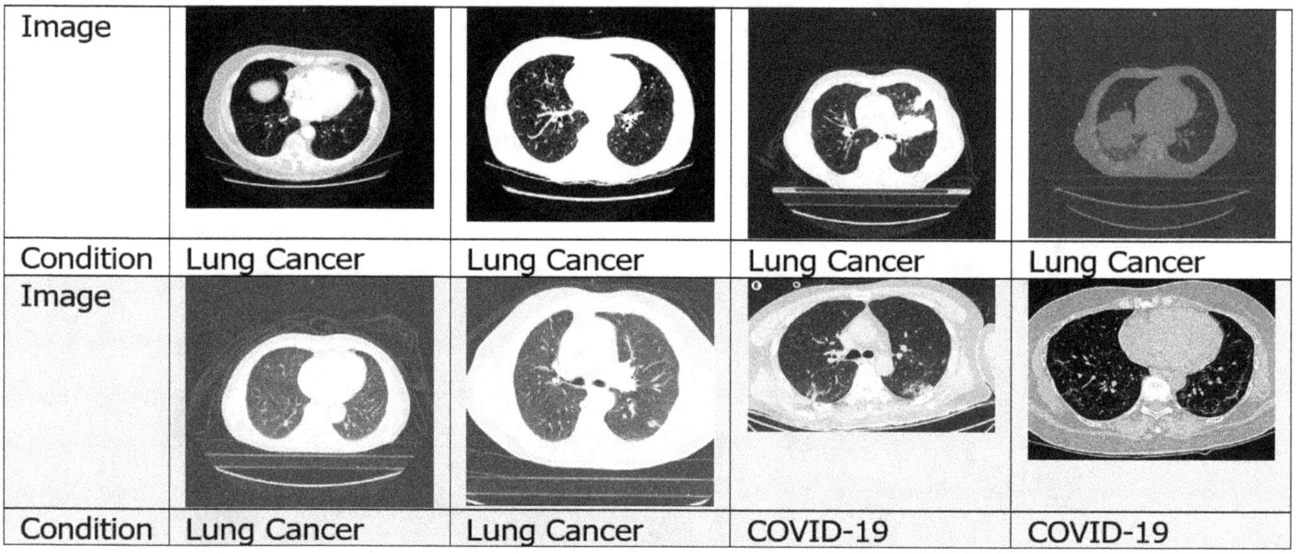

Figure 5. Examples of CT scan images.

4.1.3. Sputum Smear Microscopy Images

Sputum is a dense fluid formed in the lungs and airways leading to the lungs. To perform sputum smear examination, a very thin layer of the sputum sample is positioned on a glass slide [27]. Among the papers surveyed, only five used sputum smear microscopy image [28–32]. Figure 6 shows examples of sputum smear microscopy images.

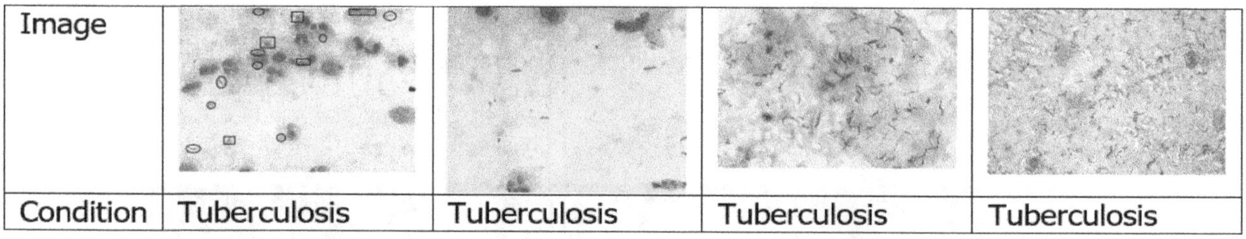

Figure 6. Examples of sputum smear microscopy images.

4.1.4. Histopathology Images

Histopathology is the study of the symptoms of a disease through microscopic examination of a biopsy or surgical specimen using glass slides. The sections are dyed with one or more stains to visualise the different components of the tissue [33]. Figure 7 shows a few examples of histopathology images. Among all the papers surveyed, only Coudray et al. [34] used histopathology images.

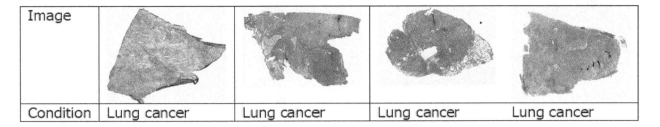

Image	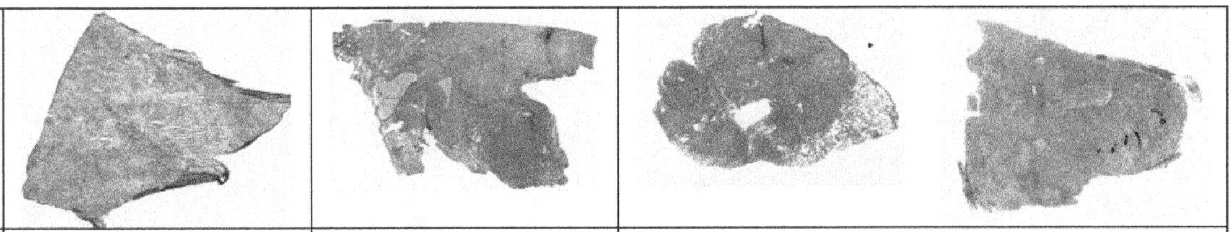			
Condition	Lung cancer	Lung cancer	Lung cancer	Lung cancer

Figure 7. Examples of histopathology images.

4.2. Features

In computer vision, features are significant information extracted from images in terms of numerical values that could be used to solve specific problem [35]. Features might be in the form of specific structures in the image such as points, edges, colour, sizes, shapes or objects. Logically, the types of images affect the quality of the features.

Feature transformation is a process that creates new features using the existing features. These new features may not have the same representation as to the original features, but they may have more discriminatory power in a different space than the original space. The purpose of feature transformation is to provide a more useful feature for the machine learning algorithm for object identification. The features used in the surveyed papers include: Gabor, GIST, Local binary patterns (LBP), Tamura texture descriptor, colour and edge direction descriptor (CEDD) [36], Hu moments, colour layout descriptor (CLD) edge histogram descriptor (EHD) [37], primitive length, edge frequency, autocorrelation, shape features, size, orientation, bounding box, eccentricity, extent, centroid, scale-invariant feature transform (SIFT), regional properties area and speeded up robust features (SURF) [38]. Other feature representations in terms of histograms include pyramid histogram of oriented gradients (PHOG), histogram of oriented gradients (HOG) [39], intensity histograms (IH), shape descriptor histograms (SD), gradient magnitude histograms (GM), curvature descriptor histograms (CD) and fuzzy colour and texture histogram (FCTH). Some studies even performed lung segmentations before training their models (e.g., [13,14,36]).

From the literature, a majority of the works surveyed used features that are automatically extracted from CNN. CNN can automatically learn and extract features, discarding the need for manual feature generation [40].

4.3. Data Augmentation

In deep learning, it is very important to have a large training dataset, as the community agrees that having more images can help improve training accuracy. Even a weak algorithm with a large amount of data can be more accurate than a strong algorithm with a modest amount of data [41]. Another obstacle is imbalanced classes. When doing binary classification training, if the number of samples of one class is a lot higher than the other class, the resulting model would be biased [6]. Deep learning algorithms perform optimally when the amount of samples in each class is equal or balanced.

One way to increase the training dataset without obtaining new images is to use image augmentation. Image augmentation creates variations of the original images. This is achieved by performing different methods of processing, such as rotations, flips, translations, zooms and adding noise [42]. Figure 8 shows various examples of images after image augmentation.

Data augmentation can also help increase the amount of relevant data in the dataset. For example, consider a car dataset with two labels, X and Y. One subset of the dataset contains images of cars of label X, but all the cars are facing left. The other subset contains images of cars of label Y, but all the cars are facing right. After training, a test image of a label Y car facing left is fed into the model, and the model labels that the car as X. The prediction is wrong as the neural network search for the most obvious features that distinguish one class from another. To prevent this, a simple solution is to flip the images in the existing dataset horizontally such that they face the other side. Through augmentation, we may introduce relevant features and patterns, essentially boosting overall performance.

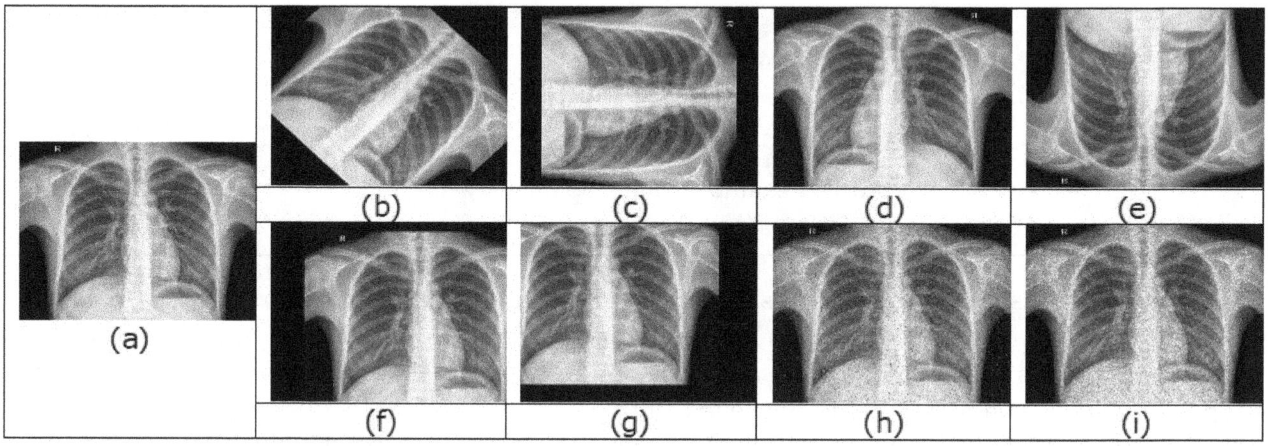

Figure 8. Examples of image augmentation: (**a**) original; (**b**) 45° rotation; (**c**) 90° rotation; (**d**) horizontal flip; (**e**) vertical flip; (**f**) positive x and y translation; (**g**) negative x and y translation; (**h**) salt and pepper noise; and (**i**) speckle noise.

Data augmentation also helps prevent overfitting. Overfitting refers to a case where a network learns a very high variance function, such as the perfect modelling of training results. Data augmentation addresses the issue of overfitting by introducing the model with more diverse data [43]. This diversity in data reduces variance and improves the generalisation of the model.

However, data augmentation cannot overcome all biases present in a small dataset [43]. Other disadvantages of data augmentation include additional training time, transformation computing costs and additional memory costs.

4.4. *Types of Deep Learning Algorithm*

The most common deep learning algorithm, CNN, is especially useful to find patterns in images. Similar to the neural networks of the human brain, CNNs consist of neurons with trainable biases and weights. Each neuron receives several inputs. Then, a weighted sum over the inputs is computed. The weighted sum is then passed to an activation function, and an output is produced. The difference between CNN and other neural networks is that CNN has convolution layers. Figure 9 shows an example of a CNN architecture [44]. A CNN consists of multiple layers, and the four main types of layers are convolutional layer, pooling layer and fully-connected layer. The convolutional layer performs an operation called a "convolution". Convolution is a linear operation involving the multiplication of a set of weights with the input. The set of weights is called a kernel or a filter. The input data are larger than the filter. The multiplication between a filter-sized section of the input and the filter is a dot product. The dot product is then summed, resulting in a single value. The pooling layer gradually reduces the spatial size of the representation to lessen the number of parameters and computations in the network, thus controlling overfitting. A rectified linear unit (ReLu) is added to the CNN to apply an elementwise activation function such as sigmoid to the output of the activation produced by the previous layer. More details of CNN can be found in [44,45].

CNN generally has two components when learning, which are feature extraction and classification. In the feature extraction stage, convolution is implemented on the input data using a filter or kernel. Then, a feature map is subsequently generated. In the classification stage, the CNN computes a probability of the image belongs to a particular class or label. CNN is especially useful for image classification and recognition as it automatically learns features without needing manual feature extraction [40]. CNN also can be retrained and applied to a different domain using transfer learning [46]. Transfer learning has been shown to produce better classification results [19].

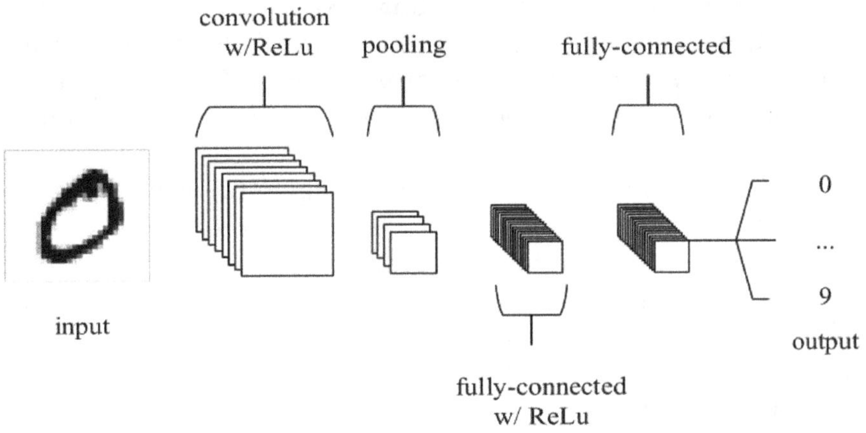

Figure 9. Example of a CNN structure.

Another deep learning algorithm is DBN. DBN can be defined as a stack of restricted Boltzmann machines (RBM) [47]. The layer of the DBN has two functions, except for the first and final layers. The layer serves as the hidden layer for the nodes that come before it, and as the input layer for the nodes that come after it. The first RBM is designed to reproduce as accurately as possible the input to train a DBN. Then, the hidden layer of the first RBM is treated as the visible layer for the second one, and the second RBM is trained using the outputs from the first RBM. This process keeps repeating until every layer of the network is trained. After this initial training, the DBN has created a model that can detect patterns in the data. DBN can be used to recognise objects in images, video sequences and motion-capture data. More details of DBN can be found in [31,48].

One more example of a deep learning algorithm used in the papers surveyed is a bag of words (BOW) model. BOW is a method to extract features from the text for use in modelling. In BOW, the number of the appearance of each word in a document is counted, then the frequency of each word was examined to identify the keywords of the document, and a frequency histogram is made. This concept is similar to the bag of visual words (BOVW), sometimes referred to as bag-of-features. In BOVW, image features are considered as the "words". Image features are unique patterns that were found in an image. The general idea of BOVW is to represent an image as a set of features, where each feature contains keypoints and descriptors. Keypoints are the most noticeable points in an image, such that, even if the image is rotated, shrunk or enlarged, its keypoints are always the same. A descriptor is the description of the keypoint. Keypoints and descriptors are used to construct vocabularies and represent each image as a frequency histogram of features. From the frequency histogram, one can find other similar images or predict the class of the image. Lopes and Valiati proposed Bag of CNN features to classify tuberculosis [19].

4.5. Transfer Learning

Transfer learning emerged as a popular method in computer vision because it allows accurate models to be built [49]. With transfer learning, a model learned from a domain can be re-used on a different domain. Transfer learning can be performed with or without a pre-trained model.

A pre-trained model is a model developed to solve a similar task. Instead of creating a model from scratch to solve a similar task, the model trained on other problem is used as a starting point. Even though a pre-trained model is trained on a task which is different from the current task, the features learned, in most cases, found to be useful for the new task. The objective of training a deep learning model is to find the correct weights for the network by numerous forward and backward iterations. By using pre-trained models that have been previously trained on large datasets, the weights and architecture obtained can be used and applied to the current problem. One of the advantages of a pre-trained model is the reduced cost of training for the new model [50]. This is because pre-trained weights were used, and the model only has to learn the weights of the last few layers.

Many CNN architectures are pre-trained on ImageNet [51]. The images were gathered from the internet and labelled by human labellers using Amazon's Mechanical Turk crowd-sourcing tool. ILSVRC uses a subset of ImageNet with approximately 1000 images in each of 1000 classes. Altogether, there are approximately 1.2 million training images, 50,000 validation images and 150,000 testing images.

Transfer learning can be used in two ways: (i) fine-tuning; or (ii) using CNN as a feature extractor. In fine-tuning, the weights of the pre-trained CNN model are preserved on some of the layers and tuned in the others [52]. Usually, the weights of the initial layers of the model are frozen while only the higher layers are retrained. This is because the features obtained from the first layers are generic (e.g., edge detectors or colour blob detectors) and applicable to other tasks. The top-level layers of the pre-trained models are retrained so that the model learned high-level features specific to the new dataset. This method is typically recommended if the training dataset is huge and very identical to the original dataset that the pre-trained model was trained on. On the other hand, CNN is used as a feature extractor. This is conducted by removing the last fully-connected layer (the one which outputs the probabilities for being in each of the 1000 classes from ImageNet) and then using the network as a fixed feature extractor for the new dataset [53]. For tasks where only a small dataset is available, it is usually recommended to take advantage of features learned by a model trained on a larger dataset in the same domain. Then, a classifier is trained from the features extracted.

There are several issues that need to be considered when using transfer learning: (i) ensuring that the pre-trained model selected has been trained on a similar dataset as the new target dataset; and (ii) using a lower learning rate for CNN weights that are being fine-tuned, because the CNN weights are expected to be relatively good, and we do not wish to distort them too quickly and too much [53].

4.6. Ensemble of Classifiers

When more than one classifier is combined to make a prediction, this is known as ensemble classification [16]. Ensemble decreases the variance of predictions, therefore making predictions that are more accurate than any individual model. From work found in the literature, the ensemble techniques used include majority voting, probability score averaging and stacking.

In majority voting, every model makes a prediction for each test instance, or, in other words, votes for a class label, and the final prediction is the label that received the most votes [54]. An alternate version of majority voting is weighted majority voting, in which the votes of certain models are deemed more important than others. For example, majority voting was used by Chouhan et al. [55].

In probability score averaging, the prediction scores of each model are added up and divided by the number of models involved [56]. An alternate version of this is weighted averaging, where the prediction score of each model is multiplied by the weight, and then their average is calculated. Examples of works which used probability score averaging are found in [15,57].

In stacking ensemble, an algorithm receives the outputs of weaker models as input and tries to learn how to best combine the input predictions to provide a better output prediction [58]. For example, stacking ensemble was used by Rajaraman et al. [12].

4.7. Type of Disease

In this section, the deep learning techniques applied for detecting tuberculosis, pneumonia, lung cancer and COVID-19 are discussed in greater detail in Sections 4.7.1–4.7.4, respectively. The first three diseases were considered as they are the most common causes of critical illness and death worldwide related to lung [2], while COVID-19 is an ongoing pandemic [3]. We also found that most of the existing work was directed at detecting these specific lung-related diseases.

4.7.1. Tuberculosis

Tuberculosis is a disease caused by Mycobacterium tuberculosis bacteria. According to the World Health Organisation, tuberculosis is among the ten most common causes of death in the world [59].

Tuberculosis infected 10 million people and killed 1.6 million in 2017. Early detection of tuberculosis is essential to increase the chances of recovery [5].

Two studies used Computer-Aided Detection for Tuberculosis (CAD4TB) for tuberculosis detection [60,61]. CAD4TB is a tool developed by Delft Imaging Systems in cooperation with the Radboud University Nijmegen and the Lung Institute in Cape Town. CAD4TB works by obtaining the patient's chest X-ray, analysing the image via CAD4TB cloud server or CAD4TB box computer, generating a heat map of the patient's lung and displaying an abnormality score from 0 to 100. Murphy et al. [60] showed that CAD4TB v6 is an accurate system, reaching the level of expert human readers. A technique for automated tuberculosis screening by combining X-ray-based computer-aided detection (CAD) and clinical information was introduced by Melendez et al. [61]. They combined automatic chest X-ray scoring by CAD with clinical information. This combination improved accuracies and specificities compared to the use of either type of information alone.

In the literature, several works use CNN to classify tuberculosis. A method that incorporated demographic information, such as age, gender and weight, to improve CNN's performance was presented by Heo et al. [62]. Results indicate that CNN, including the demographic variables, has a higher area under the receiver operating characteristic curve (AUC) score and greater sensitivity then CNN based on chest X-rays images only. A simple convolutional neural network developed for tuberculosis detection was proposed by Pasa et al. [63]. The proposed approach is found to be more efficient than previous models but retains their accuracy. This method significantly reduced the memory and computational requirement, without sacrificing the classification performance. Another CNN-based model has been presented to classify different categories of tuberculosis [64]. A CNN model is trained on the region-based global and local features to generate new features. A support vector machine (SVM) classifier was then applied for tuberculosis manifestations recognition. CNN has also been used to classify tuberculosis [65–67]. Ul Abideen et al. [68] used a Bayesian-based CNN that exploits the model uncertainty and Bayesian confidence to improve the accuracy of tuberculosis identification. In other work, a deep CNN algorithm named deep learning-based automatic detection (DLAD), was developed for tuberculosis classification that contains 27 layers with 12 residual connections [69]. DLAD shows outstanding performance in tuberculosis detection when applied on chest X-rays, obtaining results better than physicians and thoracic radiologists.

Lopes and Valiati proposed Bag of CNN features to classify tuberculosis [19] where feature extraction is performed by ResNet, VggNet and GoogLenet. Then, each chest X-ray is separated into subregions whose size is equal to the input layer of the networks. Each subregion is regarded as a "feature", while each X-ray is a "bag".

Several works that utilised transfer learning are described in this paragraph. Hwang et al. obtained an accuracy of 90.3% and AUC of 0.964 using transfer learning from ImageNet and training on a dataset of 10848 chest X-rays [70]. Pre-trained GoogLeNet and AlexNet were used to perform pulmonary tuberculosis classification by Lakhani and Sundaram [57], who concluded that higher accuracy was achieved when using the pre-trained model. Their pre-trained AlexNet achieved an AUC of 0.98 and their pre-trained GoogLeNet achieved an AUC of 0.97. Lopes and Valiati used pre-trained GoogLenet, ResNet and VggNet architectures as features extractors and the SVM classifier to classify tuberculosis [19]. They achieved AUC of 0.900–0.912. Fine-tuned ResNet-50, ResNet-101, ResNet-512, VGG16, VGG19 and AlexNet were used by Islam et al. to classify tuberculosis. These models achieved an AUC of 0.85–0.91 [71]. Instead of using networks pre-trained from ImageNet, pre-training can be performed on other datasets, such as the NIH-14 dataset [72]. This dataset contains an assortment of diseases (which does not include tuberculosis) and is from the same modality as that of the data under consideration for tuberculosis. Experiments show that the features learned from the NIH dataset are useful for identifying tuberculosis. A study performed data augmentation and then compared the performances of three different pre-trained models to classify tuberculosis [73]. The results show that suitable data augmentation methods were able to rise the accuracies of CNNs. Transfer learning was also used by Abbas and Abdelsamea [74], Karnkawinpong and Limpiyakorn [75] and Liu et al. [76]. A coarse-to-fine transfer learning was applied by Yadav et al. [77]. First, the datasets are split according to the resolution and quality of the images. Then, transfer learning is applied to the low-resolution dataset first, followed by the high-resolution dataset. In this case, the model was first trained on the low-resolution NIH dataset, and then trained on the high-resolution Shenzen and Montgomery datasets. Sahlol et al. [78] used CNN as fixed feature extractor and Artificial Ecosystem-Based Optimisation to select the optimal subset of relevant features. KNN was used as the classifier.

Several works that utilised ensemble are described in this paragraph. An ensemble method using the weighted averages of the probability scores for the AlexNet and GoogLeNet algorithms was used by Lakhani and Sundaram [57]. In [79], ensemble by weighted averages of probability scores is used. An ensemble of six CNNs was developed by Islam et al. [71]. The ensemble models were generated by calculating the simple averaging of the probability predictions given by every single model. Another ensemble classifier was created by combining the classifier from the Simple CNN Feature Extraction and a classifier from Bag of CNN features proposals [19]. Three classifiers were trained, using the features from ResNet, GoogLenet and VggNet, respectively. The Simple Features Ensemble combines all three classifiers, and the output is obtained through a simple soft-voting scheme. A stacking ensemble for tuberculosis detection was proposed by Rajaraman et al. [12]. An ensemble generated via a feature-level fusion of neural network models was also used to classify tuberculosis [80]. Three models were employed: the DenseNet, ResNet and Inception-ResNet. As such, the ensemble was called RID network. Features were extracted using the RID network, and SVM was used as a classifier. Tuberculosis classification was also executed using another ensemble of three regular architectures: ResNet, AlexNet and GoogleNet [79]. Each architecture was trained from scratch, and different optimal hyper-parameter values were used. The sensitivity, specificity and accuracy of the ensemble were higher than when each of the regular architecture was used independently. The authors of [15,81] performed a probability score averaging ensemble of CNNs trained on features extracted from a different type of images; the enhanced chest X-ray images and the edge detected images of the chest X-ray. Rajaraman and Antani [82] studied and compared various ensemble methods that include majority voting and stacking. Results show that stacking ensemble achieved the highest classification accuracy.

Other techniques used to classify tuberculosis images include k-Nearest Neighbour (kNN), sequential minimal optimisation and simple linear regression [38]. A Multiple-Instance Learning-based approach was also attempted [83]. The advantage of this method is the lower labelling detail required during optimisation. In addition, the minimal supervision required allows easy retraining of a previously optimised system. One tuberculosis detection system uses ViDi Systems for image analysis of chest X-rays [84]. ViDi is an industrial-grade deep learning image analysis software developed by COGNEX. ViDi has shown feasible performance in the detection of tuberculosis. The authors of [36] introduced a fully automatic frontal chest screening system that is capable of detecting tuberculosis-infected lungs. This method begins with the segmentation of the lung. Then, features are extracted from the segmented images. Examples of features include shape and curvature histograms. Finally, a classifier was used to detect the disease.

For CT scans related tuberculosis detection works, a method called AECNN was proposed [85]. An AE-CNN block was formed by combining the feature extraction of CNN and the unsupervised features of AutoEncoder. The model then analyses the region of interest within the image to perform the classification of tuberculosis. A research study explores the use of CT pulmonary images to diagnose and classify tuberculosis at five levels of severity to track treatment effectiveness [24]. The tuberculosis abnormalities only occupy limited regions in the CT image, and the dataset is quite small. Therefore, depth-ResNet was proposed. Depth-ResNet is a 3D block-based ResNet combined with the injection of depth information at each layer. As an attempt to automate tuberculosis related lung deformities without sacrificing accuracy, advanced AI algorithms were studied to draw clinically actionable hypotheses [86]. This approach involves thorough image processing, subsequently performing feature extraction using TensorFlow and 3D CNN to further augment the metadata with the features extracted from the image data, and finally perform six class binary classification using the random forest. Another attempt for this problem was proposed by Zunair et al. [87]. They proposed a 16-layer 3D convolutional neural network with a slice selection. The goal is to estimate the tuberculosis severity based on the CT image. An integrated method based on optical flow and a characterisation method called Activity Description Vector (ADV) was presented to take care of the classification of chest CT scan images affected by different types of tuberculosis [88]. The important point of this technique is the interpretation of the set of cross-sectional chest images produced by CT scan, not as a volume but as a series of video images. This technique can extract movement descriptors capable of classifying tuberculosis affections by analysing deformations or movements generated in these video series. The idea of optical flow refers to the approximation of displacements of intensity patterns. In short, the ADV vector describes the activity in image series by counting for each region of the image the movements made in four directions of the 2D space.

For sputum microscopy images-related tuberculosis detection works, CNN was used for the detection and localisation of drug-sensitive tuberculosis bacilli in sputum microscopy images [29]. This method automatically localises bacilli in each view-field (a patch of the whole slide). A study found that, when training a CNN on three different image versions, namely RGB, R-G and grayscale, the best performance was achieved when using R-G images [28]. Image binarisation can also be used for preprocessing before the data were fed into a CNN [30]. Image binarisation is a segmentation method to classify the foreground and background of the microscopic sputum smear images. The segmented foreground consists of single bacilli, touching bacillus and other artefacts. A trained CNN is then given the foreground objects, and the CNN will classify the objects into bacilli and non-bacilli. Another tuberculosis detection system automatically attains all view-fields using a motorised microscopic stage [32]. After that, the data are delivered to the recognition system. A customised Inception V3 DeepNet model is used to learn from the pre-trained weights of Inception V3. Afterwards, the data were classified using SVM. DBN was also used to detect tuberculosis bacillus present in the stained microscopic images of sputum [31]. For segmentation, the Channel Area Thresholding algorithm is used. Location-oriented histogram and speed up robust feature (SURF) algorithm were used to extract the intensity-based local bacilli features. DBN is then used to classify the bacilli objects. Table 1 shows the summary of papers for tuberculosis detection using deep learning.

Table 1. Summary of papers for tuberculosis detection using deep learning.

Authors	Deep Learning Technique	Features	Dataset
[74]	CNN with transfer learning and data augmentation	Features extracted from CNN	Montgomery
[38]	K-nearest neighbour, Simple Linear Regression and Sequential Minimal Optimisation (SMO) Classification	Area, major axis, minor axis, eccentricity, mean, kurtosis, skewness and entropy	Shenzhen
[84]	ViDi	Features extracted from CNN	Unspecified
[64]	CNN	Gabor, LBP, SIFT, PHOG and Features extracted from CNN	Private dataset
[24]	CNN	Features extracted from CNN	ImageCLEF 2018 dataset
[62]	CNN with transfer learning, with demographic information	Features extracted from CNN + demographic information	Private dataset
[79]	CNN with data augmentation, and ensemble by weighted averages of probability scores	Features extracted from CNN	Montgomery, Shenzhen, Belarus, JSRT
[70]	CNN with transfer learning and data augmentation	Features extracted from CNN	Private dataset, Montgomery, Shenzhen

Table 1. *Cont.*

Authors	Deep Learning Technique	Features	Dataset
[69]	CNN	Features extracted from CNN	Private datasets, Montgomery, Shenzhen
[71]	CNN with transfer learning and ensemble by simple linear probabilities averaging	Features extracted from CNN + rule-based features	Indiana, JSRT, Shenzhen
[29]	CNN	HoG features	ZiehlNeelsen Sputum smear Microscopy image DataBase
[75]	CNN and shuffle sampling	Features extracted from CNN	Private datasets
[81]	CNN with transfer learning and ensemble by averaging	CNN extracted features from edge images	Montgomery, Shenzhen
[57]	CNN with transfer learning, data augmentation and ensemble by weighted probability scores average	Features extracted from CNN	Private dataset, Montgomery, Shenzhen, Belarus
[85]	AutoEncoder-CNN	Features extracted from CNN	Private dataset
[76]	CNN with transfer learning and shuffle sampling	Features extracted from CNN	Private dataset
[65]	End-to-end CNN	Features extracted from CNN	Montgomery, Shenzhen
[88]	Optical flow model	Activity Description Vector on optical flow of video sequences	ImageCLEF 2019 dataset
[28]	CNN	Colours	TBimages dataset
[83]	Modified maximum pattern margin support vector machine (modified miSVM)	First four moments of the intensity distributions	Private datasets
[61]	CAD4TB with clinical information	Features extracted from CNN + clinical features	Private dataset
[31]	DBN	LoH + SURF features	ZiehlNeelsen Sputum smear Microscopy image DataBase
[60]	CAD4TB	Features extracted from CNN	Private dataset
[72]	CNN with transfer learning and data augmentation	Features extracted from CNN	Montgomery, Shenzhen, NIH-14 dataset
[30]	CNN	Features extracted from CNN	TBimages dataset
[63]	CNN from scratch and data augmentation	Features extracted from CNN	Montgomery, Shenzhen, Belarus
[86]	3D CNN	Features extracted from CNN + lung volume + patient attribute metadata	ImageCLEF 2019 dataset
[12]	CNN with transfer learning and ensemble by stacking	local and global feature descriptors + features extracted from CNN	Private dataset, Montgomery, Shenzhen, India
[80]	CNN with transfer learning and feature level ensemble	Features extracted from CNN	Shenzhen
[15]	CNN with transfer learning and ensemble by averaging	CNN extracted features from edge images	Montgomery, Shenzhen
[32]	CNN with transfer learning	Features extracted from CNN	ZiehlNeelsen Sputum smear Microscopy image DataBase
[66]	CNN with data augmentation	Features extracted from CNN	Shenzhen
[73]	CNN with transfer learning and data augmentation	Features extracted from CNN	NIH-14, Montgomery, Shenzhen
[19]	CNN with transfer learning, Bag of CNN Features and ensemble by a simple soft-voting scheme	Features extracted from CNN + BOW	Private dataset, Montgomery, Shenzhen
[36]	Neural network	Shape, curvature descriptor histograms, eigenvalues of Hessian matrix	Montgomery, Shenzhen

Table 1. *Cont.*

Authors	Deep Learning Technique	Features	Dataset
[77]	CNN with transfer learning and data augmentation	Features extracted from CNN	Montgomery, Shenzhen, NIH-14
[87]	3D CNN	Features extracted from CNN	ImageCLEF 2019 dataset
[78]	CNN and Artificial Ecosystem-based Optimisation algorithm	Features extracted from CNN	Shenzhen
[67]	CNN	Features extracted from CNN	Shenzhen
[68]	Bayesian based CNN	Features extracted from CNN	Montgomery, Shenzhen
[82]	CNN with transfer learning, and ensemble by majority voting, simple averaging, weighted averaging, and stacking	Features extracted from CNN	Montgomery, Shenzhen, LDOCTCXR, 2018 RSNA pneumonia challenge dataset, Indiana dataset

4.7.2. Pneumonia

Pneumonia is a lung infection that causes pus and fluid to fill the alveoli in one or both lungs, thus making breathing difficult [89]. Symptoms include severe shortness of breath, chest pain, chills, cough, fever or fatigue. Community-acquired pneumonia is still a recurrent cause of morbidity and mortality [90]. Most of the studies used transfer learning and data augmentation. Tobias et al. [91] straightforwardly used CNN. Stephen et al. [92] trained their CNN from scratch while using rescale, rotation, width shift, height shift, shear, zoom and horizontal flip as their augmentation techniques. A pre-trained CNN was utilised by the authors of [20,55,93–97] for pneumonia detection, while the latter four also applied data augmentation on their training datasets. For data augmentation, random horizontal flipping was used by Rajpurkar et al. [96]; shifting, zooming, flipping and 40-degree angles rotation were used by Ayan and Ünver [20]; Chouhan et al. [55] used noise addition, random horizontal flip random resized crop and images intensity adjustment; and Rahman et al. [97] used rotation, scaling and translation. Hashmi et al. [98] used CNN with transfer learning, data augmentation and ensemble by weighted averaging.

In a unique study, Acharya and Satapathy [99] used Deep Siamese CNN architecture. Deep Siamese network uses the symmetric structure of the two input image for classification. Thus, the X-ray images were separated into two parts, namely the left half and the right half. Each half was then fed into the network to compare the symmetric structure together with the amount of the infection that is spread across these two regions. Training the model for both left and right parts of the X-ray images makes the classification process more robust. Elshennawy and Ibrahim [100] used CNN and Long Short-Term Memory (LSTM)-CNN for pneumonia detection. The key advantage of the LSTM is that it can model both long and short-term memory and can deal with the vanishing gradient problem by training on long strings and storing them in memory. Emhamed et al. [101] studied and compared seven different deep learning algorithms: Decision Tree, Random Forest, KNN, AdaBoost, Gradient Boost, XGBboost and CNN. Their results show CNN obtained the highest accuracy for pneumonia classification, followed by Random forest and XGBboost. Hashmi et al. [98] used CNN with transfer learning, data augmentation and ensemble by weighted averaging.

In addition, Kumar et al. [102] attempted not only pneumonia classification, but also ROI identification. Pneumonia was detected by looking at lung opacity, and Mask-RCNN based model was used to identify lung opacity that is likely to depict pneumonia. They also performed ensemble by combining confidence scores and bounding boxes. In addition to pneumonia detection, Hurt et al. [103] proposed an approach that provides a probabilistic map on the chest X-ray images to assist in the diagnosis of pneumonia. Table 2 shows the summary of papers for pneumonia detection using deep learning.

Table 2. Summary of papers for pneumonia detection using deep learning

Reference	Deep Learning Technique	Features	Dataset
[99]	Deep Siamese based neural network	CNN extracted features from the left half and right half of the lungs	Unspecified Kaggle dataset
[20]	CNN with transfer learning and data augmentation	Features extracted from CNN	LDOCTCXR
[55]	CNN with transfer learning, data augmentation and ensemble by majority voting.	Features extracted from CNN	LDOCTCXR
[93]	CNN with transfer learning	Features extracted from CNN	LDOCTCXR
[102]	CNN with transfer learning, data augmentation and ensemble by combining confidence scores and bounding boxes.	Features extracted from CNN	Radiological Society of North America (RSNA) pneumonia dataset
[96]	CNN with transfer learning and data augmentation	Features extracted from CNN	NIH Chest X-ray Dataset
[92]	CNN from scratch and data augmentation	Features extracted from CNN	LDOCTCXR
[95]	CNN with transfer learning	Features extracted from CNN	LDOCTCXR
[91]	CNN	Features extracted from CNN	Mooney's Kaggle dataset
[100]	CNN and LSTM-CNN, with transfer learning and data augmentation	Features extracted from CNN	Mooney's Kaggle dataset
[103]	CNN with probabilistic map of pneumonia	Features extracted from CNN	2018 RSNA pneumonia challenge dataset
[101]	Decision Tree, Random Forest, K-nearest neighbour, AdaBoost, Gradient Boost, XGBboost, CNN	Multiple features	Mooney's Kaggle dataset
[98]	CNN with transfer learning, data augmentation and ensemble by weighted averaging	Features extracted from CNN	LDOCTCXR
[97]	CNN with transfer learning and data augmentation	Features extracted from CNN	Mooney's Kaggle dataset
[94]	CNN with transfer learning	Features extracted from CNN	Private dataset

4.7.3. Lung Cancer

One key characteristic of lung cancer is the presence of pulmonary nodules, solid clumps of tissue that appear in and around the lungs [104]. These nodules can be seen in CT scan images and can be malignant (cancerous) in nature or benign (not cancerous) [23].

As early as 2015, Hua et al. [105] used models of DBN and CNN to perform nodule classification in CT scans. They showed that, using deep learning, it is possible to seamlessly extract features for lung nodules classification into malignant or benign without computing the morphology and texture features. Rao et al. [25] and Kurniawan et al. [106] used CNN in a straightforward way to detect lung cancer in CT scans. Song et al. [23] compared the classification performance of CNN, deep neural network and stacked autoencoder (a multilayer sparse autoencoder of a neural network) and concluded that CNN has the highest accuracy among them. Ciompi et al. [107] used multi-stream multi-scale CNNs to classify lung nodules into six different classes: solid, non-solid, part-solid, calcified, perifissural and spiculated nodules. Specifically, they presented a multi-stream multi-scale architecture, in which CNN concurrently handles multiple triplets of 2D views of a nodule at multiple scales and then calculates the probability for the nodule in each of the six classes. Yu et al. [14] performed bone elimination and lung segmentation before training with CNN. Shakeel et al. [108] performed image denoising and enhanced the quality of the images, and then segmented the lungs by using the improved profuse clustering technique. Afterwards, a neural network is trained to detect lung cancer. The approach of Ardila et al. [13] consists of four components: lung segmentation, cancer region of interest detection model, full-volume model and cancer risk prediction model. After lung segmentation, the region of interest detection model proposes the most nodule-like regions, while the full-volume model was trained to predict cancer probability. The outputs of these two models were considered to generates the final prediction. Chen et al. [109] performed nodule enhancement and nodule segmentation before performing nodule detection.

For the works that employed transfer learning, Hosny et al. [110] and Xu et al. [111] both used CNN with data augmentation. For augmentations, both studies used flipping, translation and rotation. The authors of [112] leveraged the LUNA16 dataset to train a nodule detector and then refined that detector with the KDSB17 dataset to provide global features. Combining that and local features from a separate nodule classifier, they were able to detect lung cancer with high accuracy. The authors of [113] used transfer learning by training the model multiple times. It commenced using the more general images from the ImageNet dataset, followed by detecting nodules from chest X-rays in the ChestX-ray14 dataset, and finally detecting lung cancer nodules from the JSRT dataset. The authors of [34] is the only study surveyed to do lung cancer detection on histopathology images. Adenocarcinoma (LUAD) and squamous cell carcinoma (LUSC) are the most frequent subtypes of lung cancer, and visual examination by an experienced pathologist is needed to differentiate them. In this work, CNN was trained on histopathology slides images to automatically and accurately classify them into LUAD, LUSC or normal lung tissue. Xu et al. [114] used a CNN-long short-term memory network (LSTM) to detect lesions on chest X-ray images. Long short-term memory is an extension of RNN. This CNN-LSTM network offers probable clinical relationships between lesions to assist the model to attain better predictions. Table 3 shows the summary of papers for lung cancer detection using deep learning.

Table 3. Summary of papers for lung cancer detection using deep learning.

Reference	Deep Learning Technique	Features	Dataset
[13]	CNN	Features extracted from CNN	LUNA, LIDC, NLST
[113]	CNN with transfer learning	Features extracted from CNN	JSRT Dataset, NIH-14 dataset
[107]	Multi-stream multi-scale convolutional networks	Features extracted from CNN	MILD dataset DLCST dataset
[34]	CNN with transfer learning	Features extracted from CNN	NCI Genomic Data Commons
[110]	CNN with transfer learning and data augmentation	Features extracted from CNN	NSCLC-Radiomics, NSCLC-Radiomics-Genomics, RIDER Collections and several private datasets
[105]	CNN and DBN	Features extracted from CNN and DBN	LIDC-IDRI
[112]	CNN with transfer learning	Features extracted from CNN	Kaggle Data Science Bowl 2017 dataset, Lung Nodule Analysis 2016 (LUNA16) dataset
[25]	CNN	Features extracted from CNN	LIDC-IDRI
[108]	CNN	Features extracted from CNN	LIDC-IDRI
[23]	CNN with data augmentation	Features extracted from CNN	LIDC-IDRI database
[111]	CNN with transfer learning and data augmentation	Features extracted from CNN	Private dataset
[14]	Bone elimination and lung segmentation before training with CNN	Features extracted using CNN from bone eliminated lung images and segmented lung images	JSRT dataset
[114]	CNN-long short-term memory network	Features extracted from CNN	NIH-14 dataset

Table 3. *Cont.*

Reference	Deep Learning Technique	Features	Dataset
[109]	CNN with transfer learning and data augmentation	Features extracted from CNN	JSRT database
[106]	CNN with data augmentation	Features extracted from CNN	Cancer Imaging Archive

4.7.4. COVID-19

COVID-19 is an infectious disease caused by a recently discovered coronavirus [115]. Senior citizens are those at high risk to develop severe sickness, along with those that have historical medical conditions such as cardiovascular disease, chronic respiratory disease, cancer and diabetes [116].

A straightforward approach to detect COVID-19 using CNN with transfer learning and data augmentation was used by Salman et al. [21]. For transfer learning, they used InceptionV3 as a fixed feature extractor. Other works that implemented the similar approach of transfer learning for COVID-19 detection can be found in [117–122].

The authors of [123,124] performed 3-class classification using CNN with transfer learning, classifying X-ray images into normal, COVID-19 and viral pneumonia cases. Chowdhury et al. [125] utilised CNN with transfer learning and data augmentation to classify classifying X-ray images into normal, COVID-19 and viral pneumonia cases. The augmentation techniques used were rotation, scaling and translation. Wang et al. [126] trained a CNN from scratch and data augmentation to perform three-class classification. The augmentation technique used were translation, rotation, horizontal flip and intensity shift. Other work performing three-class classification can be found in [4,127–130]. Studies that employ data augmentation to increase the amount of data available can be found in [131,132]. In addition to COVID-19 detection on X-ray images, Alazab et al. [131] managed to perform prediction on the number of COVID-19 confirmations, recoveries and deaths in Jordan and Australia.

For works utilising ensemble, Ouyang et al. [133] implemented weighted averaging ensemble. Mahmud et al. [134] implemented stacking ensemble, whereby the images were classified into four categoriesL normal, COVID-19, viral pneumonia and bacterial pneumonia.

Shi et al. [135] utilised VB-Net for image segmentation and feature extraction and used a modified random decision forests method for classification. Several handcrafted features were also calculated and used to train the random forest model. More information about random forest can be found in [136].

A system that receives thoracic CT images and points out suspected COVID-19 cases was proposed by Gozes et al. [26]. The system analyses CT images at two distinct subsystems. Subsystem A performed the 3D analysis of the case volume for nodules and focal opacities, while Subsystem B performed the 2D analysis of each slice of the case to detect and localise larger-sized diffuse opacities. In Subsystem A, nodules and small opacities detection were conducted using a commercial software. Besides the detection of abnormalities, the software also provided measurements and localisation. For Subsystem B, lung segmentation was first performed, and then COVID-19 related abnormalities detection was conducted using CNN with transfer learning and data augmentation. If an image is classified as positive, a localisation map was generated using the Grad-cam technique. To provide a complete review of the case, Subsystems A and B were combined. The final outputs include per slice localisation of opacities (2D), 3D volumetric presentations of the opacities throughout the lungs and a Corona score, which is a volumetric measurement of the opacities burden.

The authors of [137] focused on location-attention classification mechanism. First, the CT images were preprocessed. Second, a 3D CNN model was employed to segment several candidate image patches. Third, an image classification model was trained and employed to categorise all image patches into one of three classes: COVID-19, Influenza-A-viral-pneumonia and irrelevant-to-infection. A location-attention mechanism was embedded in the image classification model to differentiate the structure and appearance of different infections. Finally, the overall analysis report for a single CT sample was generated using the Noisy-or Bayesian function. The results show that the proposed approach could more accurately detect COVID-19 cases than without the location-attention model. Several other studies modified the CNN for COVID-19 detection. In [138], a multi-objective differential evolution-based CNN was utilised. Sedik et al. [139] implemented CNN and LSTM with data augmentation, while Ahsan et al. [140] employed MLP-CNN based model. The authors of [141] employed capsule network-based framework with transfer learning. Table 4 shows the summary of papers for COVID-19 detection using deep learning.

Table 4. Summary of papers for COVID-19 detection using deep learning.

Authors	Deep Learning Technique	Features	Dataset
[137]	CNN with transfer learning and location-attention classification mechanism	Features extracted from CNN	Private dataset
[125]	CNN with transfer learning and data augmentation	Features extracted from CNN	SIRM database, Cohen's Github dataset, Chowdhury's Kaggle dataset
[26]	RADLogics Inc., CNN with transfer learning and data augmentation	Features extracted from RADLogics Inc and CNN	Chainz Dataset, A dataset from a hospital in Wenzhou, China, Dataset from El-Camino Hospital (CA) and Lung image database consortium (LIDC)
[123]	CNN with transfer learning	Features extracted from CNN	Cohen's Github dataset and LDOCTCXR
[21]	CNN with transfer learning and data augmentation	Features extracted from CNN	Cohen's Github dataset and unspecified Kaggle dataset
[135]	VB-Net and modified random decision forests method	96 handcrafted image features	Dataset obtained from Tongji Hospital of Huazhong University of Science and Technology, Shanghai Public Health Clinical Center of Fudan University, and China-Japan Union Hospital of Jilin University.
[126]	CNN from scratch and data augmentation	Features extracted from CNN	COVIDx Dataset
[127]	CNN with transfer learning	Features extracted from CNN	Cohen's Github dataset, Andrew's Kaggle dataset, LDOCTCXR
[117]	CNN with transfer learning	Features extracted from CNN	Cohen's Github dataset, RSNA pneumonia dataset, COVIDx
[131]	CNN with transfer learning and data augmentation	Features extracted from CNN	Sajid's Kaggle dataset
[4]	CNN with transfer learning and data augmentation	Features extracted from CNN	Cohen's Github dataset, Mooney's Kaggle dataset
[118]	CNN with transfer learning	Features extracted from CNN	COVID-CT-Dataset
[128]	CNN as feature extractor and long short-term memory (LSTM) network as classifier	Features extracted from CNN	GitHub, Radiopaedia, The Cancer Imaging Archive, SIRM, Kaggle repository, NIH dataset, Mendeley dataset
[132]	CNN with transfer learning and synthetic data generation and augmentation	Features extracted from CNN	Cohen's Github, Chowdhury's Kaggle dataset, COVID-19 Chest X-ray Dataset, Initiative
[129]	CNN with transfer learning, data augmentation and ensemble by majority voting	Features extracted from CNN	Cohen's Github, LDOCTCXR

Table 4. *Cont.*

Authors	Deep Learning Technique	Features	Dataset
[134]	CNN with transfer learning and stacking ensemble	Features extracted from CNN	Private dataset, LDOCTCXR
[130]	CNN	Features extracted from CNN	Private dataset
[138]	Multi-objective differential evolution-based CNN	Features extracted from CNN	Unspecified
[119]	CNN with transfer learning	Features extracted from CNN	Cohen's Github
[139]	CNN and ConvLSTM with data augmentation	Features extracted from CNN	Cohen's Github, COVID-CT-Dataset
[120]	CNN with transfer learning	Features extracted from CNN	Cohen's Github
[133]	CNN with ensemble by weighted averaging	Features extracted from CNN	Private hospital datasets
[121]	CNN with transfer learning	Features extracted from CNN	Cohen's Github, Mooney's Kaggle dataset, Shenzhen and Montgomery datasets
[140]	MLP-CNN based model	Features extracted from CNN	Cohen's Github
[122]	CNN with transfer learning	Features extracted from CNN	Cohen's Github, unspecified Kaggle dataset
[141]	Capsule Network-based framework with transfer learning	Features extracted from CNN	Cohen's Github, Mooney's Kaggle dataset

4.8. Dataset

The datasets used by the surveyed works are reported in this section. Tables 5–8 show the summary of datasets used for tuberculosis, pneumonia, lung cancer and COVID-19 detection, respectively. This is done to provide readers with relevant information on the datasets. Note that only public datasets are included in the tables because they are available to the public, whereas private datasets are inaccessible without permission.

According to Table 5, among the twelve datasets used for tuberculosis detection works, five of them do not contain tuberculosis medical images: JSRT dataset, Indiana dataset, NIH-14 dataset, LDOCTCXR and RSNA pneumonia dataset. JSRT dataset contains lung cancer images, while the Indiana and NIH-14 datasets contain multiple different diseases. LDOCTCXR and RSNA pneumonia datasets both contain pneumonia and normal lung images. These five datasets were used for transfer learning in several studies. Models were first trained to identify abnormalities in chest X-ray, and then they were trained to identify tuberculosis. The India, Montgomery and Shenzhen datasets contain X-ray images of tuberculosis; ImageCLEF 2018 and ImageCLEF 2019 datasets contain CT images of tuberculosis; and the Belarus dataset contains both X-ray and CT images of tuberculosis. Two of the datasets contain sputum smear microscopy images of tuberculosis: the TBimages dataset and ZiehlNeelsen Sputum smear Microscopy image DataBase.

For detection works related to pneumonia, only four public datasets are available, as shown in Table 6. All four datasets contain X-ray images only. Even though the number of datasets is low, the number of images within these datasets is high. Future studies utilising these datasets should have sufficient data.

Table 5. Summary of datasets used for tuberculosis detection.

Name	Disease	Image Type	Reference	Number of Images	Link
Belarus dataset	Tuberculosis	X-ray and CT	[142]	1299	http://tuberculosis.by
ImageCLEF 2018 dataset	Tuberculosis	CT		2287	https://www.imageclef.org/2018/tuberculosis
ImageCLEF 2019 dataset	Tuberculosis	CT	[143]	335	https://www.imageclef.org/2019/medical/tuberculosis
India	Tuberculosis	X-ray	[39]	78 tuberculosis and 78 normal	https://sourceforge.net/projects/tbxpredict/
Indiana Dataset	Multiple diseases with annotations	X-ray	[144]	7284	https://openi.nlm.nih.gov
JSRT dataset	Lung nodules and normal	X-ray and CT	[145]	154 nodule and 93 non-nodule	http://db.jsrt.or.jp/eng.php
Montgomery and Shenzhen datasets	Tuberculosis and normal	X-ray	[146]	394 tuberculosis and 384 normal	https://lhncbc.nlm.nih.gov/publication/pub9931
NIH-14 dataset	Pneumonia and 13 other diseases	X-ray	[147]	112120	https://www.kaggle.com/nih-chest-xrays/data
TBimages dataset	Tuberculosis	Sputum smear microscopy image	[148]	1320	http://www.tbimages.ufam.edu.br/
ZiehlNeelsen Sputum smear Microscopy image DataBase	Tuberculosis	Sputum smear microscopy image	[27]	620 tuberculosis and 622 normal	http://14.139.240.55/znsm/
Large Dataset of Labeled Optical Coherence Tomography (OCT) and Chest X-Ray Images (LDOCTCXR)	Pneumonia and normal	X-ray	[93]	3883 pneumonia and 1349 normal	https://data.mendeley.com/datasets/rscbjbr9sj/3
Radiological Society of North America (RSNA) pneumonia dataset	Pneumonia and normal	X-ray		5528	https://www.kaggle.com/c/rsna-pneumonia-detection-challenge/data

Table 6. Summary of datasets used for pneumonia detection.

Name	Disease	Image Type	Reference	Number of Images	Link
LDOCTCXR	X-ray	[93]	3883 pneumonia and 1349 normal	https://data.mendeley.com/datasets/rscbjbr9sj/3	
NIH Chest X-ray Dataset	Pneumonia and 13 other diseases	X-ray	[147]	112,120	https://www.kaggle.com/nih-chest-xrays/data
Radiological Society of North America (RSNA) pneumonia dataset	Pneumonia and normal	X-ray		5528	https://www.kaggle.com/c/rsna-pneumonia-detection-challenge/data
Mooney's Kaggle dataset	Pneumonia and normal	X-ray		5863	https://www.kaggle.com/paultimothymooney/chest-xray-pneumonia

According to Table 7, among the ten datasets used for lung cancer detection works, only one contains histopathology images, which is the NCI Genomic Data Commons dataset. The NIH-14 dataset contains X-ray images, while the JSRT dataset contains a mix of X-ray and CT images. The rest of the datasets all contain CT images.

Table 7. Summary of datasets used for lung cancer detection.

Name	Disease	Image Type	Reference	Number of Images	Link
JSRT dataset	Lung nodules and normal lungs	X-ray and CT	[145]	154 nodule and 93 non-nodule	http://db.jsrt.or.jp/eng.php
Kaggle Data Science Bowl 2017 dataset	Lung Cancer	CT scans		601	https://www.kaggle.com/c/data-science-bowl-2017/overview
LIDC-IDRI	Lung Cancer	CT	[149]	1018	https://wiki.cancerimagingarchive.net/display/Public/LIDC-IDRI
Lung Nodule Analysis 2016 (LUNA16) dataset	Location and size of lung nodules	CT scans	[8]	888	https://luna16.grand-challenge.org/download/
NCI Genomic Data Commons	Lung Cancer	histopa- thology images	[150]	More than 575,000	https://portal.gdc.cancer.gov/
NIH-14 dataset	14 lung diseases	X-ray	[147]	112,120	https://www.kaggle.com/nih-chest-xrays/data
NLST	Lung Cancer	CT		Approximately 200,000	https://biometry.nci.nih.gov/cdas/learn/nlst/images/
NSCLC-Radiomics	Lung Cancer	CT		422	https://wiki.cancerimagingarchive.net/display/Public/NSCLC-Radiomics
NSCLC- Radiomics -Genomics	Lung Cancer	CT		89	https://wiki.cancerimagingarchive.net/display/Public/NSCLC-Radiomics-Genomics
RIDER Collections	Lung Cancer	CT		Approximately 280,000	https://wiki.cancerimagingarchive.net/display/Public/RIDER+Collections

Table 8 shows that there are thirteen public datasets related to COVID-19. With the rise of the COVID-19 pandemic, multiple datasets have been made available to the public. Many of these datasets still have a rising number of images. Therefore, the number of images within the datasets might be different from the number reported in this paper. Take note that some of the images might be contained in multiple datasets. Therefore, future studies should check for duplicate images.

Table 9 summarises the works surveyed based on the taxonomy. This allows readers to quickly refer to the articles according to their interested attributes. The analysis of the distribution of works based on the identified attributes of the taxonomy is given in the following section.

Table 8. Summary of datasets used for COVID-19 detection.

Name	Disease	Image Type	Reference	Number of Images	Link
Andrew's Kaggle dataset	COVID-19	X-ray and CT		79	https://www.kaggle.com/andrewmvd/convid19-x-rays
Chainz Dataset	COVID-19 and normal	CT		50 COVID-19, 51 normal	www.ChainZ.cn
Chowdhury's Kaggle dataset	COVID-19, normal and pneumonia	X-ray	[125]	219 COVID-19, 1341 normal and 1345 pneumonia	https://www.kaggle.com/tawsifurrahman/covid19-radiography-database
Cohen's Github dataset	COVID-19	X-ray and CT	[151]	123	https://github.com/ieee8023/covid-chestxray-dataset

Table 8. *Cont.*

Name	Disease	Image Type	Reference	Number of Images	Link
COVIDx Dataset	COVID-19, normal and pneumonia	X-ray	[126]	573 COVID-19, 8066 normal and 5559 pneumonia	https://github.com/lindawangg/COVID-Net/blob/master/docs/COVIDx.md
Italian Society Of Medical And Interventional Radiology (SIRM) COVID-19 Database	COVID-19	X-ray and CT		68	https://www.sirm.org/category/senza-categoria/covid-19/
LDOCTCXR	Pneumonia and normal	X-ray	[93]	3883 pneumonia and 1349 normal	https://data.mendeley.com/datasets/rscbjbr9sj/3
Lung image database consortium (LIDC)	Lung Cancer	CT	[149]	1018	https://wiki.cancerimagingarchive.net/display/Public/LIDC-IDRI
Sajid's Kaggle dataset	COVID-19 and normal	X-ray		28 normal, 70 COVID-19	https://www.kaggle.com/nabeelsajid917/covid-19-x-ray-10000-images
Mooney's Kaggle dataset	Pneumonia and normal	X-ray		5863	https://www.kaggle.com/paultimothymooney/chest-xray-pneumonia
COVID-CT Dataset	COVID-19 and normal	CT		349 COVID-19 and 463 non-COVID-19	https://github.com/UCSD-AI4H/COVID-CT
Mendeley Augmented COVID-19 X-ray Images Dataset	COVID-19 and normal	X-ray		912	https://data.mendeley.com/datasets/2fxz4px6d8/4
COVID-19 Chest X-Ray Dataset Initiative	COVID-19	X-ray		55	https://github.com/agchung/Figure1-COVID-chestxray-dataset

Table 9. Summary of the works surveyed based on the taxonomy.

Attributes	Subattributes	References
Image types	X-Ray	[4,12,14,15,19–21,24,36,38,55,57,60–85,91–103,109,113,114,117,119–129,131,132,134,139–141]
	CT Scans	[13,23,25,26,86–88,105–108,110–112,118,130,133,135,137–139]
	Sputum Smear Microscopy Images	[28–32]
	Histopathology images	[34]
Features	Extracted from CNN	[4,12–15,19–21,23–26,30,32,34,55,57,60–82,84–87,91–103,105–114,117–134,137–141]
	Others	[12,15,26,28,29,31,36,38,61,62,64,71,81,83,86,88,105,135]
Data augmentation	Yes	[4,20,21,23,26,55,57,63,66,70,73,74,77,79,92,96–98,100,102,106,109–111,114,122,125,126,128,129,131,132,139]
Types of deep learning algorithm	CNN	[4,12–15,19–21,23–26,28–30,32,34,55,57,60–69,72,74,76–82,84–86,91–103,105–114,117–134,137–141]
	Non-CNN	[19,26,31,36,38,83,88,105,135]
Transfer learning	Fixed feature extractor	[12,15,19,21,62,70,76,78,80,81,93,94,96,100,102,117,127,128,137]
	Fine-tuning CNN	[4,20,26,32,34,55,57,71–74,76,77,79,82,95,97,98,102,109–113,118–125,129,131,132,134,141]
Ensemble	Majority voting	[19,55,82,129]
	Probability score averaging	[15,57,71,79,81,82,98,102,133]
	Stacking	[12,82,134]
	Other	[80]
Disease types	Tuberculosis	[12,15,19,24,28–32,36,38,57,60–88]
	Pneumonia	[20,55,91–103]
	Lung cancer	[13,14,23,25,34,105–114]
	COVID-19	[4,21,26,117–135,137–141]

5. Analysis of Trend, Issues and Future Directions of Lung Disease Detection Using Deep Learning

In this section, the broad analysis of the existing work is presented, which is the last contribution outlined in this paper. The analysis of the trend of each attribute identified in the foregoing section is described, whereby the aim is to show the progress of the works and the direction the researchers are heading over the last five years. The shown trend could be useful to suggest the future direction of the work in this domain. Section 5.1 presents the analysis of the trend of the articles considered. The issues and potential future work to address the identified issues are described in Section 5.2.

5.1. An Analysis of the Trend of Lung Disease Detection in Recent Years

This subsection presents the analysis of lung disease detection works in recent years for each attribute of the taxonomy described in the foregoing section.

5.1.1. Trend Analysis of the Image Type Used

Figure 10a shows that the usage of X-ray images increases linearly over the years. The usage of CT images also increases over the years, with a slight dip in 2018. The sputum smear microscopy and histopathology images are combined into one as 'Others' due to the low number of previous work using them to detect lung diseases. The usage of other image types slowly increases until 2018, and then drops. This indicates that deep learning aided lung disease detection works are heading towards the direction of using X-ray images and CT images.

Figure 10b shows that the majority of the studies used X-ray images at 71%, while CT images followed second with 23%. Such observation could be due to the availability, accessibility and mobility of X-ray machines over the CT scanner. Due to the COVID-19 pandemic that has spread to all types of geographical locations, it is anticipated that the X-ray images will still be the dominant choice of medical images used to detect lung-related diseases over CT images. CT images may remain the second choice because they provide more detailed information than X-rays.

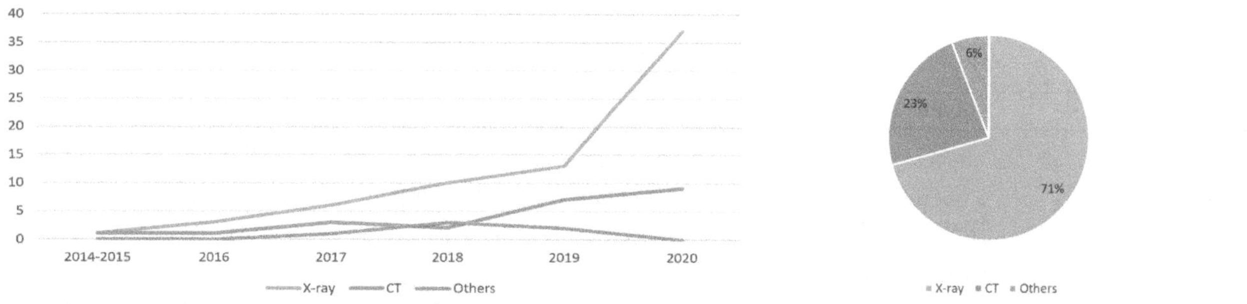

(a) **(b)**

Figure 10. (**a**) The trend of the usage of image types in lung disease detection works in recent years; and (**b**) the distribution of the image type used in deep learning aided lung disease detection in recent years.

5.1.2. Trend Analysis of the Features Used

From the perspective of features used for lung disease detection in recent years, as shown in Figure 11a, the usage of CNN extracted features is steadily increasing, while the usage of other features and the combination of CNN extracted features plus other features remain low. This is because CNN allows automated feature extraction, discarding the need for manual feature generation [40]. The usage of other features was less preferred due to the fact that most recent works showed the superiority of CNN extracted features in detecting lung diseases. Figure 11b shows the distribution of work by type of features used. CNN extracted features were used in 79% of the works. The combination of CNN extracted features plus some other features were used in 13% of the recent works, while the remaining works utilised other types of features.

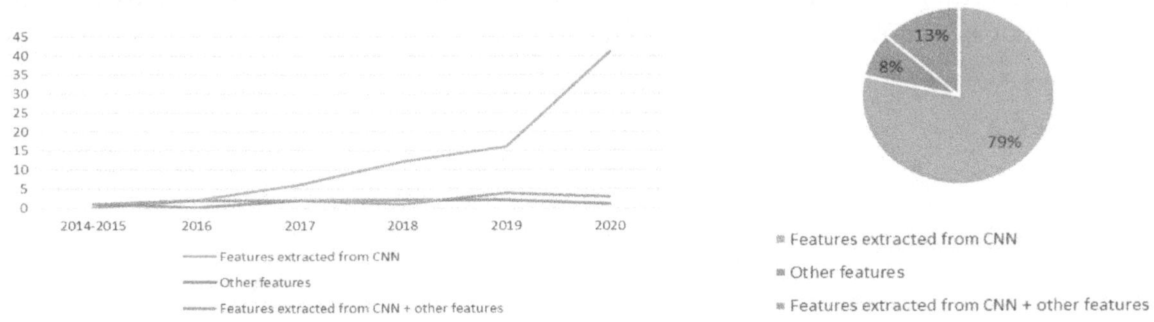

(a) (b)

Figure 11. (**a**) The trend of the usage of features in lung disease detection works in recent years; and (**b**) the distribution of usage of data augmentation in deep learning aided lung disease detection in recent years.

5.1.3. Trend Analysis of the Usage of Data Augmentation

Figure 12a shows the trend of the usage of data augmentation. Although implementing data augmentation increased the complexity of the data pre-processing, the number of works employing data augmentation increases steadily over the years. Such trend signifies that more researchers have realised how beneficial data augmentation is to train the lung disease detection models.

Figure 12b shows the distribution of data augmentation usage in deep learning aided lung disease detection. Only about one-third of the studies used data augmentation. While it is reported that data augmentation improved the classification accuracy, the majority of works did not use data augmentation. One reason for this might be that data augmentation is not that simple to implement. As mentioned in Section 4.3, the disadvantages of data augmentation include additional memory costs, transformation computing costs and training time.

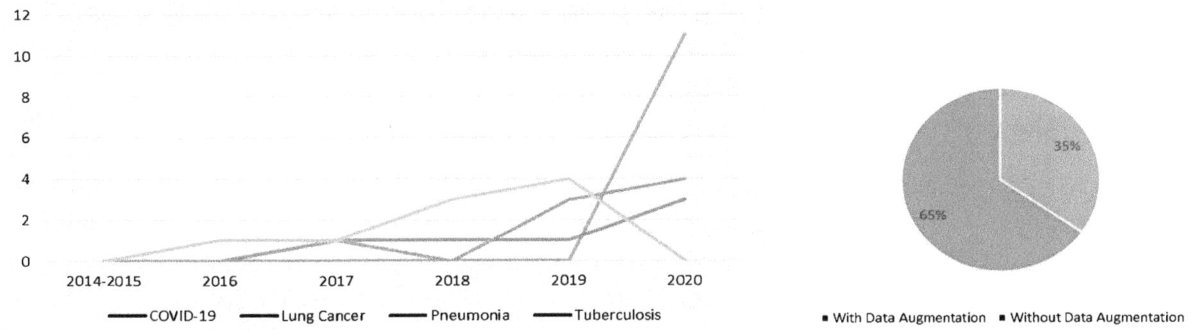

(a) (b)

Figure 12. (**a**) The trend of the usage of data augmentation in lung disease detection works in recent years; and (**b**) the distribution of usage of data augmentation in deep learning aided lung disease detection in recent years.

5.1.4. Trend Analysis of the Types of Deep Learning Algorithm Used

Figure 13a shows the trend of the usage of deep learning algorithms in lung disease detection works in recent years. As shown in Figure 13, CNN was the most preferred deep learning algorithm for the last five years. Future works will likely follow this trend, whereby more work may prefer CNN for lung disease detection over other deep learning algorithms.

Figure 13b visualises the analysis of the usage of CNN in deep learning aided lung disease detection in recent years. The majority of the papers surveyed used CNN. This is because CNN is robust and can achieve high classification accuracy. Many of the works surveyed indicate that CNN has superior performance [74]. Other benefits of using CNN include automatic feature extraction and utilising the advantages of transfer learning, which is further analysed in the following subsection.

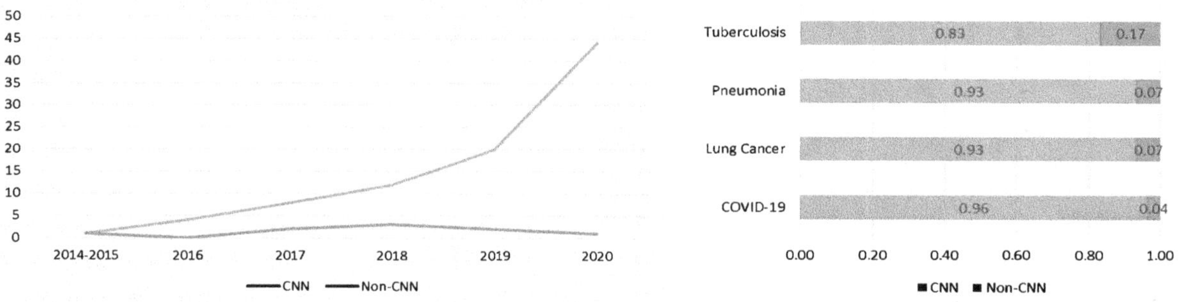

(a) (b)

Figure 13. (**a**) The trend of the usage of deep learning algorithms in lung disease detection works in recent years; and (**b**) the distribution of the usage of CNN in deep learning aided lung disease detection in recent years.

5.1.5. Trend Analysis of the Usage Of Transfer Learning

Figure 14a shows the trend of the usage of transfer learning. As time goes on, more works employed transfer learning. With transfer learning, there is no need to define a new model. Transfer learning also allows the usage features learned while training from an old task for the new task, often increasing the classification accuracy. This could be due to the model used being more generalised as it has been trained with a greater number of images.

Figure 14b shows the usage of transfer learning among the works which used CNN. According to the figure, 57% of the recent works utilised transfer learning. Even though the number of works utilising transfer learning increased over the years, as shown in Figure 14a, the percentage of works using transfer learning is just 57%. For example, in 2020, out of 44 studies that used CNN, 28 implemented transfer learning. This suggests that works in this domain are moving towards the direction of using transfer learning, but not at a high pace. Transfer learning remains a strong approach to lung disease detection, with respect to the detection performance. Hence, the distribution of work may be skewed towards transfer learning in the near future.

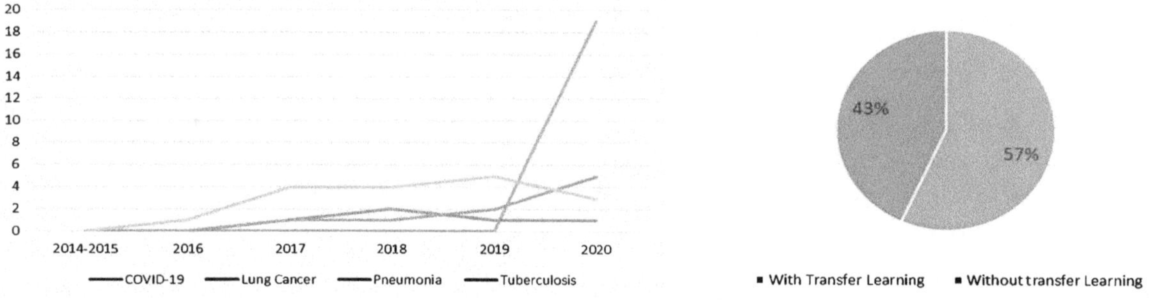

(a) (b)

Figure 14. (**a**) The trend of the usage of transfer learning in lung disease detection works in recent years; and (**b**) the usage of transfer learning in lung disease detection works using CNN.

5.1.6. Trend Analysis of the Usage Of Ensemble

Based on Figure 15a, it seems that the ensemble was only applied on COVID-19, pneumonia and tuberculosis detection. It is observed that the usage of the ensemble is slowly growing in popularity for pneumonia and COVID-19 detection. Although less popular, the works that deployed an ensemble classifier reported better detection performance than when not using ensemble.

Figure 15b shows the distribution of the usage of the ensemble in deep learning aided lung disease detection. Only 15% of the studies used ensemble. This suggests that ensemble classifier is still less explored for lung disease detection. Only three types of ensemble techniques were found in the papers surveyed, which were majority voting, probability score averaging and stacking. The challenge to implement ensemble may be the caused of such low application. Using ensemble, the performance could only improve if the errors of the base classifiers have a low correlation. When using similar data, which may occur when the size of the datasets and the number of datasets itself are limited, the correlation of errors of the base classifiers tends to be high.

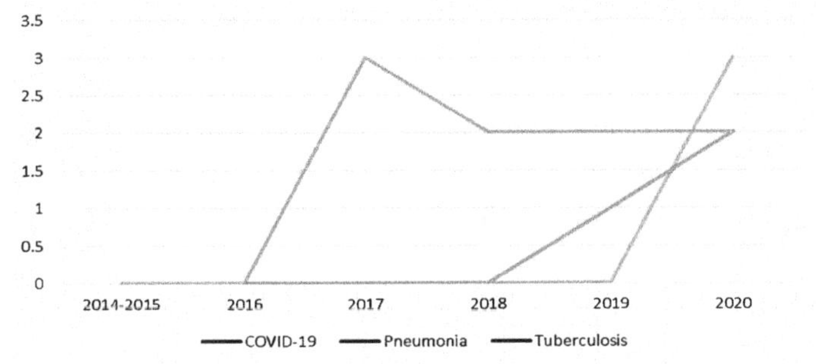

(a)

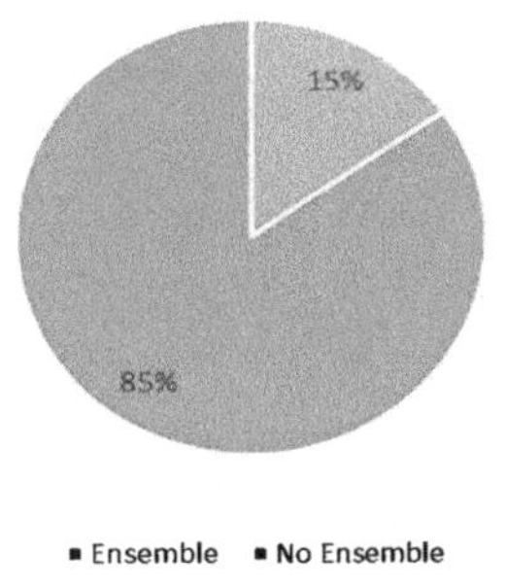

(b)

Figure 15. (**a**) The trend of the usage of ensemble classifier in lung disease detection works in recent years; and (**b**) the distribution of the usage of the ensemble in deep learning aided lung disease detection in recent years.

5.1.7. Trend Analysis of the Type Of Lung Disease Detected using Deep Learning

Based on the trend shown in Figure 16a, the total number of lung disease detection works using deep learning increased steadily over the years, with most work related to tuberculosis detection. As more lung disease medical image datasets become public, researchers have access to more data. Thus, more extensive studies were conducted. Towards 2020, the works on COVID-19 detection emerged while work conducted to detect other diseases decreased tremendously. This signifies that using deep learning to detect lung disease is still an active field of study. This also shows that much effort was directed towards easing the burden of detecting COVID-19 using the existing manual screening test, which is already anticipated.

Figure 16b shows the distribution of the diseases detected using deep learning in recent years. The majority of works were directed at tuberculosis detection, followed by COVID-19, lung cancer and pneumonia. The reason that works of tuberculosis are high is because the majority of tuberculosis-infected inhabitants were from resource-poor regions with poor healthcare infrastructure [61]. Therefore, tuberculosis detection using deep learning provides the opportunity to accelerate tuberculosis diagnosis among these communities. The reason that works of COVID-19 detection are second highest is because researchers all over the world are trying to reduce the burden of detecting COVID-19, and thus many works have been published, even though COVID-19 is a relatively new disease.

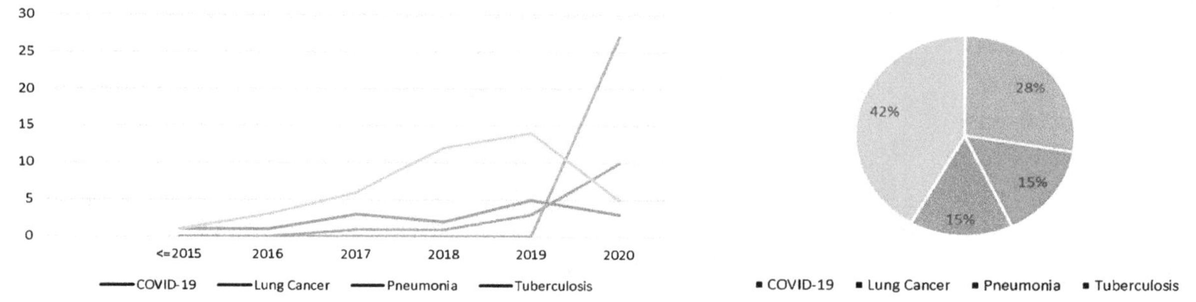

(a) (b)

Figure 16. (**a**) The trend of the deep learning aided lung disease detection works in recent years; and (**b**) the distribution of the diseases detected using deep learning in recent years.

5.2. Issues and Future Direction of Lung Disease Detection Using Deep Learning

This subsection presents the remaining issues and corresponding future direction of lung disease detection using deep learning, which are the final contributions of this paper. The state-of-the-art lung disease detection field is suffering from several issues that can be found in the papers considered. Some of the proposed future works are designed to deal with the issues found. Details of the issues and potential future works are presented in Sections 5.2.1 and 5.2.2, respectively.

5.2.1. Issues

This section presents the issues of lung disease detection using deep learning found in the literature. Four main issues were identified: (i) data imbalance; (ii) handling of huge image size; (iii) limited available datasets; and (iv) high correlation of errors when using ensemble techniques.

(i) Data imbalance: When doing classification training, if the number of samples of one class is a lot higher than the other class, the resulting model would be biased. It is better to have the same number of images in each class. However, oftentimes that is not the case. For example, when performing a multiclass classification of COVID-19, pneumonia and normal lungs, the number of images for pneumonia far exceeds the number of images for COVID-19 [126].
(ii) Handling of huge image size: Most researchers reduced the original image size during training to reduce computational cost. It is extremely computationally expensive to train with the original image size, and it is also time-consuming to train a deeply complex model even with the aid of the most powerful GPU hardware.
(iii) Limited available datasets: Ideally, thousands of images of each class should be obtained for training. This is to produce a more accurate classifier. However, due to the limited number of datasets, the number of available training data is often less than ideal. This causes researchers to search for other alternatives to produce a good classifier.
(iv) High correlation of errors when using ensemble techniques: It requires a variety of errors for an ensemble of classifiers to perform the best. The base classifiers used should have a very low correlation. This, in turn, will ensure the errors of those classifiers also will be varied. In other words, it is expected that the base classifiers will complement each other to produce better classification results. Most of the studies surveyed only combine classifiers that were trained on similar features. This causes the correlation error of the base classifiers to be high.

5.2.2. Potential Future Works

This section presents the possible future works that should be considered to improvise the performance of lung disease detection using deep learning.

(i) Make datasets available to the public: Some researchers used private hospital datasets. To obtain larger datasets, efforts such as de-identification of confidential patients' information can be conducted to make the data public. With more data available, the produced classifiers would be more accurate. This is because, with more data comes more diversity. This decreases the generalisation error because the model becomes more general as it was trained on more examples. Medical data are hard to come by. Therefore, if the datasets were made public, more data would be available for researchers.

(ii) Usage of cloud computing: Performing training using cloud computing might overcome the problem of handling of huge image size. On a local mid-range computer, training with large images will be slow. A high-end computer might speed up the process a little, but it might still be infeasible. However, by training the deep learning model using cloud computing, we can use multiple GPUs at a reasonable cost. This allows higher computational cost training to be conducted faster and cheaper.

(iii) Usage of more variety of features: Most researchers use features automatically extracted by CNN. Some other features such as SIFT, GIST, Gabor, LBP and HOG were studied. However, many other features are still yet to be explored, for example quadtree and image histogram. Efforts can be directed to studying different types of features. This can address the issue of the high correlation of errors when using ensemble techniques. With more features comes more variation. When combining many variations, the results are often better [41]. Feature engineering allows the extraction of more information from present data. New information is extracted in terms of new features. These features might have a better ability to describe the variance in the training data, thus improving model accuracy.

(iv) Usage of the ensemble learning: Ensemble techniques show great potentials. Ensemble methods often improve detection accuracy. An ensemble of several features might provide better detection results. An ensemble of different deep learning techniques could also be considered because ensembles perform better if the errors of the base classifiers have a low correlation.

6. Limitation of the Survey

The survey presented has a limitation whereby the primary source of work considered were those indexed in the Scopus database, due to the reason described in Section 2. Exceptions were given on COVID-19 related works, as most of the articles were still at the preprint level when this survey was conducted. Concerning the publication years considered, the latest publication included were those published prior to October 2020. Therefore, the findings put forward in this survey paper did not consider contributions of works that are non-Scopus indexed and those that are published commencing October 2020 and onwards.

7. Conclusions

As time goes on, more works on lung disease detection using deep learning have been published. However, there was a lack of systematic survey available on the current state of research and application. This paper is thus produced to offer an extensive survey of lung disease detection using deep learning, specifically on tuberculosis, pneumonia, lung cancer and COVID-19, published from 2016 to September 2020. In total, 98 articles on this topic were considered in producing this survey.

To summarise and provide an organisation of the key concepts and focus of the existing work on lung disease detection using deep learning, a taxonomy of state-of-the-art deep learning aided lung disease detection was constructed based on the survey on the works considered. Analyses of the trend on recent works on this topic, based on the identified attributes from the taxonomy, are also presented. From the analyses of the distribution of works, the usage of both CNN and transfer learning is high. Concerning the trend of the surveyed work, all the identified attributes in the taxonomy observed, on average, a linear increase over the years, with an exception to the ensemble attribute. The remaining issues and future direction of lung disease detection using deep learning were subsequently established and described. Four issues of lung disease detection using deep learning were identified: data imbalance, handling of huge image size, limited available datasets and high correlation of errors when using ensemble techniques. Four potential works for lung disease detection using deep learning are suggested to resolve the identified issues: making datasets available to the public, usage of cloud computing, usage of more features and usage of the ensemble.

To conclude, investigating how deep learning was employed in lung disease detection is highly significant to ensure future research will concentrate on the right track, thereby improving the performance of disease detection systems. The presented taxonomy could be used by other researchers to plan their research contributions and activities. The potential future direction suggested could further improve the efficiency and increase the number of deep learning aided lung disease detection applications.

Author Contributions: All authors contributed to the study conceptualisation and design. Material preparation and analysis were performed by S.T.H.K. and M.H.A.H. The first draft of the manuscript was written by S.T.H.K., supervised by M.H.A.H., A.B. and H.K. All authors provided critical feedback and helped shape the manuscript. All authors have read and agreed to the published version of the manuscript.

References

1. Bousquet, J. *Global Surveillance, Prevention and Control of Chronic Respiratory Diseases*; World Health Organization: Geneva, Switzerland, 2007; pp. 12–36.
2. Forum of International Respiratory Societies. *The Global Impact of Respiratory Disease*, 2nd ed.; European Respiratory Society, Sheffield, UK, 2017; pp. 5–42.
3. World Health Organization. *Coronavirus Disease 2019 (COVID-19) Situation Report*; Technical Report March; World Health Organization: Geneva, Switzerland, 2020.
4. Rahaman, M.M.; Li, C.; Yao, Y.; Kulwa, F.; Rahman, M.A.; Wang, Q.; Qi, S.; Kong, F.; Zhu, X.; Zhao, X. Identification of COVID-19 samples from chest X-Ray images using deep learning: A comparison of transfer learning approaches. *J. X-Ray Sci. Technol.* **2020**, *28*, 821–839. [CrossRef]
5. Yahiaoui, A.; Er, O.; Yumusak, N. A new method of automatic recognition for tuberculosis disease diagnosis using support vector machines. *Biomed. Res.* **2017**, *28*, 4208–4212.
6. Hu, Z.; Tang, J.; Wang, Z.; Zhang, K.; Zhang, L.; Sun, Q. Deep learning for image-based cancer detection and diagnosis-A survey. *Pattern Recognit.* **2018**, *83*, 134–149. [CrossRef]
7. American Thoracic Society. Diagnostic Standards and Classification of Tuberculosis in Adults and Children. *Am. J. Respir. Crit. Care Med.* **2000**, *161*, 1376–1395. [CrossRef]
8. Setio, A.A.A.; Traverso, A.; de Bel, T.; Berens, M.S.; van den Bogaard, C.; Cerello, P.; Chen, H.; Dou, Q.; Fantacci, M.E.; Geurts, B.; et al. Validation, comparison, and combination of algorithms for automatic detection of pulmonary nodules in computed tomography images: The LUNA16 challenge. *Med. Image Anal.* **2017**, *42*, 1–13. [CrossRef]
9. Shen, D.; Wu, G.; Suk, H.I. Deep Learning in Medical Image Analysis. *Annu. Rev. Biomed. Eng.* **2017**, *19*, 221–248. [CrossRef]
10. Wu, C.; Luo, C.; Xiong, N.; Zhang, W.; Kim, T.H. A Greedy Deep Learning Method for Medical Disease Analysis. *IEEE Access* **2018**, *6*, 20021–20030. [CrossRef]
11. Ma, J.; Song, Y.; Tian, X.; Hua, Y.; Zhang, R.; Wu, J. Survey on deep learning for pulmonary medical imaging. *Front. Med.* **2019**, *14*, 450–469. [CrossRef]
12. Rajaraman, S.; Candemir, S.; Xue, Z.; Alderson, P.O.; Kohli, M.; Abuya, J.; Thoma, G.R.; Antani, S.; Member, S. A novel stacked generalization of models for improved TB detection in chest radiographs. In Proceedings of the 2018 40th Annual International Conference the IEEE Engineering in Medicine and Biology Society (EMBC), Honolulu, HI, USA, 17–21 July 2018; pp. 718–721. [CrossRef]

13. Ardila, D.; Kiraly, A.P.; Bharadwaj, S.; Choi, B.; Reicher, J.J.; Peng, L.; Tse, D.; Etemadi, M.; Ye, W.; Corrado, G.; et al. End-to-end lung cancer screening with three-dimensional deep learning on low-dose chest computed tomography. *Nat. Med.* **2019**, *25*, 954–961. [CrossRef]
14. Gordienko, Y.; Gang, P.; Hui, J.; Zeng, W.; Kochura, Y.; Alienin, O.; Rokovyi, O.; Stirenko, S. Deep Learning with Lung Segmentation and Bone Shadow Exclusion Techniques for Chest X-Ray Analysis of Lung Cancer. *Adv. Intell. Syst. Comput.* **2019**, 638–647. [CrossRef]
15. Kieu, S.T.H.; Hijazi, M.H.A.; Bade, A.; Yaakob, R.; Jeffree, S. Ensemble deep learning for tuberculosis detection using chest X-Ray and canny edge detected images. *IAES Int. J. Artif. Intell.* **2019**, *8*, 429–435. [CrossRef]
16. Dietterich, T.G. Ensemble Methods in Machine Learning. *Int. Workshop Mult. Classif. Syst.* **2000**, 1–15._1. [CrossRef]
17. Webb, A. *Introduction To Biomedical Imaging*; John Wiley & Sons, Inc.: Hoboken, NJ, USA, 2003. [CrossRef]
18. Kwan-Hoong, N.; Madan M, R. X ray imaging goes digital. *Br. Med J.* **2006**, *333*, 765–766. [CrossRef]
19. Lopes, U.K.; Valiati, J.F. Pre-trained convolutional neural networks as feature extractors for tuberculosis detection. *Comput. Biol. Med.* **2017**, *89*, 135–143. [CrossRef] [PubMed]
20. Ayan, E.; Ünver, H.M. Diagnosis of Pneumonia from Chest X-Ray Images using Deep Learning. *Sci. Meet. Electr.-Electron. Biomed. Eng. Comput. Sci.* **2019**, 1–5. [CrossRef]
21. Salman, F.M.; Abu-naser, S.S.; Alajrami, E.; Abu-nasser, B.S.; Ashqar, B.A.M. COVID-19 Detection using Artificial Intelligence. *Int. J. Acad. Eng. Res.* **2020**, *4*, 18–25.
22. Herman, G.T. *Fundamentals of Computerized Tomography*; Springer: London, UK, 2009; Volume 224. [CrossRef]
23. Song, Q.Z.; Zhao, L.; Luo, X.K.; Dou, X.C. Using Deep Learning for Classification of Lung Nodules on Computed Tomography Images. *J. Healthc. Eng.* **2017**, *2017*. [CrossRef]
24. Gao, X.W.; James-reynolds, C.; Currie, E. Analysis of tuberculosis severity levels from CT pulmonary images based on enhanced residual deep learning architecture. *Neurocomputing* **2019**, *392*, 233–244. [CrossRef]
25. Rao, P.; Pereira, N.A.; Srinivasan, R. Convolutional neural networks for lung cancer screening in computed tomography (CT) scans. In Proceedings of the 2016 2nd International Conference on Contemporary Computing and Informatics, IC3I 2016, Noida, India, 14–17 December 2016 ; pp. 489–493. [CrossRef]
26. Gozes, O.; Frid, M.; Greenspan, H.; Patrick, D. Rapid AI Development Cycle for the Coronavirus (COVID-19) Pandemic: Initial Results for Automated Detection & Patient Monitoring using Deep Learning CT Image Analysis Article. *arXiv* **2020**, arXiv:2003.05037.
27. Shah, M.I.; Mishra, S.; Yadav, V.K.; Chauhan, A.; Sarkar, M.; Sharma, S.K.; Rout, C. Ziehl–Neelsen sputum smear microscopy image database: A resource to facilitate automated bacilli detection for tuberculosis diagnosis. *J. Med. Imaging* **2017**, *4*, 027503. [CrossRef]
28. López, Y.P.; Filho, C.F.F.C.; Aguilera, L.M.R.; Costa, M.G.F. Automatic classification of light field smear microscopy patches using Convolutional Neural Networks for identifying Mycobacterium Tuberculosis. In Proceedings of the 2017 CHILEAN Conference on Electrical, Electronics Engineering, Information and Communication Technologies (CHILECON), Pucon, Chile, 18–20 October 2017 .
29. Kant, S.; Srivastava, M.M. Towards Automated Tuberculosis detection using Deep Learning. In Proceedings of the 2018 IEEE Symposium Series on Computational Intelligence (SSCI), Bengaluru, India, 18–21 November 2018; pp. 1250–1253. [CrossRef]
30. Oomman, R.; Kalmady, K.S.; Rajan, J.; Sabu, M.K. Automatic detection of tuberculosis bacilli from microscopic sputum smear images using deep learning methods. *Integr. Med. Res.* **2018**, *38*, 691–699. [CrossRef]
31. Mithra, K.S.; Emmanuel, W.R.S. Automated identification of mycobacterium bacillus from sputum images for tuberculosis diagnosis. *Signal Image Video Process.* **2019**. [CrossRef]
32. Samuel, R.D.J.; Kanna, B.R. Tuberculosis (TB) detection system using deep neural networks. *Neural Comput. Appl.* **2019**, *31*, 1533–1545. [CrossRef]
33. Gurcan, M.N.; Boucheron, L.E.; Can, A.; Madabhushi, A.; Rajpoot, N.M.; Yener, B. Histopathological Image Analysis: A Review. *IEEE Rev. Biomed. Eng.* **2009**, *2*, 147–171. [CrossRef]
34. Coudray, N.; Ocampo, P.S.; Sakellaropoulos, T.; Narula, N.; Snuderl, M.; Fenyö, D.; Moreira, A.L.; Razavian, N.; Tsirigos, A. Classification and mutation prediction from non–small cell lung cancer histopathology images using deep learning. *Nat. Med.* **2018**, *24*, 1559–1567. [CrossRef]

35. O'Mahony, N.; Campbell, S.; Carvalho, A.; Harapanahalli, S.; Hernandez, G.V.; Krpalkova, L.; Riordan, D.; Walsh, J. Deep Learning vs . Traditional Computer Vision. *Adv. Intell. Syst. Comput.* **2020**, 128–144. [CrossRef]
36. Vajda, S.; Karargyris, A.; Jaeger, S.; Santosh, K.C.; Candemir, S.; Xue, Z.; Antani, S.; Thoma, G. Feature Selection for Automatic Tuberculosis Screening in Frontal Chest Radiographs. *J. Med Syst.* **2018**, *42*. [CrossRef]
37. Jaeger, S.; Karargyris, A.; Candemir, S.; Folio, L.; Siegelman, J.; Callaghan, F.; Xue, Z.; Palaniappan, K.; Singh, R.K.; Antani, S.; et al. Automatic tuberculosis screening using chest radiographs. *IEEE Trans. Med. Imaging* **2014**, *33*, 233–245. [CrossRef]
38. Antony, B.; Nizar Banu, P.K. Lung tuberculosis detection using x-ray images. *Int. J. Appl. Eng. Res.* **2017**, *12*, 15196–15201.
39. Chauhan, A.; Chauhan, D.; Rout, C. Role of gist and PHOG features in computer-aided diagnosis of tuberculosis without segmentation. *PLoS ONE* **2014**, *9*, e112980. [CrossRef]
40. Al-Ajlan, A.; Allali, A.E. CNN—MGP: Convolutional Neural Networks for Metagenomics Gene Prediction. *Interdiscip. Sci. Comput. Life Sci.* **2019**, *11*, 628–635. [CrossRef] [PubMed]
41. Domingos, P. A Few Useful Things to Know About Machine Learning. *Commun. ACM* **2012**, *55*, 78–87. [CrossRef]
42. Mikołajczyk, A.; Grochowski, M. Data augmentation for improving deep learning in image classification problem. In Proceedings of the 2018 International Interdisciplinary PhD Workshop, Swinoujscie, Poland, 9–12 May 2018; pp. 117–122. [CrossRef]
43. Shorten, C.; Khoshgoftaar, T.M. A survey on Image Data Augmentation for Deep Learning. *J. Big Data* **2019**, *6*. [CrossRef]
44. O'Shea, K.; Nash, R. An Introduction to Convolutional Neural Networks. *arXiv* **2015**, arXiv:1511.08458v2.
45. Ker, J.; Wang, L. Deep Learning Applications in Medical Image Analysis. *IEEE Access* **2018**, *6*, 9375–9389. [CrossRef]
46. Pan, S.J.; Yang, Q. A Survey on Transfer Learning. *IEEE Trans. Knowl. Data Eng.* **2010**, *22*, 1345–1359. [CrossRef]
47. Lanbouri, Z.; Achchab, S. A hybrid Deep belief network approach for Financial distress prediction. In Proceedings of the 2015 10th International Conference on Intelligent Systems: Theories and Applications (SITA), Rabat, Morocco, 20–21 October 2015; pp. 1–6. [CrossRef]
48. Hinton, G.E.; Osindero, S. A fast learning algorithm for deep belief nets. *Neural Comput.* **2006**, *18*, 1527–1554. [CrossRef]
49. Cao, X.; Wipf, D.; Wen, F.; Duan, G.; Sun, J. A practical transfer learning algorithm for face verification. In Proceedings of the IEEE International Conference on Computer Vision, Sydney, Australia, 1–8 December 2013; pp. 3208–3215. [CrossRef]
50. Wang, C.; Chen, D.; Hao, L.; Liu, X.; Zeng, Y.; Chen, J.; Zhang, G. Pulmonary Image Classification Based on Inception-v3 Transfer Learning Model. *IEEE Access* **2019**, *7*, 146533–146541. [CrossRef]
51. Krizhevsky, A.; Sutskeve, I.; Hinton, G.E. ImageNet Classification with Deep Convolutional Neural Networks. *Adv. Neural Inf. Process. Syst.* **2012**. [CrossRef]
52. Tajbakhsh, N.; Shin, J.Y.; Gurudu, S.R.; Hurst, R.T.; Kendall, C.B.; Gotway, M.B.; Liang, J. Convolutional Neural Networks for Medical Image Analysis: Full Training or Fine Tuning? *IEEE Trans. Med. Imaging* **2016**, *35*, 1299–1312. [CrossRef]
53. Nogueira, K.; Penatti, O.A.; dos Santos, J.A. Towards better exploiting convolutional neural networks for remote sensing scene classification. *Pattern Recognit.* **2017**, *61*, 539–556. [CrossRef]
54. Kabari, L.G.; Onwuka, U. Comparison of Bagging and Voting Ensemble Machine Learning Algorithm as a Classifier. *Int. J. Adv. Res. Comput. Sci. Softw. Eng.* **2019**, *9*, 1–6.
55. Chouhan, V.; Singh, S.K.; Khamparia, A.; Gupta, D.; Albuquerque, V.H.C.D. A Novel Transfer Learning Based Approach for Pneumonia Detection in Chest X-ray Images. *Appl. Sci.* **2020**, *10*, 559. [CrossRef]
56. Lincoln, W.P.; Skrzypekt, J. Synergy of Clustering Multiple Back Propagation Networks. *Adv. Neural Inf. Process. Syst.* **1990**, *2*, 650–659.
57. Lakhani, P.; Sundaram, B. Deep Learning at Chest Radiography: Automated Classification of Pulmonary Tuberculosis by Using Convolutional Neural Networks. *Radiology* **2017**, *284*, 574–582. [CrossRef]

58. Divina, F.; Gilson, A.; Goméz-Vela, F.; Torres, M.G.; Torres, J.F. Stacking Ensemble Learning for Short-Term Electricity Consumption Forecasting. *Energies* **2018**, *11*, 949. [CrossRef]
59. World Health Organisation. *Global Health TB Report*; World Health Organisation: Geneva, Switzerland, 2018; p. 277.
60. Murphy, K.; Habib, S.S.; Zaidi, S.M.A.; Khowaja, S.; Khan, A.; Melendez, J.; Scholten, E.T.; Amad, F.; Schalekamp, S.; Verhagen, M.; et al. Computer aided detection of tuberculosis on chest radiographs: An evaluation of the CAD4TB v6 system. *Sci. Rep.* **2019**, *10*, 1–11. [CrossRef]
61. Melendez, J.; Sánchez, C.I.; Philipsen, R.H.; Maduskar, P.; Dawson, R.; Theron, G.; Dheda, K.; Van Ginneken, B. An automated tuberculosis screening strategy combining X-ray-based computer-aided detection and clinical information. *Sci. Rep.* **2016**, *6*, 1–8. [CrossRef]
62. Heo, S.J.; Kim, Y.; Yun, S.; Lim, S.S.; Kim, J.; Nam, C.M.; Park, E.C.; Jung, I.; Yoon, J.H. Deep Learning Algorithms with Demographic Information Help to Detect Tuberculosis in Chest Radiographs in Annual Workers' Health Examination Data. *Int. J. Environ. Res. Public Health* **2019**, *16*, 250. [CrossRef]
63. Pasa, F.; Golkov, V.; Pfeiffer, F.; Cremers, D.; Pfeiffer, D. Efficient Deep Network Architectures for Fast Chest X-Ray Tuberculosis Screening and Visualization. *Sci. Rep.* **2019**, *9*, 2–10. [CrossRef]
64. Cao, Y.; Liu, C.; Liu, B.; Brunette, M.J.; Zhang, N.; Sun, T.; Zhang, P.; Peinado, J.; Garavito, E.S.; Garcia, L.L.; et al. Improving Tuberculosis Diagnostics Using Deep Learning and Mobile Health Technologies among Resource-Poor and Marginalized Communities. In Proceedings of the 2016 IEEE 1st International Conference on Connected Health: Applications, Systems and Engineering Technologies, CHASE, Washington, DC, USA, 27–29 June 2016 ; pp. 274–281. [CrossRef]
65. Liu, J.; Liu, Y.; Wang, C.; Li, A.; Meng, B. An Original Neural Network for Pulmonary Tuberculosis Diagnosis in Radiographs. In *Lecture Notes in Computer Science, Proceedings of the International Conference on Artificial Neural Networks, Rhodes, Greece, 4–7 October 2018*; Springer: Berlin/Heidelberg, Germany, 2018; pp. 158–166._16. [CrossRef]
66. Stirenko, S.; Kochura, Y.; Alienin, O. Chest X-Ray Analysis of Tuberculosis by Deep Learning with Segmentation and Augmentation. In Proceedings of the 2018 IEEE 38th International Conference on Electronics andNanotechnology (ELNANO), Kiev, Ukraine, 24–26 April 2018; pp. 422–428.
67. Andika, L.A.; Pratiwi, H.; Sulistijowati Handajani, S. Convolutional neural network modeling for classification of pulmonary tuberculosis disease. *J. Phys. Conf. Ser.* **2020**, *1490*. [CrossRef]
68. Ul Abideen, Z.; Ghafoor, M.; Munir, K.; Saqib, M.; Ullah, A.; Zia, T.; Tariq, S.A.; Ahmed, G.; Zahra, A. Uncertainty assisted robust tuberculosis identification with bayesian convolutional neural networks. *IEEE Access* **2020**, *8*, 22812–22825. [CrossRef] [PubMed]
69. Hwang, E.J.; Park, S.; Jin, K.N.; Kim, J.I.; Choi, S.Y.; Lee, J.H.; Goo, J.M.; Aum, J.; Yim, J.J.; Park, C.M. Development and Validation of a Deep Learning—based Automatic Detection Algorithm for Active Pulmonary Tuberculosis on Chest Radiographs. *Clin. Infect. Dis.* **2019**, *69*, 739–747. [CrossRef]
70. Hwang, S.; Kim, H.E.; Jeong, J.; Kim, H.J. A Novel Approach for Tuberculosis Screening Based on Deep Convolutional Neural Networks. *Med. Imaging* **2016**, *9785*, 1–8. [CrossRef]
71. Islam, M.T.; Aowal, M.A.; Minhaz, A.T.; Ashraf, K. Abnormality Detection and Localization in Chest X-Rays using Deep Convolutional Neural Networks. *arXiv* **2017**, arXiv:1705.09850v3.
72. Nguyen, Q.H.; Nguyen, B.P.; Dao, S.D.; Unnikrishnan, B.; Dhingra, R.; Ravichandran, S.R.; Satpathy, S.; Raja, P.N.; Chua, M.C.H. Deep Learning Models for Tuberculosis Detection from Chest X-ray Images. In Proceedings of the 2019 26th International Conference on Telecommunications (ICT), Hanoi, Vietnam, 8–10 April 2019; pp. 381–385. [CrossRef]
73. Kieu, T.; Ho, K.; Gwak, J.; Prakash, O. Utilizing Pretrained Deep Learning Models for Automated Pulmonary Tuberculosis Detection Using Chest Radiography. *Intell. Inf. Database Syst.* **2019**, *4*, 395–403. [CrossRef]
74. Abbas, A.; Abdelsamea, M.M. Learning Transformations for Automated Classification of Manifestation of Tuberculosis using Convolutional Neural Network. In Proceedings of the 2018 13th International Conference on Computer Engineering andSystems (ICCES), Cairo, Egypt, 18–19 December 2018; IEEE: New York, NY, USA, 2018; pp. 122–126.
75. Karnkawinpong, T.; Limpiyakorn, Y. Classification of pulmonary tuberculosis lesion with convolutional neural networks. *J. Phys. Conf. Ser.* **2018**, *1195*. [CrossRef]

76. Liu, C.; Cao, Y.; Alcantara, M.; Liu, B.; Brunette, M.; Peinado, J.; Curioso, W. TX-CNN: Detecting Tuberculosis in Chest X-Ray Images Using Convolutional Neural Network. In Proceedings of the 2017 IEEE International Conference on Image Processing (ICIP), Beijing, China, 17–20 September 2017.
77. Yadav, O.; Passi, K.; Jain, C.K. Using Deep Learning to Classify X-ray Images of Potential Tuberculosis Patients. In Proceedings of the 2018 IEEE International Conference on Bioinformatics and Biomedicine(BIBM), Madrid, Spain, 3–6 December 2018; IEEE: New York, NY, USA, 2018; pp. 2368–2375.
78. Sahlol, A.T.; Elaziz, M.A.; Jamal, A.T.; Damaševičius, R.; Hassan, O.F. A novel method for detection of tuberculosis in chest radiographs using artificial ecosystem-based optimisation of deep neural network features. *Symmetry* **2020**, *12*, 1146. [CrossRef]
79. Hooda, R.; Mittal, A.; Sofat, S. Automated TB classification using ensemble of deep architectures. *Multimed. Tools Appl.* **2019**, *78*, 31515–31532. [CrossRef]
80. Rashid, R.; Khawaja, S.G.; Akram, M.U.; Khan, A.M. Hybrid RID Network for Efficient Diagnosis of Tuberculosis from Chest X-rays. In Proceedings of the 2018 9th Cairo International Biomedical Engineering Conference(CIBEC), Cairo, Egypt, 20–22 December 2018; IEEE: New York, NY, USA, 2018; pp. 167–170.
81. Kieu, S.T.H.; Hijazi, M.H.A.; Bade, A.; Saffree Jeffree, M. Tuberculosis detection using deep learning and contrast-enhanced canny edge detected x-ray images. *IAES Int. J. Artif. Intell.* **2020**, *9*. [CrossRef]
82. Rajaraman, S.; Antani, S.K. Modality-Specific Deep Learning Model Ensembles Toward Improving TB Detection in Chest Radiographs. *IEEE Access* **2020**, *8*, 27318–27326. [CrossRef] [PubMed]
83. Melendez, J.; Ginneken, B.V.; Maduskar, P.; Philipsen, R.H.H.M.; Reither, K.; Breuninger, M.; Adetifa, I.M.O.; Maane, R.; Ayles, H.; Sánchez, C.I. A Novel Multiple-Instance Learning-Based Approach to Computer-Aided Detection of Tuberculosis on Chest X-Rays. *IEEE Trans. Med. Imaging* **2014**, *34*, 179–192. [CrossRef] [PubMed]
84. Becker, A.S.; Bluthgen, C.; van Phi, V.D.; Sekaggya-Wiltshire, C.; Castelnuovo, B.; Kambugu, A.; Fehr, J.; Frauenfelder, T. Detection of tuberculosis patterns in digital photographs of chest X-ray images using Deep Learning: Feasibility study. *Int. J. Tuberc. Lung Dis.* **2018**, *22*, 328–335. [CrossRef] [PubMed]
85. Li, L.; Huang, H.; Jin, X. AE-CNN Classification of Pulmonary Tuberculosis Based on CT images. In Proceedings of the 2018 9th International Conference on Information Technology inMedicine and Education (ITME), Hangzhou, China, 19–21 October 2018; IEEE: New York, NY, USA, 2018; pp. 39–42. [CrossRef]
86. Pattnaik, A.; Kanodia, S.; Chowdhury, R.; Mohanty, S. *Predicting Tuberculosis Related Lung Deformities from CT Scan Images Using 3D CNN*; CEUR-WS: Lugano, Switzerland, 2019; pp. 9–12.
87. Zunair, H.; Rahman, A.; Mohammed, N. *Estimating Severity from CT Scans of Tuberculosis Patients using 3D Convolutional Nets and Slice Selection*; CEUR-WS: Lugano, Switzerland, 2019; pp. 9–12.
88. Llopis, F.; Fuster-Guillo, A.; Azorin-Lopez, J.; Llopis, I. Using improved optical flow model to detect Tuberculosis; CEUR-WS: Lugano, Switzerland, 2019; pp. 9–12.
89. Wardlaw, T.; Johansson, E.W.; Hodge, M. *Pneumonia: The Forgotten Killer of Children*; United Nations Children's Fund (UNICEF): New York, NY, USA, 2006; p. 44.
90. Wunderink, R.G.; Waterer, G. Advances in the causes and management of community acquired pneumonia in adults. *BMJ* **2017**, 1–13. [CrossRef]
91. Tobias, R.R.; De Jesus, L.C.M.; Mital, M.E.G.; Lauguico, S.C.; Guillermo, M.A.; Sybingco, E.; Bandala, A.A.; Dadios, E.P. CNN-based Deep Learning Model for Chest X-ray Health Classification Using TensorFlow. In Proceedings of the 2020 RIVF International Conference on Computing and Communication Technologies, RIVF 2020, Ho Chi Minh, Vietnam, 14–15 October 2020 .
92. Stephen, O.; Sain, M.; Maduh, U.J.; Jeong, D.U. An Efficient Deep Learning Approach to Pneumonia Classification in Healthcare. *J. Healthc. Eng.* **2019**, *2019*. [CrossRef]
93. Kermany, D.S.; Goldbaum, M.; Cai, W.; Lewis, M.A. Identifying Medical Diagnoses and Treatable Diseases by Image-Based Deep Learning. *Cell* **2018**, *172*, 1122–1131.e9. [CrossRef] [PubMed]
94. Young, J.C.; Suryadibrata, A. Applicability of Various Pre-Trained Deep Convolutional Neural Networks for Pneumonia Classification based on X-Ray Images. *Int. J. Adv. Trends Comput. Sci. Eng.* **2020**, *9*, 2649–2654. [CrossRef]
95. Moujahid, H.; Cherradi, B.; Gannour, O.E.; Bahatti, L.; Terrada, O.; Hamida, S. Convolutional Neural Network Based Classification of Patients with Pneumonia using X-ray Lung Images. *Adv. Sci. Technol. Eng. Syst.* **2020**, *5*, 167–175. [CrossRef]

96. Rajpurkar, P.; Irvin, J.; Zhu, K.; Yang, B.; Mehta, H.; Duan, T.; Ding, D.; Bagul, A.; Ball, R.L.; Langlotz, C.; et al. CheXNet: Radiologist-Level Pneumonia Detection on Chest X-Rays with Deep Learning. *arXiv* **2017**, arXiv:1711.05225v3.
97. Rahman, T.; Chowdhury, M.E.H.; Khandakar, A.; Islam, K.R.; Islam, K.F.; Mahbub, Z.B.; Kadir, M.A.; Kashem, S. Transfer Learning with Deep Convolutional Neural Network (CNN) for Pneumonia Detection Using Chest X-ray. *Appl. Sci.* **2020**, *10*, 3233. [CrossRef]
98. Hashmi, M.; Katiyar, S.; Keskar, A.; Bokde, N.; Geem, Z. Efficient Pneumonia Detection in Chest Xray Images Using Deep Transfer Learning. *Diagnostics* **2020**, 1–23. [CrossRef] [PubMed]
99. Acharya, A.K.; Satapathy, R. A Deep Learning Based Approach towards the Automatic Diagnosis of Pneumonia from Chest Radio-Graphs. *Biomed. Pharmacol. J.* **2020**, *13*, 449–455. [CrossRef]
100. Elshennawy, N.M.; Ibrahim, D.M. Deep-Pneumonia Framework Using Deep Learning Models Based on Chest X-Ray Images. *Diagnostics* **2020**, *10*, 649. [CrossRef] [PubMed]
101. Emhamed, R.; Mamlook, A.; Chen, S. Investigation of the performance of Machine Learning Classifiers for Pneumonia Detection in Chest X-ray Images. In Proceedings of the 2020 IEEE International Conference on Electro Information Technology (EIT), Chicago, IL, USA, 31 July–1 August 2020; pp. 98–104.
102. Kumar, A.; Tiwari, P.; Kumar, S.; Gupta, D.; Khanna, A. Identifying pneumonia in chest X-rays: A deep learning approach. *Measurement* **2019**, *145*, 511–518. [CrossRef]
103. Hurt, B.; Yen, A.; Kligerman, S.; Hsiao, A. Augmenting Interpretation of Chest Radiographs with Deep Learning Probability Maps. *J. Thorac. Imaging* **2020**, *35*, 285–293. [CrossRef]
104. Borczuk, A.C. Benign tumors and tumorlike conditions of the lung. *Arch. Pathol. Lab. Med.* **2008**, *132*, 1133–1148.[1133:BTATCO]2.0.CO;2. [CrossRef]
105. Hua, K.L.; Hsu, C.H.; Hidayati, S.C.; Cheng, W.H.; Chen, Y.J. Computer-aided classification of lung nodules on computed tomography images via deep learning technique. *OncoTargets Ther.* **2015**, *8*, 2015–2022. [CrossRef]
106. Kurniawan, E.; Prajitno, P.; Soejoko, D.S. Computer-Aided Detection of Mediastinal Lymph Nodes using Simple Architectural Convolutional Neural Network. *J. Phys. Conf. Ser.* **2020**, *1505*. [CrossRef]
107. Ciompi, F.; Chung, K.; Van Riel, S.J.; Setio, A.A.A.; Gerke, P.K.; Jacobs, C.; Th Scholten, E.; Schaefer-Prokop, C.; Wille, M.M.; Marchianò, A.; et al. Towards automatic pulmonary nodule management in lung cancer screening with deep learning. *Sci. Rep.* **2017**, *7*, 1–11. [CrossRef]
108. Shakeel, P.M.; Burhanuddin, M.A.; Desa, M.I. Lung cancer detection from CT image using improved profuse clustering and deep learning instantaneously trained neural networks. *Meas. J. Int. Meas. Confed.* **2019**, *145*, 702–712. [CrossRef]
109. Chen, S.; Han, Y.; Lin, J.; Zhao, X.; Kong, P. Pulmonary nodule detection on chest radiographs using balanced convolutional neural network and classic candidate detection. *Artif. Intell. Med.* **2020**, *107*, 101881. [CrossRef] [PubMed]
110. Hosny, A.; Parmar, C.; Coroller, T.P.; Grossmann, P.; Zeleznik, R.; Kumar, A.; Bussink, J.; Gillies, R.J.; Mak, R.H.; Aerts, H.J. Deep learning for lung cancer prognostication: A retrospective multi-cohort radiomics study. *PLoS Med.* **2018**, *15*, 1–25. [CrossRef] [PubMed]
111. Xu, Y.; Hosny, A.; Zeleznik, R.; Parmar, C.; Coroller, T.; Franco, I.; Mak, R.H.; Aerts, H.J. Deep learning predicts lung cancer treatment response from serial medical imaging. *Clin. Cancer Res.* **2019**, *25*, 3266–3275. [CrossRef] [PubMed]
112. Kuan, K.; Ravaut, M.; Manek, G.; Chen, H.; Lin, J.; Nazir, B.; Chen, C.; Howe, T.C.; Zeng, Z.; Chandrasekhar, V. Deep Learning for Lung Cancer Detection: Tackling the Kaggle Data Science Bowl 2017 Challenge. *arXiv* **2017**, arXiv:1705.09435
113. Ausawalaithong, W.; Thirach, A.; Marukatat, S.; Wilaiprasitporn, T. Automatic Lung Cancer Prediction from Chest X-ray Images Using the Deep Learning Approach. In Proceedings of the 2018 11th Biomedical Engineering International Conference (BMEiCON), Chiang Mai, Thailand, 21–24 November 2018 .
114. Xu, S.; Guo, J.; Zhang, G.; Bie, R. Automated detection of multiple lesions on chest X-ray images: Classification using a neural network technique with association-specific contexts. *Appl. Sci.* **2020**, *10*, 1742. [CrossRef]
115. Huang, C.; Wang, Y.; Li, X.; Ren, L.; Zhao, J.; Hu, Y.; Zhang, L.; Fan, G.; Xu, J.; Gu, X. Clinical features of patients infected with 2019 novel coronavirus in Wuhan, China. *Lancet* **2020**, *395*, 497–506. [CrossRef]
116. Velavan, T.P.; Meyer, C.G. The COVID-19 epidemic. *Trop. Med. Int. Health* **2020**, *25*, 278–280. [CrossRef]

117. Shibly, K.H.; Dey, S.K.; Islam, M.T.U.; Rahman, M.M. COVID faster R–CNN: A novel framework to Diagnose Novel Coronavirus Disease (COVID-19) in X-Ray images. *Inform. Med. Unlocked* **2020**, *20*, 100405. [CrossRef]
118. Alsharman, N.; Jawarneh, I. GoogleNet CNN neural network towards chest CT-coronavirus medical image classification. *J. Comput. Sci.* **2020**, *16*, 620–625. [CrossRef]
119. Zhu, J.; Shen, B.; Abbasi, A.; Hoshmand-Kochi, M.; Li, H.; Duong, T.Q. Deep transfer learning artificial intelligence accurately stages COVID-19 lung disease severity on portable chest radiographs. *PLoS ONE* **2020**, *15*, e0236621. [CrossRef]
120. Sethi, R.; Mehrotra, M.; Sethi, D. Deep Learning based Diagnosis Recommendation for COVID-19 using Chest X-Rays Images In Proceedings of the 2020 Second International Conference on Inventive Research in Computing Applications (ICIRCA), Coimbatore, India, 15–17 July 2020 .
121. Das, D.; Santosh, K.C.; Pal, U. Truncated inception net: COVID-19 outbreak screening using chest X-rays. *Phys. Eng. Sci. Med.* **2020**, *43*, 915–925. [CrossRef] [PubMed]
122. Panwar, H.; Gupta, P.K.; Siddiqui, M.K.; Morales-Menendez, R.; Singh, V. Application of deep learning for fast detection of COVID-19 in X-Rays using nCOVnet. *Chaos Solitons Fractals* **2020**, *138*, 109944. [CrossRef] [PubMed]
123. Narin, A.; Kaya, C.; Pamuk, Z. Automatic Detection of Coronavirus Disease (COVID-19) Using X-ray Images and Deep Convolutional Neural Networks. *arXiv* **2020**, arXiv:2003.10849..
124. Apostolopoulos, I.D.; Mpesiana, T.A. Covid—19: Automatic detection from X-ray images utilizing transfer learning with convolutional neural networks. *Phys. Eng. Sci. Med.* **2020**, 1–6. [CrossRef] [PubMed]
125. Chowdhury, M.E.H.; Rahman, T.; Khandakar, A.; Mazhar, R.; Kadir, M.A.; Reaz, M.B.I.; Mahbub, Z.B.; Islam, K.R.; Salman, M.; Iqbal, A.; et al. Can AI help in screening Viral and COVID-19 pneumonia? *arXiv* **2020**, arXiv:2003.13145.
126. Wang, L.; Lin, Z.Q.; Wong, A. COVID-Net: A Tailored Deep Convolutional Neural Network Design for Detection of COVID-19 Cases from Chest X-Ray Images. *Sci. Rep.* **2020**, 10, 1–12. [CrossRef]
127. Sethy, P.K.; Behera, S.K.; Ratha, P.K.; Biswas, P. Detection of coronavirus disease (COVID-19) based on deep features and support vector machine. *Int. J. Math. Eng. Manag. Sci.* **2020**, *5*, 643–651. [CrossRef]
128. Islam, M.Z.; Islam, M.M.; Asraf, A. A combined deep CNN-LSTM network for the detection of novel coronavirus (COVID-19) using X-ray images. *Inform. Med. Unlocked* **2020**, *20*, 100412. [CrossRef]
129. Shorfuzzaman, M.; Masud, M. On the detection of covid-19 from chest x-ray images using cnn-based transfer learning. *Comput. Mater. Contin.* **2020**, *64*, 1359–1381. [CrossRef]
130. Li, L.; Qin, L.; Xu, Z.; Yin, Y.; Wang, X.; Kong, B.; Bai, J.; Lu, Y.; Fang, Z.; Song, Q.; et al. Using Artificial Intelligence to Detect COVID-19 and Community-acquired Pneumonia Based on Pulmonary CT: Evaluation of the Diagnostic Accuracy. *Radiology* **2020**, *296*, 65–71. [CrossRef]
131. Alazab, M.; Awajan, A.; Mesleh, A.; Abraham, A.; Jatana, V.; Alhyari, S. COVID-19 prediction and detection using deep learning. *Int. J. Comput. Inf. Syst. Ind. Manag. Appl.* **2020**, *12*, 168–181.
132. Waheed, A.; Goyal, M.; Gupta, D.; Khanna, A.; Al-Turjman, F.; Pinheiro, P.R. CovidGAN: Data Augmentation Using Auxiliary Classifier GAN for Improved Covid-19 Detection. *IEEE Access* **2020**, *8*, 91916–91923. [CrossRef]
133. Ouyang, X.; Huo, J.; Xia, L.; Shan, F.; Liu, J.; Mo, Z.; Yan, F.; Ding, Z.; Yang, Q.; Song, B.; et al. Dual-Sampling Attention Network for Diagnosis of COVID-19 from Community Acquired Pneumonia. *IEEE Trans. Med. Imaging* **2020**, *39*, 2595–2605. [CrossRef]
134. Mahmud, T.; Rahman, M.A.; Fattah, S.A. CovXNet: A multi-dilation convolutional neural network for automatic COVID-19 and other pneumonia detection from chest X-ray images with transferable multi-receptive feature optimization. *Comput. Biol. Med.* **2020**, *122*, 103869. [CrossRef] [PubMed]
135. Shi, F.; Xia, L.; Shan, F.; Wu, D.; Wei, Y.; Yuan, H.; Jiang, H. Large-Scale Screening of COVID-19 from Community Acquired Pneumonia using Infection Size-Aware Classification. *arXiv* **2020**, arXiv:2003.09860..
136. Breiman, L. Random forests. *Mach. Learn.* **2001**, *45*, 5–32. [CrossRef]
137. Xu, X.; Jiang, X.; Ma, C.; Du, P.; Li, X.; Ly, S.; Yu, L.; Chen, Y; Su, J.; Lang, G.; et al. A Deep Learning System to Screen Novel Coronavirus Disease 2019 Pneumonia. *Engineering* **2020**. [CrossRef]
138. Singh, D.; Kumar, V.; Kaur, M. Classification of COVID-19 patients from chest CT images using multi-objective differential evolution–based convolutional neural networks. *Eur. J. Clin. Microbiol. Infect. Dis.* **2020**, *39*, 1379–1389. [CrossRef]

139. Sedik, A.; Iliyasu, A.M.; El-Rahiem, B.A.; Abdel Samea, M.E.; Abdel-Raheem, A.; Hammad, M.; Peng, J.; Abd El-Samie, F.E.; Abd El-Latif, A.A. Deploying machine and deep learning models for efficient data-augmented detection of COVID-19 infections. *Viruses* **2020**, *12*, 769. [CrossRef]
140. Ahsan, M.M.; Alam, T.E.; Trafalis, T.; Huebner, P. Deep MLP-CNN model using mixed-data to distinguish between COVID-19 and Non-COVID-19 patients. *Symmetry* **2020**, *12*. [CrossRef]
141. Afshar, P.; Heidarian, S.; Naderkhani, F.; Oikonomou, A.; Plataniotis, K.N.; Mohammadi, A. COVID-CAPS: A capsule network-based framework for identification of COVID-19 cases from X-ray images. *Pattern Recognit. Lett.* **2020**, *138*, 638–643. [CrossRef] [PubMed]
142. Rosenthal, A.; Gabrielian, A.; Engle, E.; Hurt, D.E.; Alexandru, S.; Crudu, V.; Sergueev, E.; Kirichenko, V.; Lapitskii, V.; Snezhko, E.; et al. The TB Portals: An Open-Access, Web- Based Platform for Global Drug-Resistant- Tuberculosis Data Sharing and Analysis. *J. Clin. Microbiol.* **2017**, *55*, 3267–3282. [CrossRef] [PubMed]
143. Cid, Y.D.; Liauchuk, V.; Klimuk, D.; Tarasau, A. *Overview of ImageCLEFtuberculosis 2019—Automatic CT—Based Report Generation and Tuberculosis Severity Assessment*: CEUR-WS: Lugano, Switzerland, 2019; pp. 9–12.
144. Demner-Fushman, D.; Kohli, M.D.; Rosenman, M.B.; Shooshan, S.E.; Rodriguez, L.; Antani, S.; Thoma, G.R.; McDonald, C.J. Preparing a collection of radiology examinations for distribution and retrieval. *J. Am. Med. Inform. Assoc.* **2016**, *23*, 304–310. [CrossRef]
145. Shiraishi, J.; Katsuragawa, S.; Ikezoe, J.; Matsumoto, T.; Kobayashi, T.; Komatsu, K.I.; Matsui, M.; Fujita, H.; Kodera, Y.; Doi, K. Development of a digital image database for chest radiographs with and without a lung nodule: Receiver operating characteristic analysis of radiologists' detection of pulmonary nodules. *Am. J. Roentgenol.* **2000**, *174*, 71–74. [CrossRef] [PubMed]
146. Jaeger, S.; Candemir, S.; Antani, S.; Wáng, Y.x.J.; Lu, P.x.; Thoma, G. Two public chest X-ray datasets for computer-aided screening of pulmonary diseases. *Quant. Imaging Med. Surg.* **2014**, *4*, 475–477. [CrossRef]
147. Xiaosong, W.; Yifan, P.; Le, L.; Lu, Z.; Mohammadhadi, B.; Summers, R.M. ChestX-ray8: Hospital-scale chest X-ray database and benchmarks on weakly-supervised classification and localization of common thorax diseases. In Proceedings of the IEEE conference on computer vision and pattern recognition, Honolulu, HI, USA, 21–26 July 2017; pp. 3462–3471.
148. Costa, M.G.; Filho, C.F.; Kimura, A.; Levy, P.C.; Xavier, C.M.; Fujimoto, L.B. A sputum smear microscopy image database for automatic bacilli detection in conventional microscopy. In Proceedings of the 2014 36th Annual International Conference of the IEEE Engineering in Medicine and Biology Society, EMBC, Chicago, IL, USA, 26–30 August 2014 ; pp. 2841–2844. [CrossRef]
149. Armato, S.G.; McLennan, G.; Bidaut, L.; McNitt-Gray, M.F.; Meyer, C.R.; Reeves, A.P.; Zhao, B.; Aberle, D.R.; Henschke, C.I.; Hoffman, E.A.; et al. The Lung Image Database Consortium (LIDC) and Image Database Resource Initiative (IDRI): A completed reference database of lung nodules on CT scans. *Med. Phys.* **2011**, *38*, 915–931. [CrossRef]
150. Grossman, R.L.; Allison, P.; Ferrentti, V.; Varmus, H.E.; Lowy, D.R.; Kibbe, W.A.; Staudt, L.M. Toward a Shared Vision for Cancer Genomic Data. *N. Engl. J. Med.* **2016**, *375*, 1109–1112. [CrossRef]
151. Cohen, J.P.; Morrison, P.; Dao, L.; Roth, K.; Duong, T.Q.; Ghassemi, M. COVID-19 Image Data Collection: Prospective Predictions Are the Future. *arXiv* **2020**, arXiv:2006.11988..

9

Automatic Pancreas Segmentation using Coarse-Scaled 2D Model of Deep Learning: Usefulness of Data Augmentation and Deep U-Net

Mizuho Nishio [1,*], Shunjiro Noguchi [1] and Koji Fujimoto [2]

[1] Department of Diagnostic Imaging and Nuclear Medicine, Kyoto University Graduate School of Medicine, 54 Kawahara-cho, Shogoin, Sakyo-ku, Kyoto 606-8507, Japan; shunjiro101@gmail.com

[2] Human Brain Research Center, Kyoto University Graduate School of Medicine, 54 Kawahara-cho, Shogoin, Sakyo-ku, Kyoto 606-8507, Japan; kfb@kuhp.kyoto-u.ac.jp

* Correspondence: nmizuho@kuhp.kyoto-u.ac.jp;

Abstract: Combinations of data augmentation methods and deep learning architectures for automatic pancreas segmentation on CT images are proposed and evaluated. Images from a public CT dataset of pancreas segmentation were used to evaluate the models. Baseline U-net and deep U-net were chosen for the deep learning models of pancreas segmentation. Methods of data augmentation included conventional methods, mixup, and random image cropping and patching (RICAP). Ten combinations of the deep learning models and the data augmentation methods were evaluated. Four-fold cross validation was performed to train and evaluate these models with data augmentation methods. The dice similarity coefficient (DSC) was calculated between automatic segmentation results and manually annotated labels and these were visually assessed by two radiologists. The performance of the deep U-net was better than that of the baseline U-net with mean DSC of 0.703–0.789 and 0.686–0.748, respectively. In both baseline U-net and deep U-net, the methods with data augmentation performed better than methods with no data augmentation, and mixup and RICAP were more useful than the conventional method. The best mean DSC was obtained using a combination of deep U-net, mixup, and RICAP, and the two radiologists scored the results from this model as good or perfect in 76 and 74 of the 82 cases.

Keywords: pancreas; segmentation; computed tomography; deep learning; data augmentation

---

1. Introduction

Identification of anatomical structures is a fundamental step for radiologists in the interpretation of medical images. Similarly, automatic and accurate organ identification or segmentation is important for medical image analysis, computer-aided detection, and computer-aided diagnosis. To date, many studies have worked on automatic and accurate segmentation of organs, including lung, liver, pancreas, uterus, and muscle [1–5].

An estimated 606,880 Americans were predicted to die from cancer in 2019, in which 45,750 deaths would be due to pancreatic cancer [6]. Among all major types of cancers, the five-year relative survival rate of pancreatic cancer was the lowest (9%). One of the reasons for this low survival rate is the difficulty in the detection of pancreatic cancer in its early stages, because the organ is located in the retroperitoneal space and is in close proximity to other organs. A lack of symptoms is another reason for the difficulty of its early detection. Therefore, computer-aided detection and/or diagnosis using computed tomography (CT) may contribute to a reduction in the number of deaths caused by pancreatic cancer, similar to the effect of CT screenings on lung cancer [7,8]. Accurate segmentation of pancreas is the first step in the computer-aided detection/diagnosis system of pancreatic cancer.

Compared with conventional techniques of organ segmentation, which use hand-tuned filters and classifiers, deep learning, such as convolutional neural networks (CNN), is a framework, which lets computers learn and build these filters and classifiers from a huge amount of data. Recently, deep learning has been attracting much attention in medical image analysis, as it has been demonstrated as a powerful tool for organ segmentation [9]. Pancreas segmentation using CT images is challenging because the pancreas does not have a distinct border with its surrounding structures. In addition, pancreas has a large shape and size variability among people. Therefore, several different approaches to pancreas segmentation using deep learning have been proposed [10–15].

Previous studies designed to improve the deep learning model of automatic pancreas segmentation [10–15] can be classified using three major aspects: (i) dimension of the convolutional network, two-dimensional model (2D) versus three-dimensional model (3D); (ii) use of coarse-scaled model versus fine-scaled model; (iii) improvement of network architecture. In (i), the accuracy of pancreas segmentation was improved in a 3D model and compared with a 2D model; the 3D model makes it possible to fully utilize the 3D spatial information of pancreas, which is useful for grasping the large variability in pancreas shape and size. In (ii), an initial coarse-scaled model was used to obtain a rough region of interest (ROI) of the pancreas, and then the ROI was used for segmentation refinement using a fine-scaled model of pancreas segmentation. The difference in mean dice similarity coefficient (DSC) between the coarse-scaled and find-scaled models ranged from 2% to 7%. In (iii), the network architecture of a deep learning model was modified for efficient segmentation. For example, when an attention unit was introduced in a U-net, the segmentation accuracy was better than in a conventional U-net [12].

In previous studies, the usefulness of data augmentation in pancreas segmentation was not fully evaluated; only conventional methods of data augmentation were utilized. Recently proposed methods of data augmentation, such as mixup [16] and random image cropping and patching (RICAP) [17], were not evaluated.

In conventional data augmentation, horizontal flipping, vertical flipping, scaling, rotation, etc., are commonly used. It is necessary to find an effective combination of these, since among the possible combinations, some degrade the performance. Due to the number of the combinations, it is relatively cumbersome to eliminate the counterproductive combinations in conventional data augmentation. For this purpose, AutoAugment finds the best combination of data augmentation [18]. However, it is computationally expensive due to its use of reinforcement learning. In this regard, mixup and RICAP are easier to adjust than conventional data augmentation because they both have only one parameter.

The purpose of the current study is to evaluate and validate the combinations of different types of data augmentation and network architecture modification of U-net [19]. A deep U-net was used, to evaluate the usefulness of network architecture modification of U-net.

2. Materials and Methods

The current study used anonymized data extracted from a public database. Therefore, institutional review board approval was waived.

2.1. Dataset

The public dataset (Pancreas-CT) used in the current study includes 82 sets of contrast-enhanced abdominal CT images, where pancreas was manually annotated slice-by-slice [20,21]. This dataset is publicly available from The Cancer Imaging Archive [22]. The Pancreas-CT dataset is commonly used to benchmark the segmentation accuracy of pancreas on CT images. The CT scans in the dataset were obtained from 53 male and 27 female subjects. The age of the subjects ranged from 18 to 76 years with a mean age of 46.8 ± 16.7. The CT images were acquired with Philips and Siemens multi-detector CT scanners (120 kVp tube voltage). Spatial resolution of the CT images is 512 × 512 pixels with varying pixel sizes, and slice thickness is between 1.5–2.5 mm. As a part of image preprocessing, the pixel values for all sets of CT images were clipped to [−100, 240] Hounsfield units, then rescaled to the range [0, 1]. This preprocessing was commonly used for the Pancreas-CT dataset [15].

2.2. Deep Learning Model

U-net was used as a baseline model of deep learning in the current study [19]. U-net consists of encoding–decoding architecture. Downsampling and upsampling are performed in the encoding and decoding parts of U-net, respectively. The most important characteristic of U-net is the presence of shortcut connections between the encoding part and the decoding part at equal resolution. While the baseline U-net performs downsampling and upsampling 4 times [19], deep U-net performs downsampling and upsampling 6 times. In addition to the number of downsampling and upsampling, the number of feature maps in the convolution layer and the use of dropout were changed in the deep U-net; the number of feature maps in the first convolution layer equaled to 40 and dropout probability to 2%. In the baseline U-net, 64 feature maps and no dropout were used. In both, the baseline U-net and the deep U-net, the number of feature maps in the convolution layer was doubled after each downsampling. Figure 1 presents the deep U-net model of the proposed method. Both the baseline U-net and deep U-net utilized batch normalization. Keras (https://keras.io/) with Tensorflow (https://www.tensorflow.org/) backends was used for the implementation of the U-net models. Image dimension of the input and output in the two U-net models was 512 × 512 pixels.

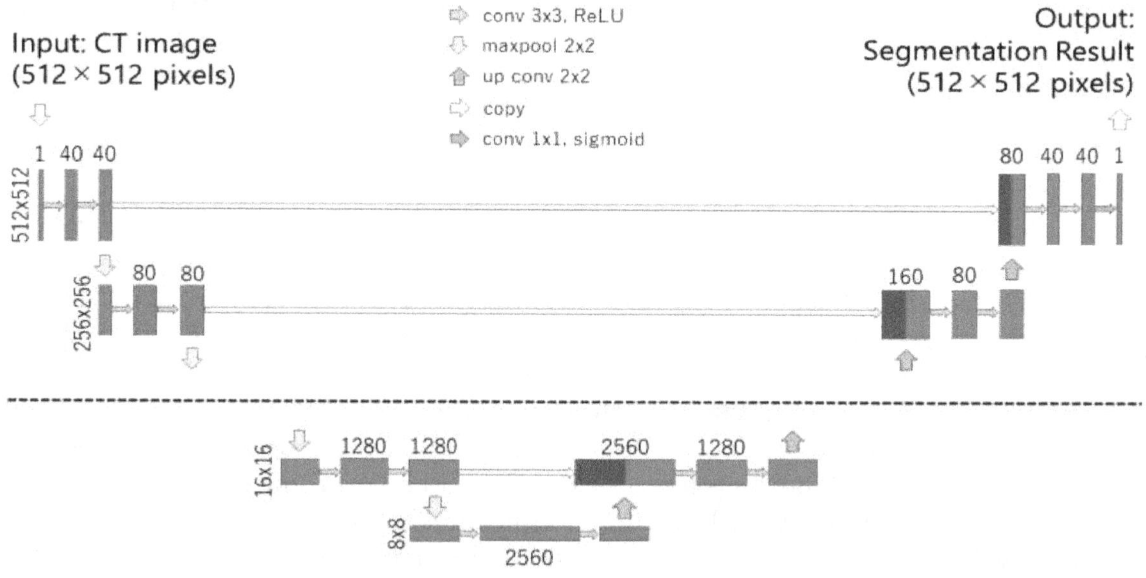

Figure 1. Illustration of the deep U-net model. The number of downsampling and upsampling is 6 in the deep U-net. Except for the last convolution layer, dropout and convolution layer are coupled. Abbreviations: convolution layer (conv), maxpooling layer (maxpool), upsampling and convolution layer (up conv), rectified linear unit (ReLU).

2.3. Data Augmentation

To prevent overfitting in the training of the deep learning model, we utilized the following three types of data augmentation methods: conventional method, mixup [16], and RICAP [17]. Although mixup and RICAP were initially proposed for image classification tasks, we utilized them for segmentation by merging or cropping/patching labels in the same way as is done for images.

Conventional augmentation methods included ±5° rotation, ±5% x-axis shift, ±5% y-axis shift, and 95%–105% scaling. Both image and label were changed by the same transformation when using a conventional augmentation method.

Mixup generates a new training sample from linear combination of existing images and their labels [16]. Here, two sets of training samples are denoted by (x, y) and (x', y'), where x and x' are images, and y and y' are their labels. A generated sample $(x^{\#}, y^{\#})$ is given by:

$$x^{\#} = \lambda x + (1 - \lambda)x' \tag{1}$$

$$y^{\#} = \lambda y + (1 - \lambda)y' \tag{2}$$

where λ ranges from 0 to 1 and is distributed according to beta distribution: $\lambda \sim Beta(\beta, \beta)$ for $\beta \in (0, \infty)$. The two samples to be combined are selected randomly from the training data. The hyperparameter β of mixup was set to 0.2 empirically.

RICAP generates a new training sample from four randomly selected images [17]. The four images are randomly cropped and patched according to a boundary position (w, h), which is determined according to beta distribution: $w \sim Beta(\beta, \beta)$ and $h \sim Beta(\beta, \beta)$. We set the hyperparameter β of RICAP to 0.4 empirically. For four images to be combined, the coordinates (x_k, y_k) (k = 1, 2, 3, and 4) of the upper left corners of the cropped areas are randomly selected. The sizes of the four cropped images are determined based on the value (w, h), such that they do not increase the original image size. A generated sample is obtained by combining the four cropped images. In the current study, the image and its label were cropped at the same coordinate and size.

2.4. Training

Dice loss function was used as the optimization target of the deep learning models. RMSprop was used as the optimizer, and its learning rate was set to 0.00004. The number of training epochs was set to 45. Following previous works on pancreas segmentation, we used 4-fold cross-validation to assess the robustness of the model (20 or 21 subjects were chosen for validation in folds). The hyperparameters related with U-net and its training were selected using random search [23]. After the random search, the hyperparameters were fixed. The following 10 combinations of deep learning models and data augmentation methods were used:

1. Baseline U-net + no data augmentation,
2. Baseline U-net + conventional method,
3. Baseline U-net + mixup,
4. Baseline U-net + RICAP,
5. Baseline U-net + RICAP + mixup,
6. Deep U-net + no data augmentation,
7. Deep U-net + conventional method,
8. Deep U-net + mixup,
9. Deep U-net + RICAP,
10. Deep U-net + RICAP + mixup.

2.5. Evaluation of Pancreas Segmentation

For each validation case of the Pancreas-CT dataset, three-dimensional CT images were processed slice-by-slice using the trained deep learning models, and the segmentation results were stacked. Except for the stacking, no complex postprocessing was utilized. Quantitative and qualitative evaluations were performed for the automatic segmentation results.

The metrics of quantitative evaluation were calculated using the three-dimensional segmentation results and annotated labels. Four types of metrics were used for the quantitative evaluation of the segmentation results: dice similarity coefficient (DSC), Jaccard index (JI), sensitivity (SE), and specificity (SP). These metrics are defined by the following equations:

$$DSC = \frac{2|P \cap L|}{|P| + |L|} \tag{3}$$

$$JI = \frac{|P \cap L|}{|P| + |L| - |P \cap L|} \tag{4}$$

$$SE = \frac{|P \cap L|}{|L|} \tag{5}$$

$$SP = 1 - \frac{|P| - |P \cap L|}{|I| - |L|} \tag{6}$$

where $|P|$, $|L|$, and $|I|$ denote the number of voxels for pancreas segmentation results, annotated label of pancreas segmentation, and three-dimensional CT images, respectively. $|P \cap L|$ represents the number of voxels where the deep learning models can accurately segment pancreas (true positive). Before calculating the four metrics, a threshold of 0.5 was used for obtaining pancreas segmentation mask from the output of the U-net [24]. The threshold of 0.5 was fixed for all the 82 cases. A Wilcoxon signed rank test was used to test statistical significance among the DSC results of 10 combinations of deep learning models and data augmentation methods. Bonferroni correction was used for controlling family wise error rate. p-values less than $0.05/45 = 0.00111$ was considered as statistical significance.

For the qualitative evaluation, two radiologists with 14 and 6 years of experience visually evaluated both the manually annotated labels and automatic segmentation results using a 5-point scale: 1, unacceptable; 2, slightly unacceptable; 3, acceptable; 4, good; 5, perfect. Inter-observer variability between the two radiologists were evaluated using weighted kappa with squared weight.

3. Results

Table 1 shows results of the qualitative evaluation of the pancreas segmentation of Deep U-net + RICAP + mixup and the manually annotated labels. The mean visual scores of manually annotated labels were 4.951 and 4.902 for the two radiologists, and those of automatic segmentation results were 4.439 and 4.268. The mean score of automatic segmentation results demonstrates that the accuracy of the automatic segmentation was good; more than 92.6% (76/82) and 87.8% (74/82) of the cases were scored as 4 or above. Notably, Table 1 shows that the manually annotated labels were scored as 4 (good, but not perfect) in four and eight cases by the two radiologists. Weighted kappa values between the two radiologists were 0.465 (moderate agreement) for the manually annotated labels and 0.723 (substantial agreement) for the automatic segmentation results.

Table 1. Results of qualitative evaluation of automatic pancreas segmentation and manually annotated labels.

Radiologist	Target	Number of Score 1	Number of Score 2	Number of Score 3	Number of Score 4	Number of Score 5
Radiologist 1	manually annotated label	0	0	0	4	78
Radiologist 1	automatic segmentation	0	3	3	31	45
Radiologist 2	manually annotated label	0	0	0	8	74
Radiologist 2	automatic segmentation	0	2	6	42	32

Table 2 shows the results of the quantitative evaluation of pancreas segmentation. Mean and standard deviation of DSC, JI, SE, and SP are calculated from the validation cases of 4-fold cross validation for the Pancreas-CT dataset. Mean DSC of the deep U-net (0.703–0.789) was better than the mean DSC of the baseline U-net (0.686–0.748) across all data augmentation methods. Because mean SP was 1.00 in all the combinations, non-pancreas lesions were not segmented by the models. Therefore, mean DSC was mainly affected by mean SE (segmentation accuracy only for pancreas lesion) as shown in Table 2. Table 2 also shows the usefulness of data augmentation. In both, the baseline U-net and deep U-net, the model combined with any of the three types of data augmentation performed better than the model with no data augmentation. In addition, mixup and RICAP were more useful than the conventional method; the best mean DSC was obtained using the combination of mixup and RICAP. The best mean DSC was obtained using the deep U-net with RICAP and mixup.

Table 2. Results of quantitative evaluation of automatic pancreas segmentation from the 82 cases using 4-fold cross validation.

Type of Model and Data Augmentation	DSC	JI	SE	SP
Baseline U-net + no data augmentation	0.686 ± 0.186	0.548 ± 0.186	0.618 ± 0.221	1.000 ± 0.000
Baseline U-net + conventional method	0.694 ± 0.182	0.556 ± 0.183	0.631±0.220	1.000 ± 0.000
Baseline U-net + mixup	0.733 ± 0.106	0.588 ± 0.122	0.698 ± 0.155	1.000 ± 0.000
Baseline U-net + RICAP	0.699 ± 0.155	0.557 ± 0.169	0.624 ± 0.200	1.000 ± 0.000
Baseline U-net + RICAP + mixup	0.748 ± 0.127	0.611 ± 0.141	0.700 ± 0.176	1.000 ± 0.000
Deep U-net + no data augmentation	0.703 ± 0.166	0.563 ± 0.169	0.645 ± 0.201	1.000 ± 0.000
Deep U-net + conventional method	0.720 ± 0.171	0.586 ± 0.176	0.685 ± 0.210	1.000 ± 0.000
Deep U-net + mixup	0.725 ± 0.125	0.582 ± 0.137	0.694 ± 0.158	1.000 ± 0.000
Deep U-net + RICAP	0.740 ± 0.160	0.609 ± 0.169	0.691 ± 0.200	1.000 ± 0.000
Deep U-net + RICAP + mixup	0.789 ± 0.083	0.658 ± 0.103	0.762 ± 0.120	1.000 ± 0.000

Note: data are shown as mean ± standard deviation. Abbreviations: Random image cropping and patching (RICAP), dice similarity coefficient (DSC), Jaccard index (JI), sensitivity (SE), and specificity (SP).

Table A2 of Appendix B shows the results of the Wilcoxon signed rank test. After the Bonferroni correction, the DSC differences between Deep U-net + RICAP + mixup and the other six models were statistically significant.

Representative images of pancreas segmentation are shown in Figures 2 and 3. In the case of Figure 2, the manually annotated label was scored as 4 by the two radiologists because the main pancreas duct and its surrounding tissue were excluded from the label.

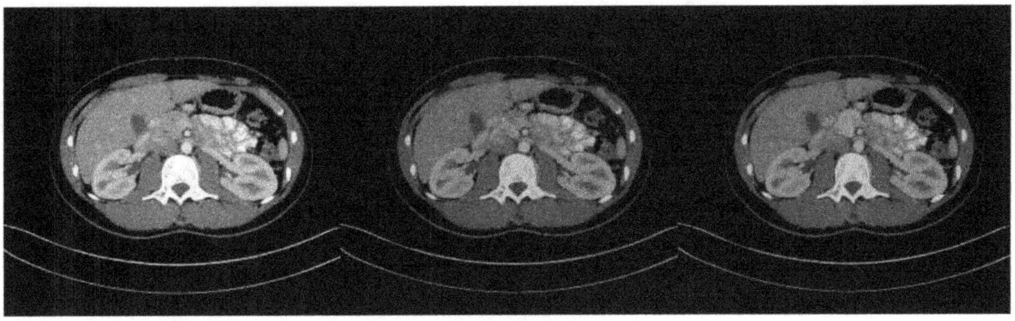

(a) (b) (c)

Figure 2. Representative image of automatic pancreas segmentation. (**a**) Original computed tomography (CT) image; (**b**) CT image with manually annotated label in red, scored as not perfect by two radiologists; (**c**) CT image with automatic segmentation in blue.

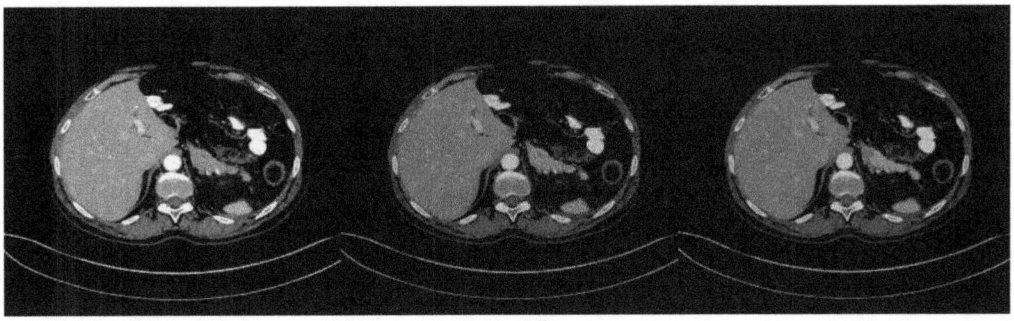

(a) (b) (c)

Figure 3. Representative image of a low-quality automatic pancreas segmentation. (**a**) Original computed tomography (CT) image; (**b**) CT image with manually annotated label in red; (**c**) CT image with automatic segmentation in blue, with part of the pancreas excluded from the segmentation.

4. Discussion

The results of the present study show that the three types of data augmentation were useful for the pancreas segmentation in both the baseline U-net and deep U-net. In addition, the deep U-net, which is characterized by additional layers, was overall more effective for automatic pancreas segmentation than the baseline U-net. In data augmentation, not only the conventional method, but also mixup and RICAP were useful for pancreas segmentation; the combination of mixup and RICAP was the most useful.

Table 3 summarizes results of previous studies using the Pancreas-CT dataset. While Table 3 includes the studies with coarse-scaled models, Table A1 includes the studies with fine-scaled models. As shown in Table 3, the coarse-scaled 2D model of the current study achieved sufficiently high accuracy, comparable to those of previous studies. While the present study focused on the 2D coarse-scaled models, the data augmentation methods used in the present study can be easily applied to 3D fine-scaled models. Therefore, it can be expected that the combination of the proposed data augmentation methods and 3D fine-scaled models might lead to further improvement of automatic pancreas segmentation.

Table 3. Summary of coarse-scaled models using the Pancreas-CT dataset.

Name of Model	2D/3D	Coarse/Fine	Mean DSC	Data Splitting
Holistically Nested 2D FCN Stage-1 [11]	2D	coarse	0.768 ± 0.111	4-fold CV
2D FCN [13]	2D	coarse	0.803 ± 0.09	4-fold CV
Coarse-scaled Model 2D FCN [14]	2D	coarse	0.757 ± 0.105	4-fold CV
Single Model 3D U-net [12] (trained from scratch)	3D	coarse	0.815 ± 0.057	61 training and 21 test sets randomly selected
Single Model 3D Attention U-net [12] (trained from scratch)	3D	coarse	0.821 ± 0.068	61 training and 21 test sets randomly selected
Coarse-scaled Model 3D U-net [15]	3D	coarse	0.819 ± 0.068	4-fold CV
Proposed model	2D	coarse	0.789 ± 0.083	4-fold CV

Data augmentation was originally proposed for the classification model, and the effectiveness of mixup was validated for segmentation on brain MRI images [25]. The results of the current study demonstrate the effectiveness of multiple types of data augmentation methods for the two models of U-net for automatic pancreatic segmentation. To the best of our knowledge, the current study is the first to validate the usefulness of multiple types of data augmentation methods in pancreas segmentation.

Table 2 shows that deep U-net was better than baseline U-net. Deep U-net included additional layers in its network architecture, compared with baseline U-net. It is speculated that these additional layers could lead to performance improvement for pancreas segmentation. Nakai et al. [26] showed that deeper U-net could efficiently denoised low-dose CT images. They also showed that deeper U-net was better than baseline U-net. Kurata et al. [4] showed that their U-net with additional layers was effective for uterine segmentation. The results of the current study are consistent with the results of these studies. The effectiveness of deep/deeper U-net has not been sufficiently investigated so far. Because U-net can be used for segmentation, image denoising, detection, and modality conversion, it is necessary to evaluate what tasks the deep/deeper U-net is effective for.

Combined use of mixup and RICAP was the best for data augmentation in the current study. The combination of mixup and RICAP was also used in the study of bone segmentation [24]. The results of bone segmentation show that effectiveness of data augmentation was observed in the dataset with limited cases, and the optimal combination was conventional method and RICAP. Based on the studies of bone and pancreas segmentation, usefulness of combination of conventional method, mixup, and RICAP should be further investigated.

Sandfort et al. used CycleGAN as data augmentation to improve generalizability in organ segmentation on CT images [27]. CycleGAN was also used for data augmentation in the classification task [28]. Because the computational cost of training CycleGAN is relatively high, the use of CycleGAN as a data augmentation method needs some consideration. In this regard, computational cost of mixup and RICAP is relatively low, and mixup and RICAP are easy to implement.

Accuracy of pancreas segmentation was visually evaluated by the two radiologists in the current study. To our knowledge, there was no study of deep learning to evaluate the segmentation accuracy of pancreas structure visually. The results of visual scores mean that automatic segmentation model of the current study was good. It is expected that the proposed model may be useful for clinical cases if the clinical CT images have similar condition and quality to those of the Pancreas-CT dataset.

In the current study, we evaluated automatic pancreas segmentation using the public dataset called Pancreas-CT. Although this dataset was used in several studies as shown in Table 3, the manually annotated labels of four or eight cases were scored as not perfect based on the visual assessment of the current study. In most of the cases, the labels for the pancreas head were assessed as low-quality. It is presumed that the low-quality labeling is caused by the fact that annotators did not fully understand the boundary between the pancreas and other organs (e.g., duodenum). To evaluate the segmentation accuracy, reliable labeling is mandatory. For this purpose, a new database for pancreas segmentation is desirable.

There were several limitations to the present study. First, we investigated the usefulness of data augmentation only in segmentation models. The usefulness of data augmentation should be evaluated for other models such as classification, detection, and image generation. Second, the 3D fine-tuned model of pancreas segmentation was not evaluated. Because U-net, mixup, and RICAP were originally suggested for 2D models, we constructed and evaluated the 2D model of pancreas segmentation. We will apply the proposed methods to the 3D fine-tuned model in future research.

5. Conclusions

The combination of deep U-net with mixup and RICAP achieved automatic pancreas segmentation, which the radiologists scored as good or perfect. We will further investigate the usefulness of the proposed method for the 3D coarse-scaled/fine-scaled models to improve segmentation accuracy.

Author Contributions: Conceptualization, M.N.; methodology, M.N.; software, M.N. and S.N.; validation, M.N. and S.N.; formal analysis, M.N.; investigation, M.N.; resources, M.N. and K.F.; data curation, M.N. and SN; writing—original draft preparation, M.N.; writing—review and editing, M.N., S.N., and K.F.; visualization, M.N.; supervision, K.F.; project administration, M.N.; funding acquisition, M.N. All authors have read and agreed to the published version of the manuscript.

Appendix A

Table A1. Summary of fine-scaled models using Pancreas-CT dataset.

Name of Model	2D/3D	Coarse/Fine	Mean DSC	Data Splitting
Holistically Nested 2D FCN Stage-2 [11]	2D	fine	0.811 ± 0.073	4-fold CV
2D FCN + Recurrent Network [13]	2D	fine	0.824 ± 0.067	4-fold CV
Fine-scaled Model 2D FCN [14]	2D	fine	0.824 ± 0.057	4-fold CV
Fine-scaled Model 3D U-net [15]	3D	fine	0.860 ± 0.045	4-fold CV

Appendix B

Table A2. Results of Statistical significance for DSC difference.

Target 1	Target 2	p-Value	Statistical Significance for DSC Difference
1	2	0.727381623	No
1	3	0.560489877	No
1	4	0.921405534	No
1	5	0.037061458	No
1	6	0.727381623	No
1	7	0.148802462	No
1	8	0.553863735	No
1	9	0.012907274	No
1	10	5.45×10^{-5}	Yes
2	3	0.85904175	No
2	4	0.87456599	No
2	5	0.080182031	No
2	6	0.958034301	No
2	7	0.211395881	No
2	8	0.856459499	No
2	9	0.029961825	No
2	10	0.000143632	Yes
3	4	0.422285602	No
3	5	0.057745373	No
3	6	0.668985055	No
3	7	0.331951771	No
3	8	0.85904175	No
3	9	0.033624033	No
3	10	3.72×10^{-5}	Yes
4	5	0.047352438	No
4	6	0.764727204	No
4	7	0.157310432	No
4	8	0.529901132	No
4	9	0.024270868	No
4	10	0.000120757	Yes
5	6	0.067465313	No
5	7	0.649935631	No
5	8	0.067465313	No
5	9	0.580595554	No
5	10	0.031228349	No
6	7	0.227439002	No
6	8	0.784877257	No
6	9	0.028739708	No
6	10	9.60×10^{-5}	Yes
7	8	0.292611693	No
7	9	0.355409719	No
7	10	0.017108607	No
8	9	0.040470933	No
8	10	5.23×10^{-5}	Yes
9	10	0.185045722	No

Note: In Target 1 and Target 2, values of cells mean the followings: (1) Baseline U-net + no data augmentation, (2) Baseline U-net + conventional method, (3) Baseline U-net + mixup, (4) Baseline U-net + RICAP, (5) Baseline U-net + RICAP + mixup, (6) Deep U-net + no data augmentation, (7) Deep U-net + conventional method, (8) Deep U-net + mixup, (9) Deep U-net + RICAP, (10) Deep U-net + RICAP + mixup. p-values less than 0.05/45 = 0.00111 was considered as statistical significance.

References

1. Nakagomi, K.; Shimizu, A.; Kobatake, H.; Yakami, M.; Fujimoto, K.; Togashi, K. Multi-shape graph cuts with neighbor prior constraints and its application to lung segmentation from a chest CT volume. *Med. Image Anal.* **2013**, *17*, 62–77. [CrossRef] [PubMed]
2. Seo, H.; Huang, C.; Bassenne, M.; Xiao, R.; Xing, L. Modified U-Net (mU-Net) with Incorporation of Object-Dependent High Level Features for Improved Liver and Liver-Tumor Segmentation in CT Images. *IEEE Trans. Med. Imaging* **2020**, *39*, 1316–1325. [CrossRef] [PubMed]
3. Asaturyan, H.; Gligorievski, A.; Villarini, B. Morphological and multi-level geometrical descriptor analysis in CT and MRI volumes for automatic pancreas segmentation. *Comput. Med. Imaging Graph.* **2019**, *75*, 1–13. [CrossRef] [PubMed]
4. Kurata, Y.; Nishio, M.; Kido, A.; Fujimoto, K.; Yakami, M.; Isoda, H.; Togashi, K. Automatic segmentation of the uterus on MRI using a convolutional neural network. *Comput. Biol. Med.* **2019**, *114*, 103438. [CrossRef] [PubMed]
5. Hiasa, Y.; Otake, Y.; Takao, M.; Ogawa, T.; Sugano, N.; Sato, Y. Automated Muscle Segmentation from Clinical CT using Bayesian U-Net for Personalized Musculoskeletal Modeling. *IEEE Trans. Med. Imaging* **2020**, *39*, 1030–1040. [CrossRef]
6. Siegel, R.L.; Miller, K.D.; Jemal, A. Cancer statistics, 2019. *CA Cancer J. Clin.* **2019**, *69*, 7–34. [CrossRef] [PubMed]
7. Ardila, D.; Kiraly, A.P.; Bharadwaj, S.; Choi, B.; Reicher, J.J.; Peng, L.; Tse, D.; Etemadi, M.; Ye, W.; Corrado, G.; et al. End-to-end lung cancer screening with three-dimensional deep learning on low-dose chest computed tomography. *Nat. Med.* **2019**, *25*, 954–961. [CrossRef] [PubMed]
8. National Lung Screening Trial Research Team; Aberle, D.R.; Adams, A.M.; Berg, C.D.; Black, W.C.; Clapp, J.D.; Fagerstrom, R.M.; Gareen, I.F.; Gatsonis, C.; Marcus, P.M.; et al. Reduced lung-cancer mortality with low-dose computed tomographic screening. *N. Engl. J. Med.* **2011**, *365*, 395–409.
9. Hesamian, M.H.; Jia, W.; He, X.; Kennedy, P. Deep Learning Techniques for Medical Image Segmentation: Achievements and Challenges. *J. Digit. Imaging* **2019**, *32*, 582–596. [CrossRef]
10. Kumar, H.; DeSouza, S.V.; Petrov, M.S. Automated pancreas segmentation from computed tomography and magnetic resonance images: A systematic review. *Comput. Methods Programs Biomed.* **2019**, *178*, 319–328. [CrossRef]
11. Roth, H.R.; Lu, L.; Lay, N.; Harrison, A.P.; Farag, A.; Sohn, A.; Summers, R.M. Spatial aggregation of holistically-nested convolutional neural networks for automated pancreas localization and segmentation. *Med. Image Anal.* **2018**, *45*, 94–107. [CrossRef] [PubMed]
12. Oktay, O.; Schlemper, J.; Folgoc, L.L.; Lee, M.; Heinrich, M.; Misawa, K.; Mori, K.; McDonagh, S.; Hammerla, N.Y.; Kainz, B.; et al. Attention U-Net: Learning Where to Look for the Pancreas. In Proceedings of the 1st Conference on Medical Imaging with Deep Learning (MIDL2018), Amsterdam, The Netherlands, 4–6 July 2018.
13. Cai, J.; Lu, L.; Xie, Y.; Xing, F.; Yang, L. Improving deep pancreas segmentation in CT and MRI images via recurrent neural contextual learning and direct loss function. In Proceedings of the MICCAI 2017, Quebec City, QC, Canada, 11–13 September 2017.
14. Zhou, Y.; Xie, L.; Shen, W.; Wang, Y.; Fishman, E.K.; Yuille, A.L. A fixed-point model for pancreas segmentation in abdominal CT scans. In Proceedings of the MICCAI 2017, Quebec City, QC, Canada, 11–13 September 2017.
15. Zhao, N.; Tong, N.; Ruan, D.; Sheng, K. Fully Automated Pancreas Segmentation with Two-stage 3D Convolutional Neural Networks. *arXiv* **2019**, arXiv:1906.01795.
16. Zhang, H.; Cisse, M.; Dauphin, Y.N.; Lopez-Paz, D. mixup: Beyond Empirical Risk Minimization. *arXiv* **2017**, arXiv:1710.09412.
17. Takahashi, R.; Matsubara, T.; Uehara, K. Data Augmentation using Random Image Cropping and Patching for Deep CNNs. *arXiv* **2018**, arXiv:1811.09030. [CrossRef]
18. Cubuk, E.D.; Zoph, B.; Mane, D.; Vasudevan, V.; Le, Q.V. AutoAugment: Learning Augmentation Policies from Data. In Proceedings of the Computer Vision and Pattern Recognition (CVPR2019), Long Beach, CA, USA, 16–20 June 2019.

19. Ronneberger, O.; Fischer, P.; Brox, T. U-net: Convolutional networks for biomedical image segmentation. In Proceedings of the International Conference on Medical Image Computing and Computer-Assisted Intervention, Munich, Germany, 5–9 October 2015; Volume 9351, pp. 234–241.
20. Roth, H.R.; Farag, A.; Turkbey, E.B.; Lu, L.; Liu, J.; Summers, R.M. Data from Pancreas-CT. The Cancer Imaging Archive. 2016. Available online: http://doi.org/10.7937/K9/TCIA.2016.tNB1kqBU (accessed on 13 February 2020).
21. Roth, H.R.; Lu, L.; Farag, A.; Shin, H.-C.; Liu, J.; Turkbey, E.B.; Summers, R.M. DeepOrgan: Multi-level Deep Convolutional Networks for Automated Pancreas Segmentation. In Proceedings of the MICCA 2015, Munich, Germany, 5–9 October 2015; Volume 9349, pp. 556–564.
22. Clark, K.; Vendt, B.; Smith, K.; Freymann, J.; Kirby, J.; Koppel, P.; Moore, S.; Phillips, S.; Maffitt, D.; Pringle, M.; et al. The Cancer Imaging Archive (TCIA): Maintaining and Operating a Public Information Repository. *J. Digit. Imaging* **2013**, *26*, 1045–1057. [CrossRef] [PubMed]
23. Bergstra, J.; Bardenet, R.; Bengio, Y.; Kégl, B. Algorithms for Hyper-Parameter Optimization. In Proceedings of the 25th Annual Conference on Neural Information Processing Systems 2011, Granada, Spain, 12–15 December 2011; Available online: http://dl.acm.org/citation.cfm?id=2986743 (accessed on 5 May 2020).
24. Noguchi, S.; Nishio, M.; Yakami, M.; Nakagomi, L.; Togashi, K. Bone segmentation on whole-body CT using convolutional neural network with novel data augmentation techniques. *Comput. Biol. Med.* **2020**, *121*, 103767. [CrossRef] [PubMed]
25. Eaton-Rosen, Z.; Bragman, F.; Ourselin, S.; Cardoso, M.J. Improving Data Augmentation for Medical Image Segmentation. In Proceedings of the 1st Conference on Medical Imaging with Deep Learning (MIDL 2018), Amsterdam, The Netherlands, 4–6 July 2018.
26. Nakai, H.; Nishio, M.; Yamashita, R.; Ono, A.; Nakao, K.K.; Fujimoto, K.; Togashi, K. Quantitative and Qualitative Evaluation of Convolutional Neural Networks with a Deeper U-Net for Sparse-View Computed Tomography Reconstruction. *Acad. Radiol.* **2020**, *27*, 563–574. [CrossRef] [PubMed]
27. Sandfort, V.; Yan, K.; Pickhardt, P.J.; Summers, R.M. Data augmentation using generative adversarial networks (CycleGAN) to improve generalizability in CT segmentation tasks. *Sci. Rep.* **2019**, *9*, 16884. [CrossRef] [PubMed]
28. Muramatsu, C.; Nishio, M.; Goto, T.; Oiwa, M.; Morita, T.; Yakami, M.; Kubo, T.; Togashi, K.; Fujita, H. Improving breast mass classification by shared data with domain transformation using a generative adversarial network. *Comput. Biol. Med.* **2020**, *119*, 103698. [CrossRef] [PubMed]

10

Full 3D Microwave Breast Imaging using a Deep-Learning Technique

Vahab Khoshdel *, Mohammad Asefi, Ahmed Ashraf and Joe LoVetri

Department of Electrical and Computer Engineering, University of Manitoba, Winnipeg, MB R3T 5V6, Canada; masefi@151research.com (M.A.); ahmed.ashraf@umanitoba.ca (A.A.); Joe.LoVetri@umanitoba.ca (J.L.)

* Correspondence: khoshdev@myumanitoba.ca

Abstract: A deep learning technique to enhance 3D images of the complex-valued permittivity of the breast obtained via microwave imaging is investigated. The developed technique is an extension of one created to enhance 2D images. We employ a 3D Convolutional Neural Network, based on the U-Net architecture, that takes in 3D images obtained using the Contrast-Source Inversion (CSI) method and attempts to produce the true 3D image of the permittivity. The training set consists of 3D CSI images, along with the true numerical phantom images from which the microwave scattered field utilized to create the CSI reconstructions was synthetically generated. Each numerical phantom varies with respect to the size, number, and location of tumors within the fibroglandular region. The reconstructed permittivity images produced by the proposed 3D U-Net show that the network is not only able to remove the artifacts that are typical of CSI reconstructions, but it also enhances the detectability of the tumors. We test the trained U-Net with 3D images obtained from experimentally collected microwave data as well as with images obtained synthetically. Significantly, the results illustrate that although the network was trained using only images obtained from synthetic data, it performed well with images obtained from both synthetic and experimental data. Quantitative evaluations are reported using Receiver Operating Characteristics (ROC) curves for the tumor detectability and RMS error for the enhancement of the reconstructions.

Keywords: microwave breast imaging; image reconstruction; tumor detection; convolutional neural networks; deep learning

---

1. Introduction

Microwave Imaging (MWI) techniques that have been applied to the detection of breast cancer come in two forms: Radar-based techniques that attempt to detect tumors within the breast's interior [1], and inverse-scattering based methods that attempt to reconstruct complex permittivity maps corresponding to the distribution of different breast tissues [2]. The quantitative techniques, which are of interest herein, rely on the fact that different breast tissues (e.g., skin, adipose, fibroglandular and cancerous tumors) have different dielectric properties in the microwave frequency band [3,4].

Successfully implementing the inverse-scattering approach requires that one has a good numerical electromagnetic field model for the MWI system being used to acquire scattered-field data, including the antennas and the breast, but more importantly, requires that one solves a non-linear ill-posed inverse scattering problem. This is usually accomplished using computationally expensive iterative methods where the inversion model consists of a numerical solution of an electromagnetic forward scattering problem [5]. One challenge in using MWI for breast imaging is that the breast is a high-contrast object-of-interest (OI) having complicated internal structures and this produces unique artifacts in the quantitative reconstructions of the complex-valued permittivity of the breast tissue.

Both the non-linearity and the ill-posedness of the inverse scattering problem become more difficult to deal with for high contrast OIs having such complicated internal structure because they lead to multiple reflections within the OI.

The MWI technique we use in the work reported herein is the Contrast Source Inversion (CSI) method [6–8]. Although this is a state-of-the-art MWI technique it still succumbs to artifacts even when prior information is utilized to try to alleviate the non-linearity and ill-posedness of the problem [9,10]. Note that all MWI techniques, qualitative and quantitative alike, currently have difficulties with imaging artifacts [1,2,5,11].

Recently, there has been intense interest in the use of deep learning techniques in a broad range of applications such as natural language processing, computer vision and speech recognition [12]. In medical imaging, utilizing deep learning techniques for segmentation [13,14], as well as detection and classification [15–17] has been well investigated, at least for the more common modalities. Studies have shown that there is significant potential in applying deep learning techniques for the purpose of removing artifacts from biomedical images generated using some common modalities. Kang et al. proposed a deep Convolutional Neural Networks (CNNs) using directional wavelets for low dose x-ray computed tomography (CT), and results illustrate that a deep CNN using directional wavelets was more efficient in removing low dose-related CT noise [18]. Han et al. [19] and Jin et al. [20] independently proposed multi-scale residual learning networks using U-Net to remove these global streaking artifacts, In addition, domain adaptation from CT to MRI has been successfully demonstrated [21].

MWI researchers are also trying to use machine learning techniques to improve the performance of microwave imaging. For instance, researchers combined a neural network with microwave imaging to learn the forward model for a complex data-acquisition system [22]. Rekanos et al. proposed radial basis function neural network to estimate the position and size of proliferated marrow inside bone tissue with microwave imaging [23]. Le et al. tried to take the benefit of a deep neural network to enhance the constructed images [24]. Their deep neural network was trained to take microwave images created using the back-projection (BP) method as an input and have the network output a much-improved image. In fact, they tried to by-pass the use of iterative techniques for solving the full nonlinear electromagnetic inverse problem. Most recently, we have investigated utilizing deep learning techniques to improve 2D microwave imaging for the breast imaging application [25]. Researchers employing radar-based techniques have also been investigating machine learning approaches for the detection of breast lesions [26].

In this paper, we utilize a deep learning technique, based on CNNs, to enhance full 3D MWI reconstructions obtained using a 3D CSI algorithm that uses the Finite Element Method (FEM) to solve the electromagnetic forward problem [27]. The enhancement removes reconstruction artifacts and improves the accuracy of the resulting images. We utilize a 3D 10-channel U-Net architecture for the CNN where the input and output are both 3D images, and each channel corresponds to the real and imaginary parts of the complex-valued permittivity images created using five different microwave frequencies.

In Section 2 we start by providing a brief description of the CSI-based methodology that we use, as well as the numerical phantoms and MWI parameters utilized to generate training images. We also provide details of our chosen deep learning approach. In Section 3 we describe the training data set as well as the parameters used for the network training. In the following, quantitative assessment and assessment of robustness for numerical experiments are described. Section 4 provides a brief description of our experimental setup and also the result of trained CNN for the experimental data. Finally, in Section 5 we give our conclusion and explain our future work.

2. 3D CSI-Deep-Learning Methodology

In microwave data acquisition processes, electromagnetic fields scatter from, and propagate through, the tissue in a three-dimensional (3D) space. However, to accelerate the image reconstruction process and reduce the computational complexity, researchers are trying to represent electromagnetic waves in 3D space as a simplified 2D model. However, studies have shown that simplifying 3D problems to 2D models can increase the level of artifacts in the recovered dielectric properties [28]. Moreover, in 2D imaging when the object of interest is small, there is a chance that it place between two consecutive imaging slice, then the reconstruction algorithm would not discover the target precisely. Hence, utilizing a viable 3D microwave image reconstruction will enhance the accuracy and quality of reconstruction [29]. While iterative methods have improved dramatically over the years, providing improved resolution and accuracy of the reconstructed properties, as well as more efficient implementations, there are still many fundamental trade-offs between these three aspects due to operational, financial, and physical constraints.

Lower resolution in comparison with other modalities, as well as the many reconstruction artifacts that are related to the nonlinearity and ill-posedness of the associated inverse problem, are the main reasons that MWI is not clinically accepted yet. Although it has been shown that using accurate prior information will reduce the Root-Mean-Squared (RMS) reconstruction error over the whole image [9,10,30–32], artifacts and reconstruction errors near the tumor can translate to poor tumor detection results [33].

2.1. Microwave Imaging via Contrast Source Inversion

The first part of the proposed 3D CSI-Deep-Learning methodology consists of quantitatively generating the complex-valued permittivity images using a MWI technique. Quantitative MWI requires that one solve a non-linear ill-posed inverse scattering problem. A plethora of algorithms have been developed during the past 40 years to solve this problem. They generally involve computationally expensive iterative methods to locally minimize a specially designed functional that incorporates a numerical inversion model approximating the relevant electromagnetic phenomena of the problem [5,11]. In the past, different MWI techniques have utilized tailored optimization algorithms with various functionals. Some of the most prominent techniques have been the Distorted Born Iterative Method [34], Gauss–Newton Inversion [35], the Levenberg–Marquardt method [36] and the Contrast Source Inversion technique [6]. Innovations on these foundational algorithms have allowed improvements to the obtainable imaging accuracy and resolution, especially in the area of breast imaging, e.g., [37,38]. Being an ill-posed problem, regularization techniques are required to solve the inverse scattering problem [39,40].

As previously mentioned, to solve the electromagnetic inverse scattering problem associated with microwave breast imaging we employ the CSI method. The numerical inversion model utilized within the CSI algorithm is based on a full-vectorial 3D electromagnetic model of the MWI system that includes a quasi-resonant flat-faceted chamber [41,42]. The 3D FEM-CSI algorithm is utilized with prior information in the form of an inhomogeneous background as was done in [27]. Breast images reconstructed from both synthetic and experimental scattered-field data are utilized in this work. The experimental data is collected using the same air-based quasi-resonant imaging chamber described in [27]. Thus, the forward model for creating the synthetic data and the inversion model, both utilize a 3D finite element model of the same imaging chamber.

We consider both synthetic and actual experimental breast phantoms with three tissue types: fat, fibroglandular and tumor. These breast phantoms are formed using a simple outer fat layer, and an interior fibroglandular region that contains one or more embedded tumors. The breast phantoms are positioned within the chamber as depicted in Figure 1.

The phantoms are interrogated using microwave energy with magnetic-field probes located on the conductive chamber walls. The same probes are used as those in receivers. As described in [42], the 24 transmitters and receivers are ϕ-polarized. Data were collected at single frequencies and for every transmitter, 23 magnetic fields were recorded at the receiver locations. Thus, 552 complex numbers (magnitude and phase) were utilized to reconstruct the breast phantom that was located within the chamber. That is, the real and imaginary parts of the complex permittivity of the breast phantom were reconstructed using the CSI algorithm.

The forward data were obtained using a 3D-FEM electromagnetic field solver. Before inverting the data using the FEM-CSI algorithm, we added 5 % noise as is usual in creating synthetic data [8]. This procedure was performed at individual frequencies and for the work considered herein, the frequency band of 1.1 GHz to 1.5 GHz was used. It has been shown that reconstruction artifacts appear at different locations of the imaging domain when different frequencies are used, whereas the tumor is typically reconstructed at approximately the same location [27]. In that work, it was shown that this feature can improve the tumor detection by using the intersection of thresholded images.

For the synthetically generated data and inversions, the permittivity was assumed to be constant over frequency. The complex permittivity values that were used are given in Table 1. For the experimental test case considered herein, the permittivities of the utilized tissue-mimicing liquids do vary with frequency (see [27] for details).

Table 1. Complex permittivity for different tissues.

Permittivity			
Air	Fat	Fibroglandular	Tumor
1 − 0.001j	3 − 0.6j	20 − 21.6j	56.3 − 30j

It has been shown that successful CSI reconstructions can be obtained if one introduces a fat and fibroglandular region as prior information in the CSI algorithm. This prior information is in the form of an inhomogeneous numerical background against which the contrast is defined. That is, if $\epsilon_n(r)$ and $\epsilon(r)$ represent the background information and the desired complex permittivity, as functions of position, then the contrast $\chi(r) = (\epsilon(r) - \epsilon_n(r))/\epsilon_n(r)$ is one of the variables solved for in the CSI algorithm (the other variable being the contrast sources generated for each transmitter). Full details of the CSI algorithm, used in this way, are provided in [9,10].

Introducing an inhomogeneous background in this way is a form of regularizing the inverse problem, but as was already mentioned, various reconstruction artifacts are still present in the CSI-reconstructed images. These artifacts increase the false-positive and reduce the true-positive tumor detection rates. For the case of 2D imaging, it was recently shown that using a deep-learning technique ameliorates this problem [25]. This has motivated the interest in using a similar deep-learning technique to improve 3D MWI. However, in addition to artifacts, 3D MWI also suffers from the problem of producing reconstructions that do not reach the maximum permittivity values of the true phantom model. This was noted in [27] and therefore the detection threshold was based on 85% of the maximum reconstructed value. Fortunately, the tumor permittivity values are at the extreme end of the scale, so such a procedure is successful. Improving the CSI reconstructions by correcting the reconstructed permittivity values, in addition to removing artifacts is the sought after goal of using a deep learning technique.

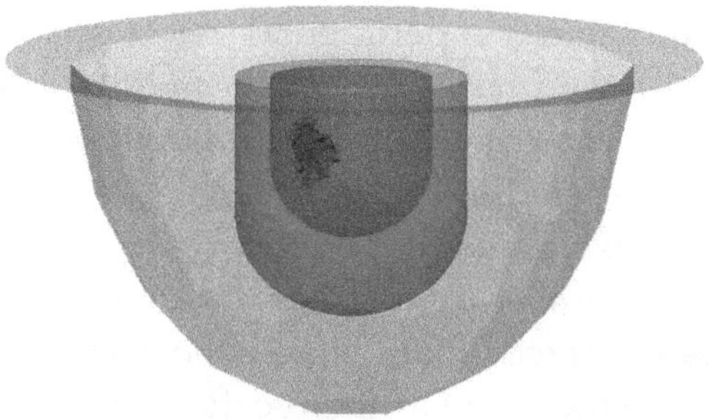

Figure 1. Simulated Breast Model. Gray, blue, green, and red regions represent air, fat, fibroglandular, and tumor, respectively.

2.2. Machine Learning Approach to Reconstruction

Combining the CSI technique with a deep learning approach is accomplished by learning a data-driven mapping, $\mathcal{G}$, from a CSI reconstruction to the true permittivity ($\mathcal{G} : \epsilon^{CSI} \rightarrow \epsilon^{true}$).

In this study, we learn a mapping from the real and imaginary parts of the permittivities in CSI reconstructions at several frequencies to a single real permittivity image. Thus, if the CSI complex permittivity map is an $L \times M \times N$ 3D image, and reconstructions at five frequencies are utilized, then each of the learned functions maps $5 \times L \times M \times N$ complex domain to $L \times M \times N$ real domain (e.g., $\mathcal{G}_R : \mathbb{C}^{5\times L\times M\times N} \mapsto \mathbb{R}^{L\times M\times N}$). The complex output of CSI at the five selected frequencies can be treated as a 10-channel image. We realized this mapping through a deep neural network as follows.

The desired mapping for our task at hand is an image-to-image transformation; there are multiple neural architectures that can implement this mapping. For instance, a naive choice could be a fully-connected single layer neural network which takes in CSI reconstruction as input and is trained to output the ground truth permittivity. However, such an architecture would be very prone to overfitting [12]. We, therefore, use a hierarchical convolutional neural network for our image-to-image transformation task. A good template for such a task is the U-Net architecture which is one of the most successful deep neural networks for image segmentation and reconstruction problems [13]. The architecture consists of successive convolutional and downsampling layers, followed by successive deconvolutional and upsampling layers. Moreover, the skip connections between the corresponding contractive and expansive layers keep the gradients from vanishing that helps in the optimization process [13,43]. To use a U-Net for reconstruction, the original objective of the U-Net is replaced with the sum of pixelwise squared reconstruction errors between the true real part of permittivity and the output of U-Net [13]. In our problem, the network input is the 3D CSI reconstructed complex images (after 500 iterations). Thus, there are two options for choosing the U-Net architecture, U-Net with complex weights and U-Net with real weights. Very few studies have been done on the training of U-Net with complex weights, although very recently Trabelsi et al. tried to train the neural network with complex weights for convolutional architectures [44]. In this paper, we decided to use a U-Net architecture having real-valued weights. A schematic representation of our architecture is shown in Figure 2. The motivation for choosing the neural network parameters (the number of convolutional layers, size and number of filters) is as follows. In a hierarchical multi-scale CNN, the effective receptive field of the convolution filters is variable at each layer, i.e., through successive sub-sampling it is possible to have a larger receptive field even by using filters of smaller kernel size [12,45]. As mentioned above, the input to our neural network is $L \times M \times N \times 10$; in particular, for each frequency, the dimension of our input image volume is $64 \times 64 \times 64$ (i.e., $L = M = N = 64$). If we start with a 3D receptive field of $3 \times 3 \times 3$, after four layers of successive convolutions and subsampling (by a factor of $1/2$), the receptive field would effectively span the entire image volume. We, therefore, use four convolutional layers with a 3D filter kernel size of $3 \times 3 \times 3$. Since after each convolutional layer the size of the image volume is reduced, we can increase the number of filters at each successive layer to enhance the representational power of the neural network [12]. In particular, we start with 32 filters for the first layer and successively double the number of filters after each layer (number of filters after the fourth layer is 512). This defines the encoder part of the U-net i.e., the part of a neural network consisting of contractive convolutions. For the decoder part, we follow a symmetric architecture consisting of expansive convolutions [13].

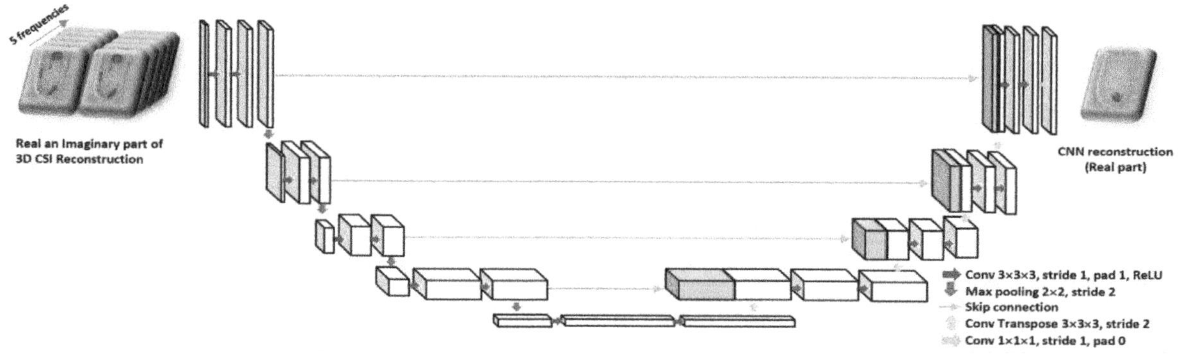

Figure 2. Schematic for the proposed U-Net to reconstruct the real part of permittivity. The input to the network is the 3D Contrast-Source Inversion (CSI) reconstruction, and the network is trained to output the corresponding true 3D permittivity map.

3. Numerical Experiments

3.1. Datasets

While we tested our neural network on both experimental and synthetic data, for training we only used a synthetically generated dataset. The training dataset consisted of 600 numerical breast phantoms; tumors were randomly generated within the fibroglandular region of the phantom. Starting from a random initial position, tumor pixels were grown randomly until the maximum diameter reached a threshold. To have variability in the dataset, the threshold for the maximum diameter was also randomly sampled from the range: 1.1–1.5 cm. One half the dataset consisted of breast phantoms with one tumor, while the other half had phantoms with two tumors. We then employed a forward solver [8] to generate the scattered field data corresponding to the phantoms. CSI reconstructions were performed at five frequencies: 1.1, 1.2, 1.3, 1.4, and 1.5 GHz. These CSI reconstructions together with the corresponding ground-truth permittivity values for the phantoms formed our training data for the U-Net input and output respectively.

3.2. Network Training

All the CNNs were implemented using Python 3.6 and Keras 2.0.6 with Tensorflow backend. We used a Windows 10 computer with a Tesla P100-PCIE-12GB graphic processor and Intel(R) CPU(3.50 GHz). We used the popular Xavier initialization for the convolutional layer weights to obtain an appropriate scale [46]. We trained with a batch size of 10, for 200 epochs with Adam optimization. Four-fold cross-validation strategy has been utilized to evaluate the proposed deep neural network for all experiments. The U-net wastrained using the real and imaginary parts for five different frequencies as inputs. With 600 phantoms in our dataset, each fold in four-fold cross-validation consisted of 150 examples. For every fold, training was done using 450 cases, while the testing set consisted of the held-out 150 examples. Thus all 600 cases featured as test examples when they were not part of the training set. For the loss function, we use pixel wise mean squared error between the ground truth 3D image and the CNN 3D reconstructed image as follows:

$$RMSError = \frac{1}{LMN} \sum_{x=1}^{L} \sum_{y=1}^{M} \sum_{z=1}^{N} (I_{x,y,z}^{GT} - I_{x,y,z}^{CNN})^2 \quad (1)$$

where $I_{x,y,z}^{CNN}$ represents a 3D image reconstructed by the CNN and $I_{x,y,z}^{GT}$ represents a 3D ground truth image.

3.3. *Quantitative Assessment*

The CNN-enhanced reconstruction performance and the subsequent tumor segmentation based on thresholding was evaluated quantitatively. The Root Mean Squared (RMS) reconstruction error between the network output and the true permittivity values was used to evaluate the reconstruction quality. The performance of a detection algorithm is often assessed in terms of two types of error i.e., False Positive Rate (FPR) and False Negative Rate (FNR). FPR and FNR will vary depending on the decision threshold used on the output score of the detection algorithm. To quantify the ability of the output score to separate the two classes, we need to analyze the two errors for all possible thresholds. In particular, we performed Receiver Operating Characteristics (ROC) analysis to assess the ability of the reconstructed complex permittivity to distinguish between tumor and non-tumor pixels. The ROC curve is a plot of True Positive Rate ($TPR = \frac{TP}{TP+FN}$) against the False Positive Rate ($FPR = \frac{FP}{FP+TN}$) for all thresholds. The Area Under the Curve (AUC) for the ROC is a metric quantifying the separability between tumor and non-tumor pixels [47]. For comparison we also computed RMS reconstruction error and performed ROC analysis on CSI-only reconstructions. ROC carries information about the relation of the true positives vs. the false positives. However, the information about the distributions of thresholds at which the different ratios fall would be lost in this curve. Therefore, the distance from any location on the ROC curve to the top-left corner of the plot is also an informative metric (we call this the "Distance-to-MaxTD" or "DMTD" plot). We use the DMTD curve as a complementary metric to display/analyze the relation between the true positive detection as well as the threshold at which a certain true positive to negative ratio happens. This will especially help us better understand the performance of the overlapping (or very similar) ROC curves for different scenarios. The depth of the curve tells us about the quality of the reconstruction; the lower the dip, the better the performance of the algorithm. The location of the dip carries information about the separation of the tumor relative to the background; for instance, the further the dip of the DMTD curve is to the left, the higher the separation between the background and tumor. Additionally, the width of the dip gives us information about the robustness of the algorithm; the wider the dip of the curve, the higher the chances of having a tumor with no artifacts (false positives) for the proper reconstruction of the tumor size and shape. The results of this quantitative evaluation by using four-fold cross-validation strategy for all 600 images are shown in Figure 3 and Table 2.

Figure 4 illustrates the performance of the trained U-Net in comparison with CSI reconstruction for an arbitrary example with two tumors. Based on the AUC and RMS error metrics, it could be concluded that the proposed CNN is successful in term of reconstruction and tumor detection. However, in a previous study [27], it was shown that taking the intersection of multi-frequency thresholded 3D images performs the best at detecting tumors. Therefore, we compared our trained CNN with the intersection of multi-frequency thresholded 3D images in terms of detection. The superiority of the trained CNN to CSI results as well as to multi-frequency thresholded results are shown in Figure 3. For this same example, the CSI reconstructions at the remaining four other frequencies are shown in Figure 5. The resulting images for the real and imaginary parts of the permittivity after taking the intersection of the reconstructions that were thresholded at 85% of the maximum reconstructed permittivity value are also shown in the figure. Note that results using a CNN trained to reconstruct the imaginary part of the complex permittivity (not shown) are very similar to those using the CNN trained to reconstruct the real part in terms of tumor detection (ROC Curve) and reconstruction performance (RMS error). Thus, the ROC curve in Figure 3 and RMS error in Table 2, were computed using only reconstructions of the real part of the permittivity.

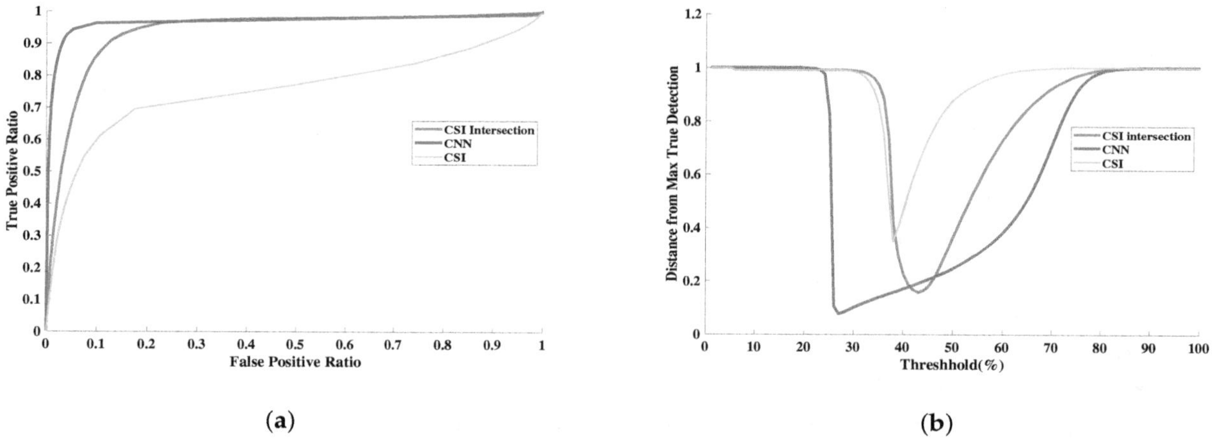

Figure 3. The detection performance using the reconstructed outputs of the Convolutional Neural Network (CNN) and CSI as well as the intersection of CSI reconstructions at the five chosen frequencies. (**a**) Receiver Operating Characteristics (ROC) curves derived from the reconstructions. (**b**) The DMTD curve.

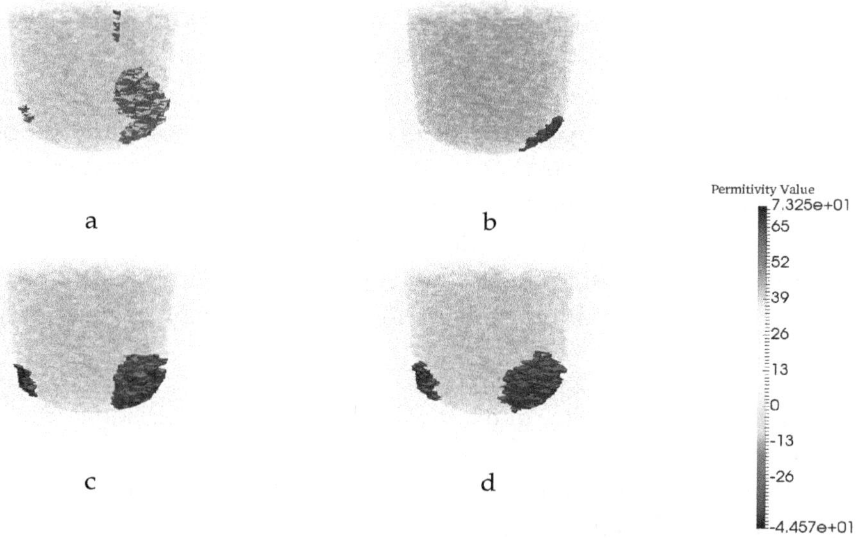

Figure 4. Reconstruction results for a particular example with two tumors. The real (**a**) and imaginary (**b**) part of CSI reconstruction at 1.1 GHz. (**c**) CNN reconstruction. (**d**) Ground truth.

Table 2. Comparison of reconstruction and tumor detection performance.

	RMS Error		**AUC**	
	CSI	CNN	CSI	CNN
Synthetic Data	1.4356	1.161	0.935	0.957
Exprimental Data	1.250	1.172	0.794	0.938

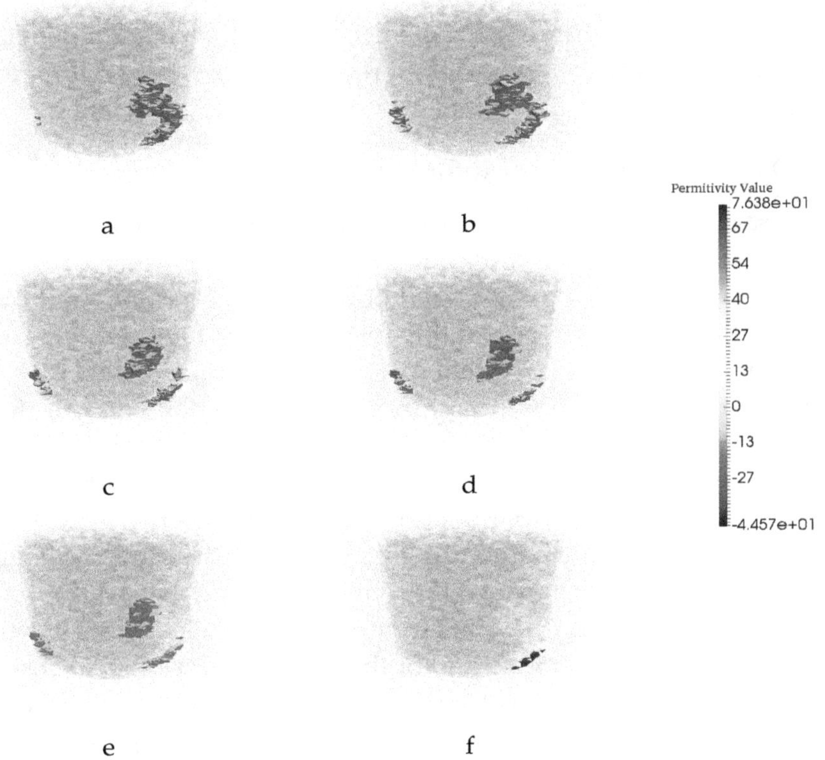

Figure 5. CSI reconstructions at four remaining frequencies for the same example as in Figure 4 and resulting images after intersecting images thresholded at 85% of the maximum reconstructed permittivity. (**a–d**) The real part of CSI reconstructions at 1.2, 1.3, 1.4, and 1.5 GHz. (**e**) Intersection of real part of CSI reconstructions. (**f**) Intersection of imaginary part of CSI reconstructions.

3.4. Assessment of Robustness

It is important to assess the robustness of our trained neural network when being tested on images different from those used during training. We investigate four aspects of variation in test data as compared to the training data: (i) changes in frequencies used to generate CSI reconstructions, (ii) changes in breast phantom geometry, (iii) changes in prior-information, and (v) breast phantom with no tumor.

3.4.1. Robustness to Changes in Frequency

First, given that the CNN was trained utilizing images created at 1.1 GHz, 1.2, 1.3, 1.4, and 1.5 GHz, the performance of the trained network was checked qualitatively by testing with CSI reconstructions that were created using data obtained at five arbitrarily chosen frequencies: 1.05, 1.15, 1.25, 1.35 and 1.45 GHz. Therefore, CSI reconstructions at chosen frequencies for five different breast phantoms have been created. These tests indicated that the trained U-Net was indeed superior to the CSI-only case. Results for one test example of the CSI and CNN outputs, from data obtained at 1.05 GHz, are shown in Figure 6. This suggests that the CNN is robust to testing images reconstructed using frequencies in the same bandwidth as used for training (one does not have to rely on using the exact same frequencies). As will be seen shortly, however, this is not the case once much higher frequencies are used.

3.4.2. Robustness to Changes in Breast Phantom Geometry

The next test for the network's robustess is to check against geometric changes of the breast phantom model. Thus, a new model which has the same dimensions for the fat region but has a smaller fibroglandular region (the height of fibroglandular region is decreased by 0.9 cm) was generated. By using this new small model, five different breast phantoms with a random tumor have been generated to evaluate the trained CNN. Figure 7 demonstrates the performance of the trained CNN for a particular example when the input images were CSI reconstructed images for this new model. As can be seen, the CNN significantly alters the CSI reconstructions (row 1) to bring them closer to the ground truth (row 2).

3.4.3. Robustness to Imperfections in Prior Information

In order to understand the U-Net's ability to remove artifacts, the next test case artificially induces artifacts into the CSI reconstructions by utilizing incorrect, or imperfect, prior information. Clearly, using perfect prior information results in very good CSI reconstructions; however, perfect prior information regarding the structural shape of the fibroglandular region as well as the permittivity of the fibroglandular tissue is difficult to obtain in practical circumstances. It is well known that using CSI with imperfect prior information produces various reconstruction artifacts. To evaluate this aspect of robustness we introduced 10% error in the permittivity of the fibroglandular tissue used as prior information. Figure 8 shows the performance of the CNN when tested with CSI reconstructions using imperfect permittivity in a structurally perfect fibroglandular region. The ROC curves created from the CSI and CNN outputs corresponding to this case shown in the plots of Figure 9. From the green colored curves we see that the CNN-enhanced reconstructions do provide an improvement over the CSI reconstructions. The distance-to-maxTD curve in Figure 9 clearly shows that the range in the threshold that could be used for good detection for the CNN-enhanced reconstructions is much wider than that could be used for the CSI reconstructions. When imperfect structural prior was used for a test case it was found that neither the CSI nor the CNN reconstructions performed well. This is the last test performed using synthetically generated images.

3.4.4. Robustness to Breast Phantom with No Tumor

Lastly, given that the CNN was trained only on breast phantom in presence of tumor, the last test in this section has been done to check the performance of the trained CNN for breast phantom with no tumor. Note that to prevent having zero scattered field data, we have to use imperfect prior information. We introduced 5% error in the permittivity of the fibroglandular tissue used as prior information. Figure 10 demonstrates the performance of the trained network when the input images were CSI reconstructed images with no tumor.

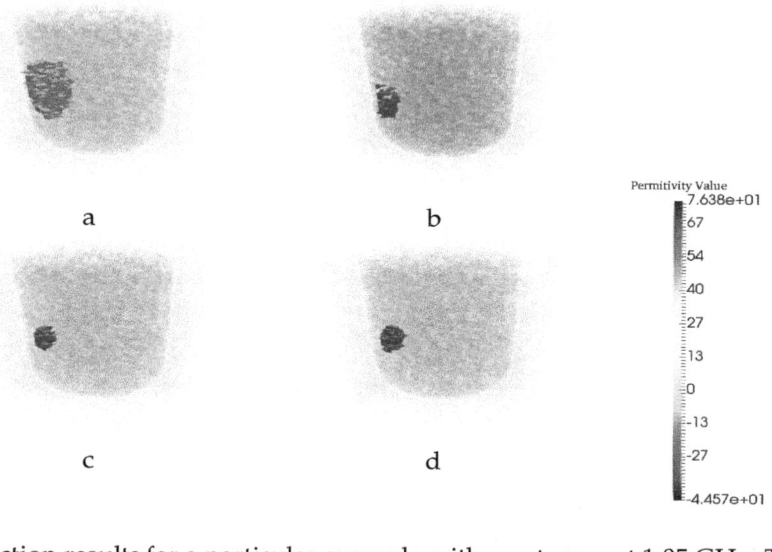

Figure 6. Reconstruction results for a particular example with one tumor at 1.05 GHz. The real (**a**) and imaginary (**b**) part of CSI reconstruction. (**c**) CNN reconstruction. (**d**) Ground truth.

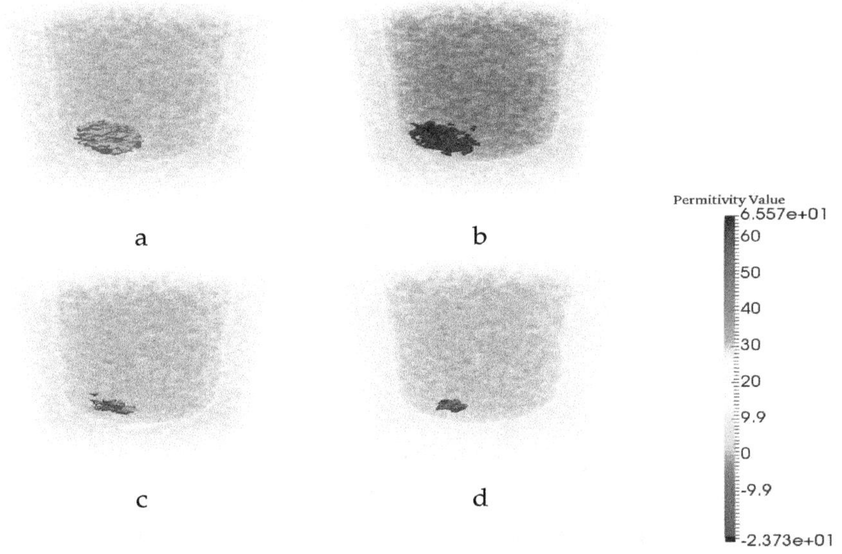

Figure 7. Reconstruction results for a particular example when the test images are CSI results for a breast phantom having a smaller fibroglandular region than those of the training set. The (**a**) real and (**b**) imaginary parts of the CSI reconstructions. (**c**) CNN reconstruction. (**d**) Ground truth.

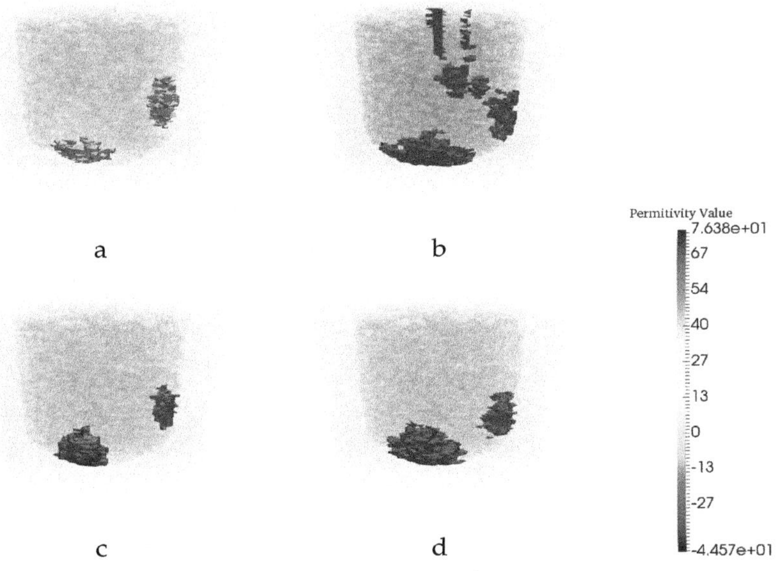

Figure 8. Reconstruction results for a particular example with two tumor when the training images are CSI results with perfect prior information, but the neural net was tested on imperfect prior information. The real (**a**) and imaginary (**b**) part of CSI reconstruction. (**c**) CNN reconstruction. (**d**) Ground truth.

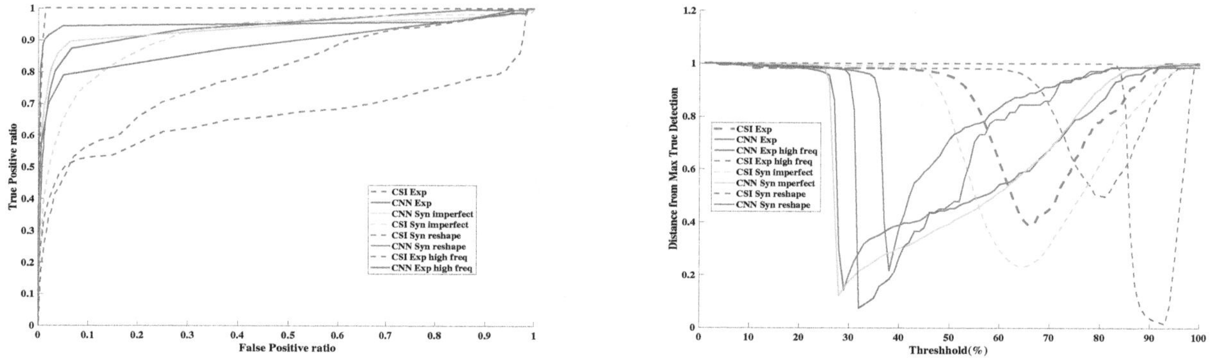

(a) (b)

Figure 9. Detection performance based on the reconstructed outputs of CNN and CSI. (**a**) ROC curves derived from the reconstructed real part of the permittivity from CSI and CNN. (**b**) The DMTD. test cases are: synthetic: imperfect permittivity prior, and true breast phantom with elongated fibroglandular region. Experimental: using data within the frequency band and much higher than the training frequency band.

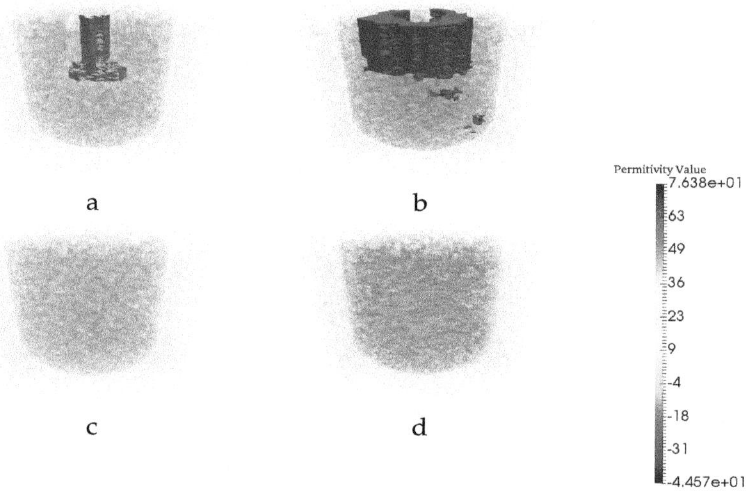

Figure 10. Reconstruction results for a particular example when the training images are CSI results with one or two tumors but the neural net was tested on a phantom with no tumor. The real (**a**) and imaginary (**b**) part of CSI reconstruction. (**c**) CNN reconstruction. (**d**) Ground truth.

4. Experimental Tests and Results

The experimental setup described in [27,42] was used to collect data to test the described neural network. A depiction of the imaging chamber and the breast phantom used in the experiment is shown in Figure 11. This chamber has 44 facets and contains 24 magnetic field probes and the breast phantom used in the chamber has three regions with similar sizes and properties to those of the numerical breast phantom described earlier for the fat and fibro regions; a 2 cm spherical phantom was used as the tumor region with properties similar to that of the tumor described in the numerical test cases. To mimic the properties close to those of a realistic breast, the fat region was filled with canola oil while a 20:80 ratio of water to glycerin is used to fill the fibroglanduar shell, and a 10:90 ratio of water to glycerin is used to fill the spherical inclusion representing a tumor. For these ratios, the permittivities of the canola oil and water/glycerin mixture are measured as $3.0 - j0.193$, $23.3 - j18.1$ and $50 - j25$ respectively for fat, fibrogladular, and tumor at 1.1 GHz [27]. It is worth noting that this simplistic phantom is used as a simple proof of concept target for inverting a high contrast multilayered medium in an air background and not testing the system against realistic breast phantoms.

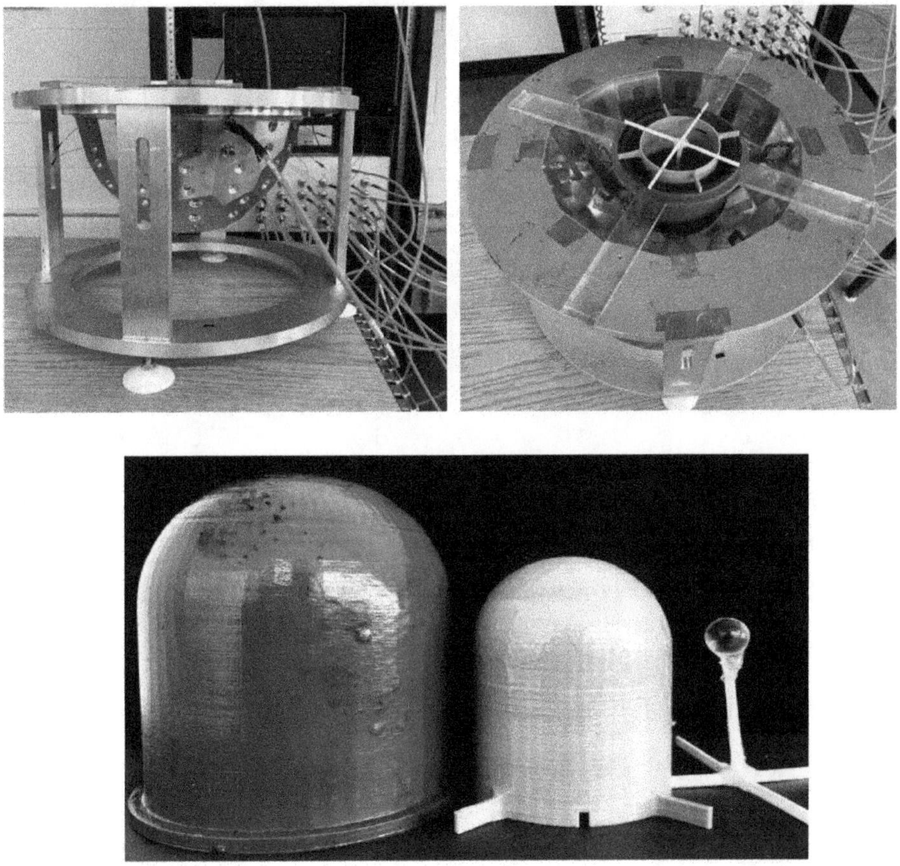

Figure 11. The experimental system including the three region breast phantom (Diameter of fat, fibroglanduar and tumor regions are 10 , 8 and 2 CM respectively).

In medical imaging, sometimes it is difficult to build a large experimental training data set. Therefore, it is desirable that a neural network trained on synthetic data generalizes well when tested on experimental data. To investigate this, we collected experimental data using a wide range of frequencies (1.1 to 2.9 GHz). The performance of the trained network for experimental data is evaluated and shown in Figure 12. Results illustrate that trained CNN improved the experimental CSI reconstructed images when frequencies similar or close to those for training data were used. However, when we tested the trained CNN with experimental images created with frequencies well beyond the band of frequencies used to create the training data, it is observed that CNN is not able to detect the tumor. Figure 13. One reason for this can be the significant change in the nature of the artifacts. In general, for the results presented in this manuscript, the artifacts at almost all lower frequency reconstructions have a lower permittivity compared to the value of the reconstructed tumor. However, the permittivities of the reconstructed artifacts at higher frequencies are higher than those of the reconstructed tumor.

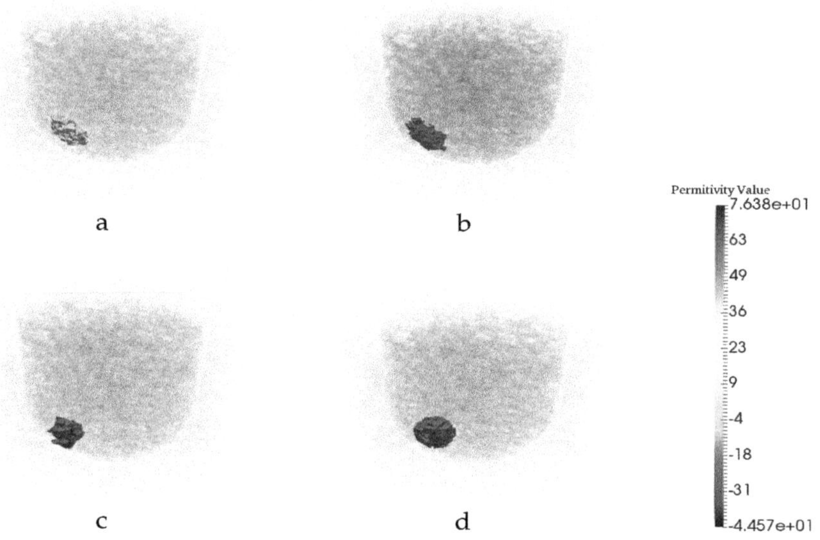

Figure 12. CNN performance for experimental result when the neural net was trained on Synthetic data. The real (**a**) and imaginary (**b**) part of CSI reconstruction. (**c**) CNN reconstruction. (**d**) Ground truth.

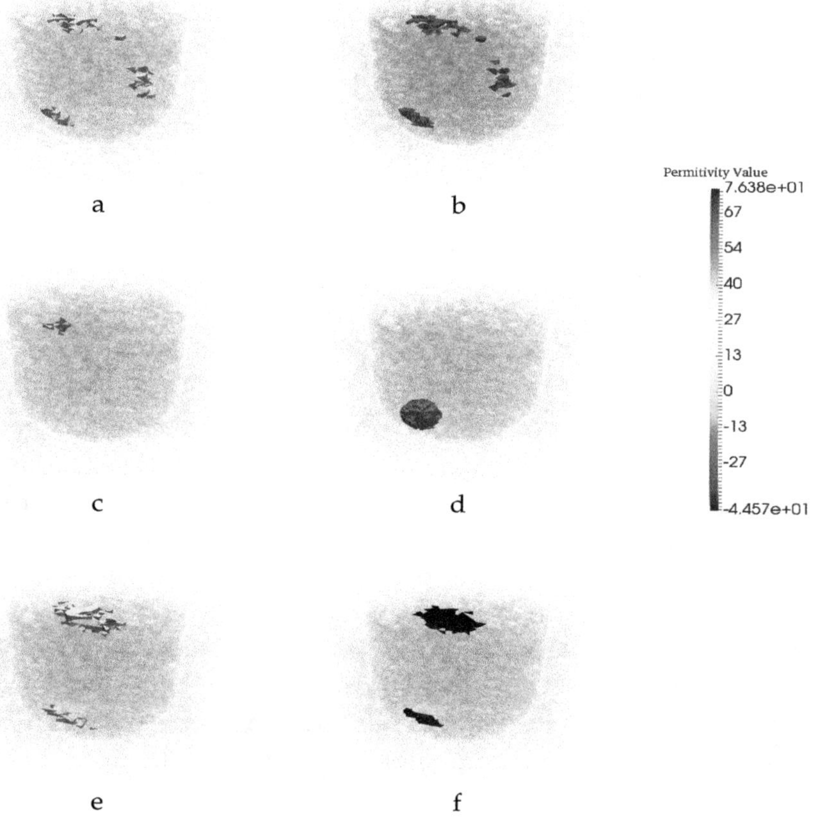

Figure 13. Reconstruction results for a particular example when the test images are CSI results in high frequencies but the neural net was trained on low frequencies. The real (**a**) and imaginary (**b**) part of CSI reconstruction. (**c**) CNN reconstruction. (**d**) Ground truth. (**e**) Intersection of real part of CSI reconstruction at all frequencies.(**f**) Intersection of imaginary part of CSI reconstruction at all frequencies(two intersection images are binary image).

5. Conclusions

A deep learning technique using a 3D CNN was developed to improve the imaging performance of 3D MWI of the breast. The improvement manifests as the removal of artifacts in the 3D reconstructions of the complex-valued permittivity of the breast being imaged. These reconstruction artifacts are specific to the MWI system wherein the microwave scattered-field data is collected as well as to the numerical inversion algorithm, in our case CSI, being used to create the images. Using synthetic 3D images that take both these factors into account, a CNN was trained with the goal to reproduce the true permittivity image of the breast from the artifact-laden 3D reconstructions. The trained CNN was tested with synthetic images as well as with images created using experimentally obtained microwave scattered-field data from an MWI system: the same MWI system for which a numerical model was utilized in the creation of the synthetic 3D images.

The RMS error between the CNN-reconstructed images and the true images are improved over the corresponding error between the CSI-only reconstructions and the true images. In addition, tumor detection was evaluated using ROC-AUC metrics and these are much improved for the CNN-reconstructed images over the ROC-AUC results for the CSI-only reconstructions. The results show that this deep learning technique has the ability to improve 3D CSI reconstructions in three interdependent ways. First, and foremost, the CNN has shown its ability to remove reconstruction artifacts which are a great challenge for quantitative MWI. Secondly, the trained CNN successfully corrects the permittivity values which tend to be undershot in the CSI reconstructions. Finally, from a qualitative perspective, the tumor location is more accurately reconstructed with respect to its true position and size.

There are several limitations of this work, but the most critical is that numerical phantoms with a single, relatively simple, fibroglandular region were utilized for training and testing. This same region was reproduced in the physical phantom utilized for the experimental results. Our experience with utilizing a similar technique with 2D images showed that this limitation can be removed by training with breast models having several types of fibroglandular regions. Similarly, this work has shown that when the artifacts are due to reconstructions obtained from data generated with MWI system parameters that were not utilized in the training set, for example artifacts generated by using microwave frequencies that are much higher than what the MWI system was designed for, then the trained CNN was not able to identify these as artifacts. In fact, some of these artifacts were identified as tumors. This result limits the robustness of the trained CNN but this study has provided a good understanding of that robustness. We further note that due to the significant level of computational resources required during the generation of forward data and inverse 3D CSI reconstructions, we generated only a moderately sized dataset consisting of 600 phantoms. Being aware of the limited number of training examples, we made extensive use of cross-validation and regularization techniques to avoid the possibility of model overfitting, which is evidenced by the generalization our CNN demonstrates on unseen examples. That said, having more training data would potentially help us to train a more robust CNN with better generalization properties. Techniques for overcoming some of these limitations will be investigated in planned future work.

Author Contributions: All four authors (V.K., M.A., A.A., J.L.) contributed to Methodology, Validation, Investigation, Writing (review and editing). V.K. and J.L. have contributed to Writing (original draft preparation), Conceptualization and Resources. J.L. contributed to Project administration and Supervision. V.K. contributed to Software and Visualization. All authors have read and agreed to the published version of the manuscript.

References

1. O'Loughlin, D.; O'Halloran, M.J.; Moloney, B.M.; Glavin, M.; Jones, E.; Elahi, M.A. Microwave Breast Imaging: Clinical Advances and Remaining Challenges. *IEEE Trans. Biomed. Eng.* **2018**, *65*, 2580–2590. [CrossRef]

2. Bolomey, J.C. Crossed Viewpoints on Microwave-Based Imaging for Medical Diagnosis: From Genesis to Earliest Clinical Outcomes. In *The World of Applied Electromagnetics: In Appreciation of Magdy Fahmy Iskander*; Lakhtakia, A., Furse, C.M., Eds.; Springer International Publishing: Cham, Switzerland, 2018; pp. 369–414.
3. Lazebnik, M.; Popovic, D.; McCartney, L.; Watkins, C.B.; Lindstrom, M.J.; Harter, J.; Sewall, S.; Ogilvie, T.; Magliocco, A.; Breslin, T.M.; et al. A large-scale study of the ultrawideband microwave dielectric properties of normal, benign and malignant breast tissues obtained from cancer surgeries. *Phys. Med. Biol.* **2007**, *52*, 6093. [CrossRef]
4. Halter, R.J.; Zhou, T.; Meaney, P.M.; Hartov, A.; Barth, R.J., Jr.; Rosenkranz, K.M.; Wells, W.A.; Kogel, C.A.; Borsic, A.; Rizzo, E.J.; et al. The correlation of in vivo and ex vivo tissue dielectric properties to validate electromagnetic breast imaging: Initial clinical experience. *Physiol. Meas.* **2009**, *30*, S121. [CrossRef]
5. Pastorino, M. *Microwave Imaging*; John Wiley & Sons: Hoboken, NJ, USA, 2010.
6. Van den Berg, P.M.; Kleinman, R.E. A contrast source inversion method. *Inverse Probl.* **1997**, *13*, 1607–1620. [CrossRef]
7. Abubakar, A.; van den Berg, P.M.; Mallorqui, J.J. Imaging of biomedical data using a multiplicative regularized contrast source inversion method. *IEEE Trans. Microw. Theory Tech.* **2002**, *50*, 1761–1771. [CrossRef]
8. Zakaria, A.; Gilmore, C.; LoVetri, J. Finite-element contrast source inversion method for microwave imaging. *Inverse Probl.* **2010**, *26*, 115010. [CrossRef]
9. Kurrant, D.; Baran, A.; LoVetri, J.; Fear, E. Integrating prior information into microwave tomography Part 1: Impact of detail on image quality. *Med. Phys.* **2017**, *44*, 6461–6481. [CrossRef] [PubMed]
10. Baran, A.; Kurrant, D.; Fear, E.; LoVetri, J. Integrating prior information into microwave tomography part 2: Impact of errors in prior information on microwave tomography image quality. *Med. Phys.* **2017**, *44*, 6482–6503.
11. Chen, X. *Computational Methods for Electromagnetic Inverse Scattering*; Wiley Online Library: Hoboken, NJ, USA, 2018.
12. Goodfellow, I.; Bengio, Y.; Courville, A. *Deep Learning*; MIT Press: Cambridge, MA, USA, 2016; Available online: http://www.deeplearningbook.org (accessed on 10 August 2020).
13. Ronneberger, O.; Fischer, P.; Brox, T. U-Net: Convolutional Networks for Biomedical Image Segmentation. *arXiv* **2015**, arXiv:1505.04597.
14. Wang, G.; Li, W.; Zuluaga, M.A.; Pratt, R.; Patel, P.A.; Aertsen, M.; Doel, T.; David, A.L.; Deprest, J.; Ourselin, S.; et al. Interactive Medical Image Segmentation Using Deep Learning With Image-Specific Fine Tuning. *IEEE Trans. Med. Imaging* **2018**, *37*, 1562–1573. [CrossRef]
15. Shin, H.; Roth, H.R.; Gao, M.; Lu, L.; Xu, Z.; Nogues, I.; Yao, J.; Mollura, D.; Summers, R.M. Deep Convolutional Neural Networks for Computer-Aided Detection: CNN Architectures, Dataset Characteristics and Transfer Learning. *IEEE Trans. Med Imaging* **2016**, *35*, 1285–1298. [CrossRef]
16. McCann, M.T.; Jin, K.H.; Unser, M. Convolutional Neural Networks for Inverse Problems in Imaging: A Review. *IEEE Signal Process. Mag.* **2017**, *34*, 85–95. [CrossRef]
17. Xie, Y.; Xia, Y.; Zhang, J.; Song, Y.; Feng, D.; Fulham, M.; Cai, W. Knowledge-based Collaborative Deep Learning for Benign-Malignant Lung Nodule Classification on Chest CT. *IEEE Trans. Med. Imaging* **2019**, *38*, 991–1004. [CrossRef] [PubMed]
18. Kang, E.; Min, J.; Ye, J.C. A deep convolutional neural network using directional wavelets for low-dose X-ray CT reconstruction. *Med. Phys.* **2017**, *44*, e360–e375. [CrossRef] [PubMed]
19. Han, Y.; Yoo, J.J.; Ye, J.C. Deep Residual Learning for Compressed Sensing CT Reconstruction via Persistent Homology Analysis. *arXiv* **2016**, arXiv:1611.06391.
20. Jin, K.H.; McCann, M.T.; Froustey, E.; Unser, M. Deep Convolutional Neural Network for Inverse Problems in Imaging. *IEEE Trans. Image Process.* **2017**, *26*, 4509–4522. [CrossRef]
21. Han, Y.; Yoo, J.; Kim, H.H.; Shin, H.J.; Sung, K.; Ye, J.C. Deep learning with domain adaptation for accelerated projection-reconstruction MR. *Magn. Reson. Med.* **2018**, *80*, 1189–1205. [CrossRef]
22. Rahama, Y.A.; Aryani, O.A.; Din, U.A.; Awar, M.A.; Zakaria, A.; Qaddoumi, N. Novel Microwave Tomography System Using a Phased-Array Antenna. *IEEE Trans. Microw. Theory Tech.* **2018**, *66*, 5119–5128. [CrossRef]
23. Rekanos, I.T. Neural-network-based inverse-scattering technique for online microwave medical imaging. *IEEE Trans. Magn.* **2002**, *38*, 1061–1064. [CrossRef]

24. Li, L.; Wang, L.G.; Teixeira, F.L.; Liu, C.; Nehorai, A.; Cui, T.J. DeepNIS: Deep Neural Network for Nonlinear Electromagnetic Inverse Scattering. *IEEE Trans. Antennas Propag.* **2019**, *67*, 1819–1825. [CrossRef]
25. Khoshdel, V.; Ashraf, A.L.J. Enhancement of Multimodal Microwave-Ultrasound Breast Imaging Using a Deep-Learning Technique. *Sensors* **2019**, *19*, 4050. [CrossRef] [PubMed]
26. Rana, S.P.; Dey, M.; Tiberi, G.; Sani, L.; Vispa, A.; Raspa, G.; Duranti, M.; Ghavami, M.; Dudley, S. Machine learning approaches for automated lesion detection in microwave breast imaging clinical data. *Sci. Rep.* **2019**, *9*, 1–12. [CrossRef] [PubMed]
27. Asefi, M.; Baran, A.; LoVetri, J. An Experimental Phantom Study for Air-Based Quasi-Resonant Microwave Breast Imaging. *IEEE Trans. Microw. Theory Tech.* **2019**, *67*, 3946–3954. [CrossRef]
28. Meaney, P.M.; Paulsen, K.D.; Geimer, S.D.; Haider, S.A.; Fanning, M.W. Quantification of 3-D field effects during 2-D microwave imaging. *IEEE Trans. Biomed. Eng.* **2002**, *49*, 708–720. [CrossRef]
29. Golnabi, A.H.; Meaney, P.M.; Epstein, N.R.; Paulsen, K.D. Microwave imaging for breast cancer detection: Advances in three–dimensional image reconstruction. In Proceedings of the 2011 Annual International Conference of the IEEE Engineering in Medicine and Biology Society, Boston, MA, USA, 30 August–3 September 2011; pp. 5730–5733.
30. Golnabi, A.H.; Meaney, P.M.; Geimer, S.D.; Paulsen, K.D. 3-D Microwave Tomography Using the Soft Prior Regularization Technique: Evaluation in Anatomically Realistic MRI-Derived Numerical Breast Phantoms. *IEEE Trans. Biomed. Eng.* **2019**, *66*, 2566–2575. [CrossRef]
31. Abdollahi, N.; Kurrant, D.; Mojabi, P.; Omer, M.; Fear, E.; LoVetri, J. Incorporation of Ultrasonic Prior Information for Improving Quantitative Microwave Imaging of Breast. *IEEE J. Multiscale Multiphys. Comput. Tech.* **2019**, *4*, 98–110. [CrossRef]
32. Gil Cano, J.D.; Fasoula, A.D.L.; Bernard, J.G. Wavelia Breast Imaging: The Optical Breast Contour Detection Subsystem. *Appl. Sci.* **2020**, *10*, 1234. [CrossRef]
33. Odle, T.G. Breast imaging artifacts. *Radiol. Technol.* **2015**, *89*, 428.
34. Chew, W.C.; Wang, Y.M. Reconstruction of two-dimensional permittivity distribution using the distorted Born iterative method. *IEEE Trans. Med. Imaging* **1990**, *9*, 218–225. [CrossRef]
35. Joachimowicz, N.; Pichot, C.; Hugonin, J.P. Inverse scattering: An iterative numerical method for electromagnetic imaging. *IEEE Trans. Antennas Propag.* **1991**, *39*, 1742–1753. [CrossRef]
36. Franchois, A.; Pichot, C. Microwave imaging-complex permittivity reconstruction with a Levenberg-Marquardt method. *IEEE Trans. Antennas Propag.* **1997**, *45*, 203–215. [CrossRef]
37. Bulyshev, A.; Semenov, S.; Souvorov, A.; Svenson, R.; Nazarov, A.; Sizov, Y.; Tatsis, G. Computational modeling of three-dimensional microwave tomography of breast cancer. *IEEE Trans. Biomed. Eng.* **2001**, *48*, 1053–1056. [CrossRef] [PubMed]
38. Meaney, P.M.; Geimer, S.D.; Paulsen, K.D. Two-step inversion with a logarithmic transformation for microwave breast imaging. *Med. Phys.* **2017**, *44*, 4239–4251. [CrossRef]
39. Mojabi, P.; LoVetri, J. Overview and classification of some regularization techniques for the Gauss-Newton inversion method applied to inverse scattering problems. *IEEE Trans. Antennas Propag.* **2009**, *57*, 2658–2665. [CrossRef]
40. Van den Berg, P.; Abubakar, A.; Fokkema, J. Multiplicative regularization for contrast profile inversion. *Radio Sci.* **2003**, *38*. [CrossRef]
41. Zakaria, A.; Jeffrey, I.; LoVetri, J.; Zakaria, A. Full-Vectorial Parallel Finite-Element Contrast Source Inversion Method. *Prog. Electromagn. Res.* **2013**, *142*, 463–483. [CrossRef]
42. Nemez, K.; Baran, A.; Asefi, M.; LoVetri, J. Modeling Error and Calibration Techniques for a Faceted Metallic Chamber for Magnetic Field Microwave Imaging. *IEEE Trans. Microw. Theory Techn.* **2017**, *65*, 4347–4356. [CrossRef]
43. He, K.; Zhang, X.; Ren, S.; Sun, J. Deep Residual Learning for Image Recognition. In Proceedings of the 2016 IEEE Conference on Computer Vision and Pattern Recognition (CVPR), Las Vegas, NV, USA, 27–30 June 2016; pp. 770–778.
44. Trabelsi, C.; Bilaniuk, O.; Zhang, Y.; Serdyuk, D.; Subramanian, S.; Santos, J.F.; Mehri, S.; Rostamzadeh, N.; Bengio, Y.; Pal, C. Deep Complex Networks. *arXiv* **2018**, arXiv:1705.09792.
45. Krizhevsky, A.; Sutskever, I.; Hinton, G.E. ImageNet Classification with Deep Convolutional Neural Networks. In *Advances in Neural Information Processing Systems 25*; Pereira, F., Burges, C.J.C., Bottou, L., Weinberger, K.Q., Eds.; Curran Associates, Inc.: Red Hook, NY, USA, 2012; pp. 1097–1105.

46. Glorot, X.; Bengio, Y. Understanding the difficulty of training deep feedforward neural networks. In Proceedings of the International Conference on Artificial Intelligence and Statistics (AISTATS'10), Society for Artificial Intelligence and Statistics, Tübingen, Germany, 21–23 April 2010.
47. Hanley, J.; McNeil, B. The meaning and use of the area under a receiver operating characteristic (ROC) curve. *Radiology* **1982**, *43*, 29–36. [CrossRef]

11

Explainable Machine Learning Framework for Image Classification Problems: Case Study on Glioma Cancer Prediction

Emmanuel Pintelas [1,*], Meletis Liaskos [2], Ioannis E. Livieris [1], Sotiris Kotsiantis [1] and Panagiotis Pintelas [1]

[1] Department of Mathematics, University of Patras, GR 265-00 Patras, Greece; livieris@upatras.gr (I.E.L.); sotos@math.upatras.gr (S.K.); ppintelas@gmail.com (P.P.)

[2] Department of Biomedical Engineering, University of West Attica, GR 122-43 Egaleo Athens, Greece; melletis@hotmail.com

* Correspondence: ece6835@upnet.gr

Abstract: Image classification is a very popular machine learning domain in which deep convolutional neural networks have mainly emerged on such applications. These networks manage to achieve remarkable performance in terms of prediction accuracy but they are considered as black box models since they lack the ability to interpret their inner working mechanism and explain the main reasoning of their predictions. There is a variety of real world tasks, such as medical applications, in which interpretability and explainability play a significant role. Making decisions on critical issues such as cancer prediction utilizing black box models in order to achieve high prediction accuracy but without provision for any sort of explanation for its prediction, accuracy cannot be considered as sufficient and ethnically acceptable. Reasoning and explanation is essential in order to trust these models and support such critical predictions. Nevertheless, the definition and the validation of the quality of a prediction model's explanation can be considered in general extremely subjective and unclear. In this work, an accurate and interpretable machine learning framework is proposed, for image classification problems able to make high quality explanations. For this task, it is developed a feature extraction and explanation extraction framework, proposing also three basic general conditions which validate the quality of any model's prediction explanation for any application domain. The feature extraction framework will extract and create transparent and meaningful high level features for images, while the explanation extraction framework will be responsible for creating good explanations relying on these extracted features and the prediction model's inner function with respect to the proposed conditions. As a case study application, brain tumor magnetic resonance images were utilized for predicting glioma cancer. Our results demonstrate the efficiency of the proposed model since it managed to achieve sufficient prediction accuracy being also interpretable and explainable in simple human terms.

Keywords: interpretable/explainable machine learning; image classification; image processing; machine learning models; white box; black box; cancer prediction

---

1. Introduction

Image classification is a very popular machine learning domain in which Convolutional Neural Networks (CNNs) [1] have been successfully applied on wide range of image classification problems. These networks are able to filter out noise and extract useful information from the initial images' pixel representation and use it as input for the final prediction model. CNN-based models are able to achieve remarkable prediction performance although in general they need very large number of input instances. Nevertheless, this model's great limitation and drawback is that it is almost totally unable to interpret and explain its predictions, since its inner workings and its prediction function is not transparent due to its high complexity mechanism [2].

In recent days, interpretability/explainability in machine learning domain has become a significant issue, since much of real-world problems require reasoning and explanation on predictions, while it is also essential to understand the model's prediction mechanism in order to trust it and make decisions on critical issues [3,4]. The European Union General Data Protection Regulation (GDPR) which was enacted in 2016 and took effect in 2018, demanded a "right to explanation" for decisions performed by automated and artificial intelligent algorithmic systems. This new regulation promotes to develop algorithmic frameworks which will ensure an explanation for every Machine Learning decision while this demand will be legally mandated by the GDPR. The term right to explanation [5] refers to the explanation that an algorithm must give, especially on decisions which affect human individual rights and critical issues. For example, a person who applies for a bank loan and was not approved may ask for an explanation which could be "The bank loan was rejected because you are underage. You need to be over 18 years old in order to apply." It is obvious that there could be plenty of other reasons for his rejection, however the explanation has to be short and comprehensive [6], presenting the most significant reason for his rejection, while it would be very helpful if the explanation provides also a fast solution for this individual in order to counter the rejection decision.

Explainability can also assist in building efficient machine learning models and secures that they are reliable in practice [6]. For example, let assume that a model classified an image as a "cat" followed by explanations like "because there is a tree in image". In this scenario, the model associated the whole image as a cat based on a tree which is indeed pictured in the image, but the explanation is obviously based on an incorrect feature (the tree). Thus, explainability revealed some hidden weaknesses that this model may have even if its testing prediction accuracy is accidentally very high. An explainable model can reveal the significant features which affect a prediction. Subsequently, humans can then determine if these features are actually correct, based on their domain knowledge, in order to make the model reliable and generalize well in every new instance in real world applications. For example, a possible "correct" feature which would prove that the model makes reliable predictions could be "this image is classified as a cat because the model identified sharp contours" this explanation would reflect that the model associated the cat with its nails which is probably a unique and correct feature that represents a cat.

Medical applications such as cancer prediction, is another example where explainability is essential since it is considered a critical and a "life or death" prediction problem, in which high forecasting accuracy and interpretation are two equally essential and significant tasks to achieve. However, this is generally a very difficult task, since there is a "trade-off" between interpretation and accuracy [4]. Imaging (Radiology) tests for cancer is a medical area in which radiologists try to identify signs of cancer utilizing imaging tests, sending forms of energy such as magnetic fields, in order to take pictures of the inner human body. A radiologist is a doctor who specializes in imaging analysis techniques and is authorized to interpret images of these tests and write a report of his/her findings. This report finally is sent to the patient's doctor while a copy of this report is sent to the patient records. CNNs have proved that they are almost as accurate as these specialists on predicting cancer from images. However, reasoning and explanation of their predictions is one of their greatest limitations in contrast to the radiologists which are able (and obligated) to analyze, interpret and explain their decision based on the features they managed to identify in an image. For example, an explanation/reasoning of a diagnosis/prediction of a case image could probably be: "This image probably is classified as cancer because the tumor area is large, its texture color is white followed by high density and irregular shape."

Developing an accurate and interpretable model at the same time is a very challenging task as typically there is a trade-off between interpretation and accuracy [7]. High accuracy often requires developing complicated black box models while interpretation requires developing simple and less complicated models, which are often less accurate. Deep neural networks are some examples of powerful, in terms of accuracy, prediction models but they are totally non-interpretable (black box models), while decision trees and logistic regression are some classic examples of interpretable models (white box models) which are usually not as accurate. In general, interpretability methods can be divided into two main categories, intrinsic and post-hoc [6]. Intrinsic methods are considered the prediction models which are by nature interpretable, such as all the white box models like decision trees and linear models, while post-hoc methods utilize secondary models in order to explain the predictions of a black box model.

Local Interpretable Model-agnostic Explanations (LIME) [8], One-variable-at-a-Time approach [9], counterfactual explanations [10] and SHapley Additive exPlanations (SHAP) [6] are some state of the art examples of post-hoc interpretable models. Grad-CAM [11] is a very popular post-hoc explanation technique applied on CNNs models making them more transparent. This algorithm aims to interpret any CNN model by "returning" the most significant pixels which contributed to the final prediction via a visual heatmap of each image. Nevertheless, explainability properties such as fidelity, stability, trust and representativeness of explanations (some essential properties which define an explanation as "good explanation") constitute some of the main issues and problems of post hoc methods in contrast to intrinsic models. Our proposed prediction framework is intrinsic model able to provide high quality explanations (good explanations).

In a recent work, Pintelas et al. [7], proposed an intrinsic interpretable Grey-Box ensemble model exploiting black-box model's accuracy and white-box model's explainability. The main objective was the enlargement of a small initial labeled dataset via a large pool of unlabeled data adding black-box's most confident predictions. Then, a decision tree model (intrinsic interpretable model) was trained with the final augmented dataset while the prediction and explanation were performed by the white box model. However, one basic limitation is that the application of a decision tree classifier or any white box classifier on raw image data without a robust feature extraction framework would be totally inefficient since it would require an enormous amount of images in order to build an accurate and robust image classification model. In addition, the interpretation of this tree would be too complicated since the explanations would rely on individual pixels. Our proposed prediction framework would be able to provide stable/robust and accurate predictions followed by explanations based on meaningful high-level features extracted from every image.

This paper proposes an explainable machine learning prediction framework for image classification problems. In short, it is composed by a feature extraction and an explanation extraction framework followed by some proposed "conditions" which aim to validate the quality of any model's predictions explanations for every application domain. The feature extraction framework is based on traditional image processing tools and provides a transparent and well-defined high level feature representation input, meaningful in human terms, while these features will be used for training a simple white box model. These extracted features aim to describe specific properties found in an image based on texture and contour analysis. The feature explanation framework aims to provide good explanations for every individual prediction by exploiting the white box model's inner function with respect to the extracted features and our defined conditions. It is worth mentioning that the proposed framework is general and can potentially be applied to any image classification task. However, this work aims to apply this framework on tasks where interpretation and explainability are vitally and significantly prominent. To this end, it was chosen to perform a case study application on Magnetic Resonance Imaging (MRI) for brain cancer prediction. In particular, we aim to diagnose and interpret glioma, which is a very dangerous type of tumor, being in most cases a malignant cancer [12], versus other tumor types, which are most of the times benign. Some examples of extracted meta-features for this case study are tumor's size, tumor's shape, texture irregularity level and tumor's color.

The contribution of this work lies on the development of an accurate and robust prediction framework, being also intrinsic interpretable, able to make high quality explanations and make reasoning and justification on its predictions for image classification tasks. For this task, it is proposed a feature extraction framework which creates transparent and meaningful high level features from images and an explanation extraction framework which exploits a linear model's inner function in order to make good explanations. Furthermore, we propose and define some conditions which aim to validate the quality of any model's explanations on every application domain. In particular, if one model verifies all these conditions, then its predictions' explanations can be considered as good. Finally, 3 types of presentation forms are also proposed for the prediction's explanations with respect to the target audience and the application domain.

The remainder of this paper is organized as follows. Section 2 presents in a very detailed way our proposed research framework while Section 3 presents our experimental results, regarding the prediction accuracy and model interpretation/explanation. In Section 4, a brief discussion regarding our proposed framework is conducted. Finally, Section 5 sketches our conclusive remarks and possible future research.

2. Materials and Methods

2.1. Proposed Explainable Prediction Framework

Figure 1 presents the abstract architecture of our model which is composed by the feature extraction framework, which will be described in next subsection, a white box linear model and an explanation extraction framework. The great advantage of lineal models is that the identification of the most important features is very easy since it naturally comes out by the interpretation of their corresponding weights. A low weight's absolute value indicates low importance while in contrast a high, indicates high importance. We have to mention that although linear models are considered intrinsic interpretable models, this does not imply that they can also provide by default good explanations. Therefore, it was developed a new explanation extraction framework that will exploit the inner linear model's prediction function in such a way that will provide an easily understandable explanation output scheme which will satisfy all the proposed conditions that verify an explanation as good.

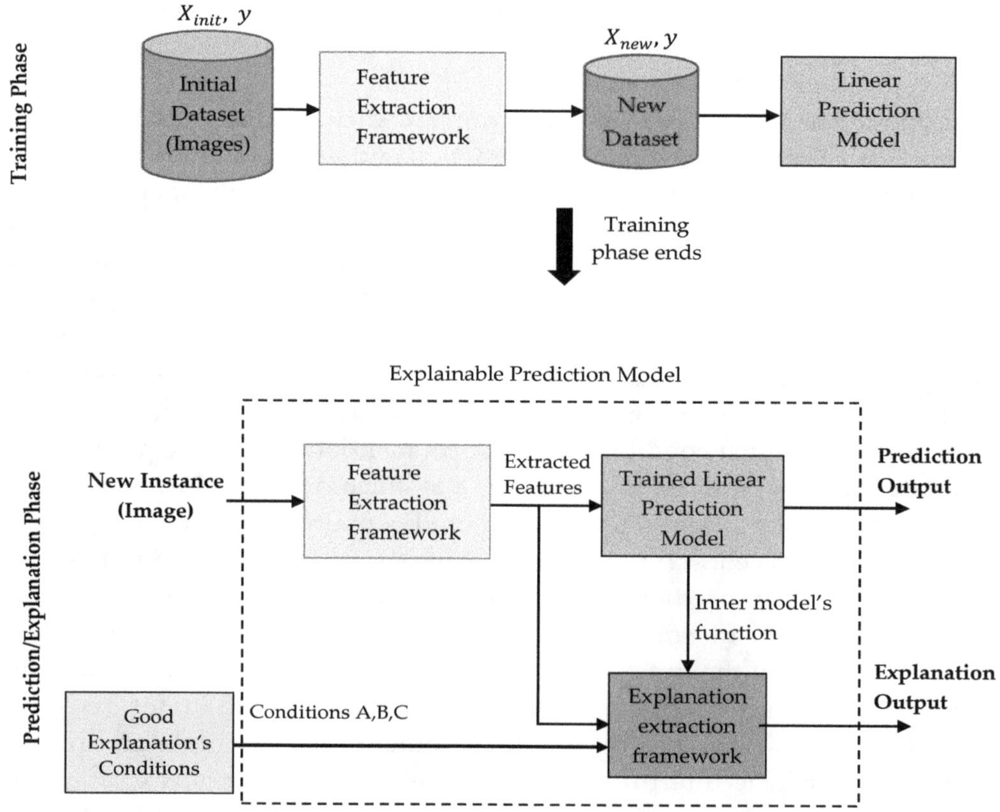

Figure 1. An abstract overview of our proposed explainable model.

2.2. *Image Feature Extraction Methodology*

In general, the input feature representation which a machine learning model uses to make predictions or the feature representation input that an explanation algorithm uses to make explanations (e.g., post hoc models) must be understandable to humans when the objective is the development of an explainable prediction model [8]. Therefore, we introduce a feature extraction framework which will create transparent and well-defined features from images by processing the pixel values from grayscale images based on traditional image analysis techniques, while these features will be also applied as an input on a prediction model. This feature extraction step is essential in order to convert the initial noisy pixel representation input of every image to a compressed, compact, robust and meaningful high-level feature representation input for the final prediction model while this representation will be meaningful to humans too. Following such approach, we can get rid of the black box approach of utilizing CNN models for image classification tasks and use instead simple, stable and intrinsic interpretable models as final predictors such as linear models.

It is worth mentioning that probably some of the utilized features will not be totally understandable to every human since the main audience domain which are directed to is for image analysts and therefore this fact points out our main approach's limitation. Based on this limitation, in Section 2.2.4 we provide a qualitative explanation in human understandable terms for some of these complex features in order to expand our model's explanations audience range. However, easily defined features such as size of object (e.g., tumor size in our case study), mean value of image pixels (e.g., tumor color tends to be black or white) and cyclic level (e.g., tumor shape tends to be cyclic or oval) are by default easily understandable to most humans but they may not be significant for the prediction problem which a machine learning model aims to solve. Therefore, identifying features understandable to humans being also informative and useful for the machine learning model, constitute a key factor for creating efficient and viable explainable prediction models.

2.2.1. Data Acquisition

As mentioned before, the main objective of this work is to apply the proposed framework on tasks where interpretation and explainability is vital and very significant. Therefore, we chose to perform a case study application on MRI for glioma tumor classification. The utilized dataset is publicly available [13]. In particular, it is consisted of 3064 head images with glioma (1426 slices), meningioma (708 slices) and pituitary (930 slices). The slices consist of 512×512 resolution, 0.49×0.49 mm^2 voxel size and tumor depicted in three planes (axial, coronal and sagittal). The main task of this case study is the identification of glioma tumor, since in most cases, the glioma lesion tends to be malignant while meningioma and pituitary (the other two main types of brain tumor) tend to be benign. Therefore, the images were separated in two groups. The first group includes glioma with 1426 instances and the other meningioma and pituitary with 1638 instances.

Our feature extraction procedure consists of two main image feature family types, texture and contour features. Texture features are extracted based on the image's pixel values intensities (e.g., gray levels) while contour features based on the shape of the Region of Interest (ROI) lied into the image. The final extracted dataset consists of 234 different features in total composed by 194 texture features and 40 contour features. Some examples of these extracted features from each image are area size of tumor, pixels mean value, intensity, variation, correlation, smoothness, coarseness and regularity [14].

The first step constitutes the identification of the ROI. The ROI was evaluated quantitatively using the manual segmentation by experts as ground truth. Figures 2 and 3 present some examples of extracted tumor areas.

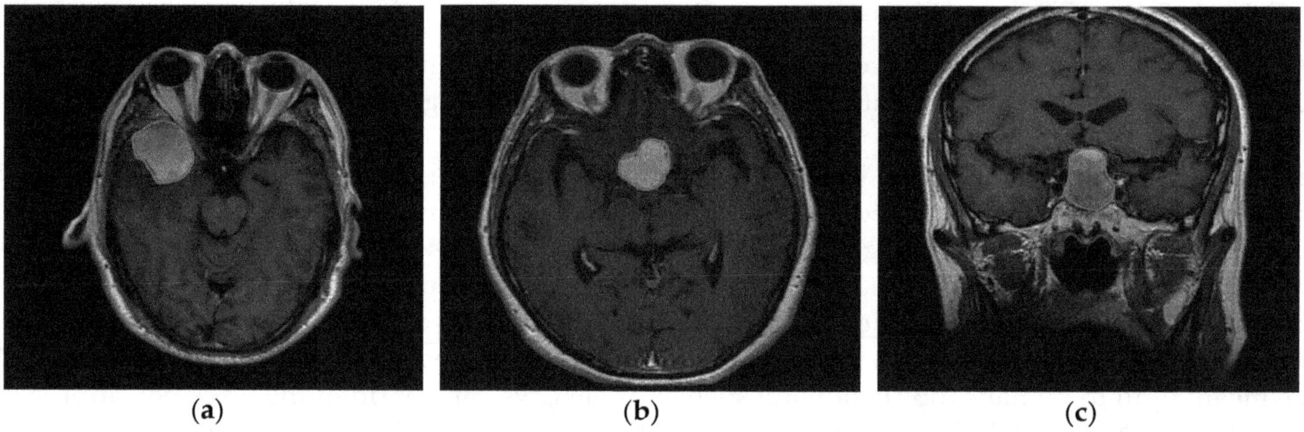

Figure 2. Head MRI examples. The red color illustrates the tumor area (**a**) glioma, (**b**) meningioma, (**c**) pituitary.

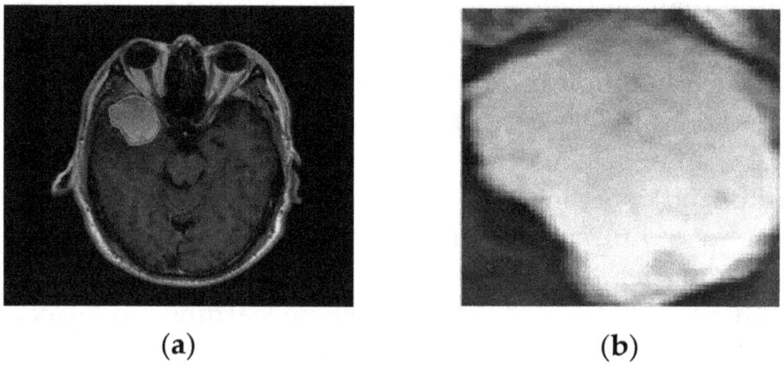

Figure 3. (**a**) Image with glioma, (**b**) Region of Interest (ROI) extraction.

The body of tumor is represented by pixels with different gray levels. Every pixel has significant information about the type of tumor. Furthermore, we normalized the images from 0 to 32 gray levels. The low values represent the dark color pixels and the high values the light white pixels.

2.2.2. Texture Features

Texture analysis is one of the high-speed feature extraction methods for image analysis and classification using the pixel's values. These methods mainly aim to describe the spatial distribution of intensities and the varying shades of pixels in images. In this study, three major approaches were utilized, the gray-level Co-Occurrence matrix, Run length and Statistical values from ROI matrix.

Co-Occurrence matrix [14] characterizes the texture of an image by capturing the gray-level values with spatial dependence from image, calculating how often pairs of pixel with specific values and in a specified spatial relationship occur in an image. In particular, we used the initial ROI matrix of every image and four more scales from wavelet transform [15] as pre-processing step, in order to find all pixel information. Then, the Co-occurrence matrices for every ROI image (initial plus four extracted filtered images) were calculated. The Co-Occurrence matrix is calculated by the following equation:

$$G = \begin{bmatrix} p(1,1) & p(1,2) & \cdots & p(1,N_g) \\ p(2,1) & p(2,2) & \cdots & p(2,N_g) \\ \vdots & \vdots & \ddots & \vdots \\ p(N_g,1) & p(N_g,2) & \cdots & p(N_g,N_g) \end{bmatrix}$$

N_g is the number of gray levels in the image and $p(i,j)$ is the probability that a pixel with value I will be found adjacent to a pixel of value j. Based on the Co-Occurrence matrix, meaningful features for every image can be extracted such as entropy, energy, contrast, homogeneity, variance and correlation. In total, we extracted 100 features via the Co-Occurrence approach. Some of the most significant identified features are presented in Table 1.

Table 1. Mathematic description of the most important identified features of Co-Occurrence approach.

Co-Occurrence Features	Formula
Correlation	$\frac{1}{\sigma_x\sigma_y}\left(\sum_{i=1}^{N_g}\sum_{j=1}^{N_g} p(i,j) - \mu_x\mu_y\right)$
Information Measure of Correlation	$(1-exp[-2(HXY_2-HXY)])^{\frac{1}{2}}$
Sum Average	$\sum_{i=2}^{2N_g} ip_{x+y}(i)$

where x and y are the coordinates (row and column) of the entry matrix, $p_{x+y}(i)$ is the probability of coordinated summing to $x+y$, μ_x, μ_y, σ_x and σ_y are the means and standard deviations of p_x and p_y which are the partial probability density functions,

$$HXY = -\sum_{i=1}^{N_g}\sum_{j=1}^{N_g} p(i,j)log\{p(i,j)\}$$

$$HXY_2 = -\sum_{i=1}^{N_g}\sum_{j=1}^{N_g} p_x(i)p_y(j)log\{p_x(i)p_y(j)\}$$

and HX, HY are the entropies of p_x and p_y.

Run-length matrix is another way to characterize the surface of a given object or region utilizing a *gray level run*. A gray level run is a set of consecutive image points computed in any direction [16]. The matrix element (i,j) specifies the number of times that the pixel value appears in every direction. These elements correspond to the number of homogeneous runs of j voxel with gray value i [17]. From run-length method were produced 39 features. The most important run-length features identified via the interpretation of the weights of our utilized white box linear prediction model are Short Run Emphasis (SRE), Run Length Non-Uniformity Normalized (RLNUN) and Low Gray Level Run Emphasis (LGLRE) as presented in Table 2.

Table 2. Mathematic description of the most important identified features of Run Length approach.

Run-Length Features	Formula
SRE	$\frac{1}{N}\sum_{i=1}^{N_g}\sum_{j=1}^{N_r}\frac{p(i,j)}{j^2}$
RLNU	$\frac{1}{N^2}\sum_{i=1}^{N_g}\left(\sum_{j=1}^{N_r} p(i,j)\right)^2$
LGLRE	$\frac{1}{N}\sum_{i=1}^{N_g}\sum_{j=1}^{N_r}\frac{p(i,j)}{i^2}$

where Nr is the number of different run-length that occurs. Higher value of SRE indicates fine textures. RLNU measures the distribution of runs over the gray values and LGLRE is the distribution of the low gray-level runs [16]. These feature values are low when runs are equally distributed along grey levels indicating higher similarity in intensity values [17].

Statistical Values are features based on first and second order statistical analysis. The texture of an image is determined by the distribution over the pixels in calculated region. These features aim to describe specific properties of an image, such as the smoothness or irregularity, homogeneity or inhomogeneous while some extracted features are mean value, standard deviation, kurtosis, entropy, correlation and contrast.

2.2.3. Contour Features

In general, contour features aim to describe the characteristics and the information lied in the shape of objects. In our case study, tumor shape constitutes the object on every image as presented in Figure 4. For example, such features can describe if the tumor shape tends to be irregular or regular, oval or cyclic, large or small and so on. In our study, tumor size was identified to be the most significant contour feature (based on formulas described in Section 2.3.4).

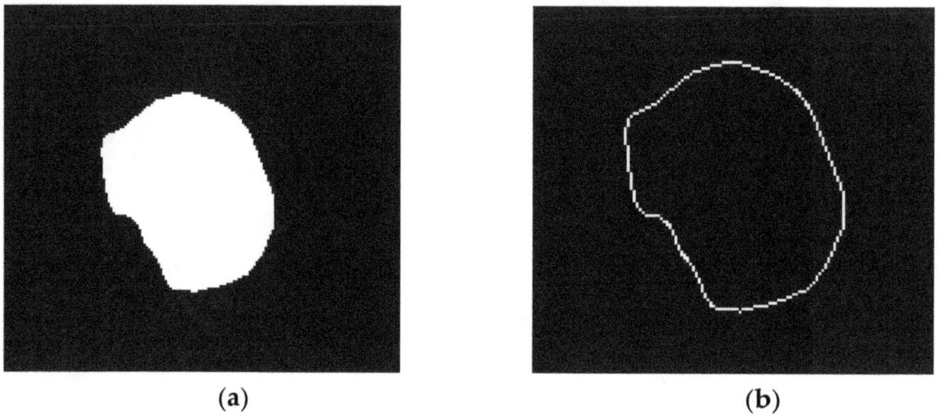

Figure 4. (**a**) Binary image, (**b**) border extraction.

This feature is described by the following formula:

$$tumor\ size = N_{in}$$

where N_{in} is the number of pixels inside the tumor object. It is worth mentioning that this is an informative feature for the final prediction model while it is also easily understandable in human terms. In general, the identification of features which are easily understandable to most humans while they are also useful for the machine learning prediction task, probably constitute some of the main research challenges and key elements in explainable machine learning domain. The identification of such useful and easily understandable features can contribute positively to this domain since the explanation of the model's decision would rely on features understandable in human terms and thus it would be able to address a much larger audience.

2.2.4. Qualitative Explanation of Extracted Features

We recall that an explainable machine learning model requires also an explainable feature representation in which the explanation output will rely on. Therefore, in the sequel it is attempted to explain in easy human understandable terms some complicated mathematically defined features of our framework. Table 3 presents a qualitative description of some of the most important identified features. For each of those features, we present two extreme example cases (high-low value comparison) in order to illustrate their main characteristics differences.

Correlation feature measures the linear relationship between two variables, which in our case, these variables are pixel coordinates. In other words, correlation measures the similarity between neighborhood sub-image's regions. In natural images, neighboring pixels tend to have similar values while a white-noise image exhibits zero (lowest value) correlation. A high correlation indicates the existence of an object, objects or some kind of structure lied in the image while a low correlation could indicate that there is no object in the image or it is not transparent enough. Regarding our case study, a correlation value can indicate how clear or not, the tumor can be seen in an image. For example, in Table 3, images on the 1st column (left) correspond to a very high correlation in contrast to images on the 2nd column (right). In the left image, a tumor (object) is clearly defined, in contrast to the right which no object can be seen at all.

Table 3. Qualitative description of some of the most important identified features.

Features	Tumor Examples (High Value)	Tumor Examples (Low Value)	Description
Correlation	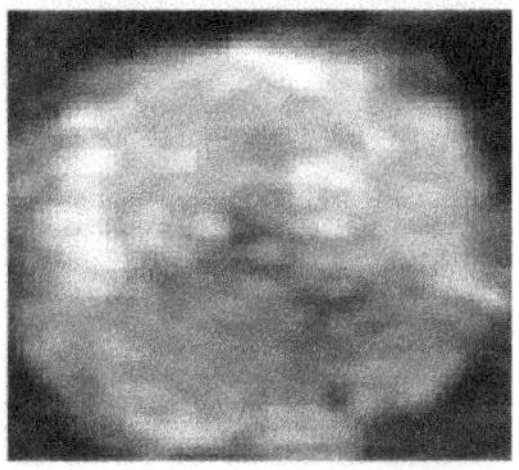		Measures the linear relationship between two variables (pixels coordinates for images). In other words, measures the similarity between neighborhood sub-image's regions.
Information Measure of Correlation		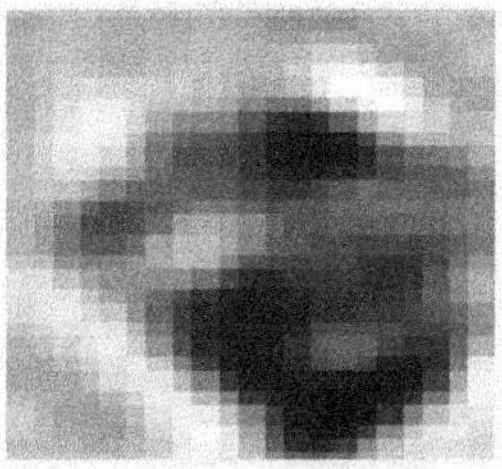	Measures the amount of information that one variable contains about another. In other words, it measures how irregular is the texture of an image.
Sum Average	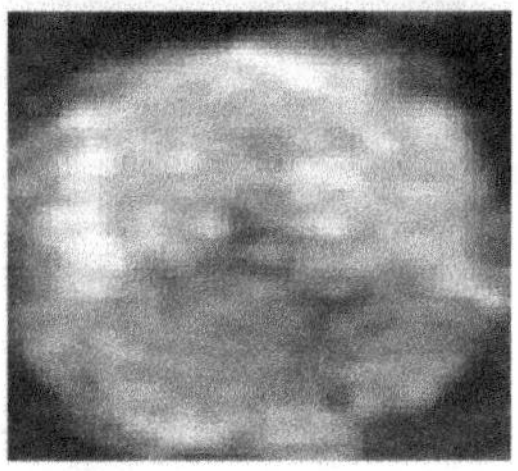		Provides the average of the grey values from ROI.

Information measure of correlation measures the amount of information which one variable contains about another (pixel coordinates for images). A high value can indicate that the pixel's intensities values of an image will tend to be smooth and regular while a low value that its pixel's intensities values will tend to irregular. This feature for our specific study can be defined also as "tumor's texture irregularity level".

Sum average feature aims to measure the average of the grey values from ROI. Although its mathematic definition in Table 1 seems to be a bit complicated, in practice it measures a very easily understandable in human terms feature. In particular, it aims to describe how light or dark is by average a gray image. In our case study, a high value indicates that the tumor's color tends to be white, a low value to be black, while an average value indicates that the tumor's color tends to be gray.

2.3. Machine Learning Prediction Explanations

Interpretable machine learning focuses on interpreting machine learning models' prediction mechanism in a reasonable form. More specifically, it aims to describe the mathematic or rule formula which an algorithm utilizes to make predictions, in a compact and meaningful form. An example is presented in Figure 5. Algorithm's interpretation mainly aims to present and interpret (e.g., via visualization of their decision boundaries) the model's decision function behavior. This can be very useful for machine learning developers, experts and data scientists in order to understand how a prediction model works, to identify its weaknesses and further improve its performance.

Explainable machine learning aims to explain machine learning models' predictions to human understandable terms. The definition of explainability is a very blur issue since it deals with humans and social aspects and thus explanations can be unclear and subjective [6]. Therefore, we have to define the properties of machine learning models' prediction explanations and clarify what should be considered as a good explanation. Our analysis below is based on the recent work of Christoph

Molnar in his book Interpretable machine learning [6], the popular research work of Ribeiro et al. [8] and the resent study of Robnik-Šikonja and Bohanec [9].

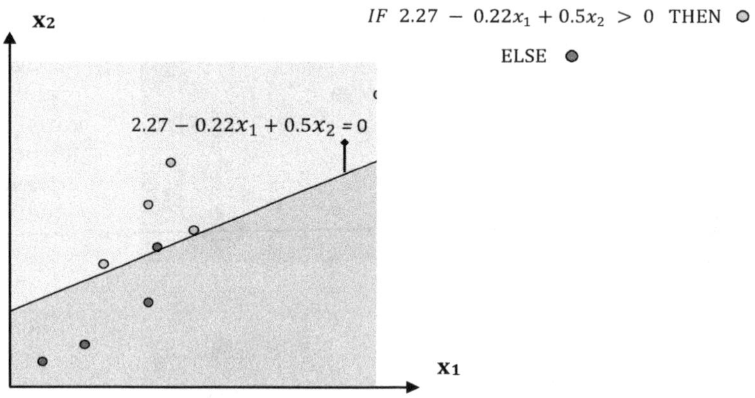

Figure 5. A visualization example presenting the decision function of a trained linear model.

2.3.1. Properties of Explanations

In general, an explanation usually has to relate in some way the features utilized by the algorithm in order to make predictions understandable to human terms. Some basic properties that explanations have, are described below.

Expressive Power is the language of the explanation output which is provided by the prediction framework. Some language examples are if-then rules, decision trees, weighted sums, finite state machines, graph diagrams, etc. This property is a very significant starting step for an explanation method since the way that this language will be defined, will determine the quality and the understandability of explanations to humans. Every machine learning algorithm has its own raw language in which makes decisions and predictions depending on its own unique computation formula and algorithm. If we just utilize the algorithm's raw output as the explanation output giving it to humans, it will be impractical, confusing and most likely not understandable at all.

For example, the raw interpretation output of a logistic regression algorithm (considered as white box model) applied on a specific dataset composed by three features could be:

$$\text{if } \frac{1}{1+e^{-(2+5x_1+7x_2-3x_3)}} > 0.5 \text{ then Output} = 1 \text{ else Output} = 0$$

which is probably not understandable and not meaningful to most humans. In contrast, decision trees models have by nature expressive power very close to human general logic since their explanation output come in an if-then-else total rule form composed by an ensemble of sub-rules which relate only one feature at a time. For example, an explanation output of a decision tree could be:

$$\text{if } \{(\text{sub-rule } 1) \text{ and } (\text{sub-rule } 2) \text{ and } (\text{sub-rule } 3)\} \text{ then } (\text{Output } = 1)\text{else } (\text{Output} = 0)$$

where sub-rules 1, 2 and 3 could be $x_1 = $ "poor", $x_2 = $ "young", $x_3 > 95$ kg where $x_3 = $ "weight", respectively.

Then this is close to human reasoning and understanding as an expressive language.

Fidelity is a property, which describes how well the explanation output approximates the actual raw decision function of the prediction algorithm. For example, a decision tree model has very high fidelity since its decision function matches exactly with the utilized explanation output. In contrast, an explanation output for a black box model utilizing post-hoc methods has to approximate the original black box decision function for example with simple intrinsic models.

However, global fidelity which describes how well the explanation output approximates the complete model's decision function providing global explanations, is almost impossible to achieve in practice and thus the explanations focus on local fidelity which deals with specific data instances or local data instances and data sub-sets, providing instance and local explanations. Individual instances and local explanations are usually more significant in practice, since humans mostly care about explanations for every individual instance at a time or for instances, which belong to the same vicinity (similar instances), instead of giving a global detailed explanation for every possible instance which could lead to information overload and very confusing explanations. Nevertheless, global explanations or explanations which cover as much more instances and data sub-sets at the same time (also called representativeness of explanations), are very significant in order to ascertain trust in the model.

Stability refers to the ability of a prediction model to provide similar explanations for similar instances. This means that slight changes in the feature values of an instance will not substantially change the explanation. High stability is desirable since it can enhance the trust and reliability of model's decisions and explanations. Notice that a beneficial side effect of the stability property is that it can also diagnose possible overfitting behavior of a prediction model since lack of explanations' stability highlights also high variance of the model's decision function. Finally, it is worth mentioning that the more complicated a model's decision function is, the more unstable this model will probably be, while its function interpretation will be more difficult. This means that simple models with simple prediction function are stable models. However, this does not mean that all white box models are stable (since white boxes are usually considered simple models). A decision tree with a very large max depth will probably lead in a very complicated prediction function being probably extremely unstable just like a common complicated black box model.

Comprehensibility refers to the ability of an explanation to be short and comprehensive being understandable by most humans. This property is very significant since it defines how informative and understandable at the same time is an explanation. Comprehensibility is highly depended on the target audience. This means that different explanations may need for example, a mathematician/statistician comparing to the manager or director of a company. Therefore, this property is highly affected by the expressive power as mentioned before, since an intelligent choice and definition of the explanation's expressive power can lead to a very high comprehensibility factor with respect to the audience that the specific explanation is directed to.

Degree of importance refers to the ability of an explanation to reflect the most important features which affect the predictions. These features can describe the model's decision function in a global way, in a local way and in individual way. Global important features are the features which highly affect the decision function of the model taking into consideration all the instances trained on. Local important features are the features which highly affect the model's decision function taking into consideration local data sub-sets, while instance's important features are the features which highly affect the prediction just only for this specific individual instance. This global–local differentiation is very crucial since *"features that are globally important may not be important in the local context, and vice versa"* [8]. Therefore, an explanation for an individual prediction mostly cares for the specific features that affect this specific instance or similar to it instances, rather than describing the global important features.

2.3.2. Fundamental Property of Explanations

Nevertheless, even if an explanation possesses all of these properties, the main fundamental property than an explanation should have, is its humanistic social property which comes from the interactive dialogue between the explainer and the audience. An explanation which covers all factors for a certain prediction is not a human friendly explanation while the explanations have to be selected and come gradually via small answers based on the questions applied. More specifically, this dialogue comes up in a "questions–answers" form, where questions are in general contrastive and answers (explanations) are selected.

It was proved that humans' questions usually are contrastive and humans most of the times expect and desire selected explanations [6]. The term contrastive question means that questions are in a counterfactual form, e.g., *"Why the model predicted output 1 instead of 2?"*, *"What the prediction would be if feature input X would be different?", "What is the minimum change required for feature input X in order the model to predict a different output result?"*. The term selected means that explainers usually select only one or two causes and present these as the explanation [6]. Therefore good explanations have to be able to answer contrastive questions and be selected, while this does not necessary imply that every other property described on previous section is not significant.

2.3.3. Proposed Conditions for Good Explanations

The definition and the validation of a good explanation can be considered in general extremely subjective and unclear. Therefore, taking into consideration the above analysis, we try to define three basic conditions that any prediction algorithm has to satisfy in order its prediction explanations to be considered good, stable, useful and easily understandable.

Condition A. Identification of features which highly determine the prediction result for the specific individual instance. This is probably the most significant and basic part of every explanation method since most of them mainly aim to identify these features. For example, the Grad-CAM method identifies and returns the pixels of an image which are important and determine a specific prediction for a black box model such as CNN. If the pixels' location, color level and volume can be considered as the raw initial features of every image, then such methods typically return the most significant features just like linear models would do via the interpretation of their weights on every feature variable.

Nevertheless, it is worth mentioning that by just returning the most significant pixels of an image which determined a specific prediction it does not always lead to useful explanations. If the objective is the identification of higher level representation features and properties that come out by pixels' grouping, such as shape and texture properties of an object lying in an image, which determine a prediction output, then relying only on pixels returns as explanations cannot reveal any useful information. For example, if a doctor classified a tumor image as malignant cancer and the main reason for this decision was just the tumor size and tumor's irregularity level, then pixels by itself are useless. Our proposed framework will be able to provide such type of explanations and this is the main difference comparing to other works which provide explanations based on image pixel returns.

However, explanations with pixels returns is very useful when the objective is the segmentation of an object (in our case tumor) or the identification of an object hidden in a noisy image, since the return of significant pixels would reveal if the model decided correctly utilizing the correct area of pixels or wrongly. For example, if a model classified an image as a cat, where this image actually illustrates a man hugging a dog and a cat, then explanations based on pixels returns would reveal if the model decided by cat's pixels (proper area) or another area e.g., dog's pixels where that would be obviously wrong.

Condition B. For a specific individual prediction identify some other instances such as local data sub-sets or instances that belong to the same vicinity (similar instances) which share the same prediction output and share at least one common explanation rule. This condition deals with the stability (robustness) and the representation property of model's explanations and as a result with the trust factor of a prediction model. An untruthful or unstable model, such as Deep Neural Network [18], probably will provide totally different explanations for similar instances. A very common example constitutes the adversarial attacks which aim to modify an original image in a way that the changes are almost undetectable to the human eye while the prediction function of an unstable model will probably be highly affected. In a very recent study, One pixel attack for fooling deep neural networks, 2019 [19] the authors revealed that the output of Deep Neural Networks can be easily altered by adding relatively small perturbations to the input pixel vector revealing that such models could be totally unstable and unreliable on image classification tasks.

Let assume a scenario in which an explanation method like Grad-CAM, identified for one new image (instance) the important pixels which determined a specific prediction. In order to ascertain some trust in the model, it would be very helpful if an explanation framework could also provide answers to questions like *"For those identified pixels, what are their volume values in which this prediction remains same*?" A possible answer (explanation) could be "If the mean value of those pixels' volume is higher than 180 then the prediction will remain stable". In practice this means that for every new image which shares the same important identified pixels (or at least close to it) and the same rule: mean volume value > 180, then the model's prediction will remain the same. Obviously, if a method can provide meaningful explanations in a global way, this is desirable too, but generally this is almost impossible in practice and as already mentioned in previous section, humans usually care for individual explanations and explanations for local or similar instances.

Condition C. Identification of the most important features' critical values in which the prediction result will change. This condition aims to validate the explanation method's ability of answering contrastive questions based on the social humanistic property for making questions in a counterfactual form, as presented in previous section. Following the same previously defined scenario, some possible contrastive questions could be *"If those identified pixels were changing color and volume, what the prediction would be, would it be still the same? If not, what is the minimum change required for those pixel's mean volume value in order the model to predict a different output result?"* A possible answer (explanation) could be "If their mean volume value increases by 30 then the prediction will change."

Final Presentation form. Merge all explanation's information in a compact, selected, comprehensive and informative form, with respect to the targeted audience and application domain (significant the proper definition of expressive power). This step deals with the explanation framework's ability to create comprehensive and selected explanations which constitute some of the most significant properties of good explanations as already described in previous section. For instance, if the explanation framework was a decision tree, by default a decision tree is an example which provides information in a comprehensive and easy to read form, since one can just follow its nodes and easily verify and obtain the prediction result [7]. Nevertheless, we have to mention that even a decision tree which is naturally interpretable and explainable model, has to provide selected explanations in the case that the tree's maximum depth is very large. This means that one has to prune and select explanation rules from the global tree in order to provide selected and comprehensive individual explanations. This is a significant limitation because this procedure is not straightforward since it must define a probably subjective threshold for this pruning procedure.

2.3.4. Explanation Extraction Framework

Let assume the Logistic Regression (LR) [20] algorithm our utilized linear prediction model (it is worth mentioning that this framework theoretically can be applied on every linear interpretable prediction model). We have to note that one basic limitation of a Logistic Regression model is that it is restricted for binary classification problems and thus this limitation applies also to the proposed total prediction framework.

The prediction function of the trained LR model is given by the following formula:

$$f_{LR} = \begin{cases} 1 & F > 0.5 \\ \text{"}unidentified\text{"} & F = 0.5 \\ 0 & F < 0.5 \end{cases} \tag{1}$$

where F is defined by the following function:

$$F = \frac{1}{1 + \mathrm{e}^{-(a_0 + \sum_{j=1}^{N} a_j x_j)}} \tag{2}$$

N is the total number of features, while if $F = 0.5$ then the prediction output f_{LR} will be *"unidentified"* meaning that the output can be either 0 or 1. In such cases, the prediction output can be chosen randomly or set by default to one value. By solving the inequality in Equation (1), the initial function can be simplified to:

$$f_{LR} = \begin{cases} 1 & G > 0 \\ \text{"}unidentified\text{"} & G = 0 \\ 0 & G < 0 \end{cases} \tag{3}$$

where G is defined by the following function:

$$G = a_0 + \sum_{j=1}^{N} a_j x_j \tag{4}$$

Let assume a new instance:

$$I_i = \left(x_{i1},\ x_{i2}, \ldots, x_{ij}, \ldots x_{iN}\right)$$

Verifying explanation Condition A. In linear models the absolute values of weights a_j of each feature x_j express the importance factors of its prediction function. A high weight value of a_j for feature x_j indicates that this feature is important because small changes of feature x_j multiplied by a large a_j weight value will highly affect the final output. The important features are chosen by the following formula:

$$Most\ important\ features:\ K = \left\{j:\ \left|a_j\right| > d_{th}\right\} \tag{5}$$

where d_{th} is a defined threshold which defines the minimum feature's importance factor.

Verifying explanation Condition C. For the features k identified as important: $k \in K$, we will compute their critical values in which the prediction result will change. These critical values are defined when the prediction output is in the "*unidentified*" region state. Based on Equations (3) and (4) the critical feature values $xcrit_k$ satisfy the following equation:

$$a_0 + \sum_{j=1}^{k-1} a_j x_{ij} + a_k xcrit_{ik} + \sum_{j=k+1}^{N} a_j x_{ij} = 0,\ \forall\ k\ \in\ K \tag{6}$$

and it turns out that:

$$xcrit_{ik} = -\frac{a_0 + \sum_{j=1}^{k-1} a_j x_{ij} + \sum_{j=k+1}^{N} a_j x_{ij}}{a_k},\quad \forall\ k\ \in\ K \tag{7}$$

Verifying explanation Condition B. If $x_k < xcrit_{ik}$ by Equation (7) it turns out that:

$$a_0 + \sum_{j=1}^{k-1} a_j x_{ij} + a_k x_k + \sum_{j=k+1}^{N} a_j x_{ij} < 0$$

while if $x_k > xcrit_{ik}$ similarly it turns out that:

$$a_0 + \sum_{j=1}^{k-1} a_j x_{ij} + a_k x_k + \sum_{j=k+1}^{N} a_j x_{ij} > 0$$

and thus by Equations (3) and (4) it turns out that:

$$y = \begin{cases} 1, & \forall\ x_k \geq\ xcrit_{ik}\ and\ x_j = x_{ij},\ \forall\ j \neq k \\ 0, & \forall\ x_k < xcrit_{ik}\ and\ x_j = x_{ij},\ \forall\ j \neq k \end{cases} \tag{8}$$

where y is the prediction output. For sake of simplicity we defined by default the prediction output to be 1 for the "*undentifined*" state.

Summarizing, the function described in Equations (3) and (4) represent the global interpretation formula of our prediction model while Equation (8) describes a local interpretation for instances similar to I_i which share the same prediction output, sharing one common explanation rule.

Final Presentation form. We have to find out a comprehensive and understandable form that will merge all information provided by conditions A, B and C while humans will be able by just following some basic rules, to easily obtain all this information. 2 main types of presentation forms are proposed for the explanation output of our prediction model: graph form since they can provide in an intelligible and compact way explanations to humans and a question–answers form since it is probably one of the most common and desirable ways that humans make explanations (Section 2.3.2). We will present it analytically in next section on our application case study scenario.

2.4. Summary of Proposed Framework

In Table 4 are summarized and described in a compact form our total proposed framework's basic steps.

Table 4. Summary of proposed framework.

Step 1. Import images $\left(X_{init}^{M\times H\times W},\ y\right)$, where M is the number of images, H and W are the number of pixels corresponding to the Height and Width of every image.
Step 2. Compute Co-Occurrence, Run-length, Statistical and Contour features and extract new dataset $\left(X_{new}^{M\times N},\ y\right)$, where N is the number of new extracted features.
Step 3. Train White Box Linear model LR with $\left(X^{M\times N},\ y\right)$.
Step 4. Define a weight threshold d_{th} and compute most important features K.
Step 7. For every new instance $X_{new}^{1\times N}$ and every feature $k \in K$ compute its critical values $xcrit_k$.
Step 8. Verify explanation Conditions A, B and C.
Step 9. Select and define the language of the explanation with respect to the targeted audience.
Step 10. Create the Final Presentation explanation output.

3. Results

In this section, we present our experimental results regarding to the proposed explainable prediction framework for image classification tasks, applying it on glioma prediction from MRI as a case study application scenario. In our experiments, all utilized machine learning models (Table 5) were trained using the new data representation which was created via our feature extraction framework and validated using a 10-fold cross-validation using the performance metrics: Accuracy *(Acc)*, F_1-score (F_1), Sensitivity *(sen)*, Specificity *(spe)*, Positive Predictive Value *(PPV)*, Negative Predictive Value *(NPV)* and the Area Under the Curve (*AUC*) [21]. It was considered not essential to conduct experiments based on the initial dataset (raw images) since such experiments were already performed by various CNN models based on transfer learning approach on previous works [22,23] managing to achieve around to 99% accuracy score. It is worth mentioning that since this work proposes an explainable intrinsic prediction model, obviously our goal is not to surpass the performance of these powerful black box models but manage to achieve a decent performance score with powerful explainability.

Table 5. Summary of utilized machine learning models.

WB Model	Basic Parameters	BB Model	Basic Parameters
DT_1	max depth = 3	NN_1	N.L.1 = 64, N.L.2 = 16
DT_2	max depth = 5	NN_2	N.L.1 = 128, N.L.2 = 32
DT_3	max depth = 10	NN_3	N.L.1 = 256, N.L.2 = 64
NB	No parameters	SVM_1	C = 1
LR_1	C = 1	SVM_2	C = 500
LR_2	C = 500	SVM_3	C = 1000
LR_3	C = 1000	*k*-NN	$k = 3$

Our experiments were performed via two phases. In the first phase, various white box (WB) models were compared while in the second phase, the best identified WB model was compared with various black box (BB) models. Table 5 depicts all the utilized machine learning models and their basic tuning parameters. All Decision Trees (DT) models were evaluated based on their max depth parameter. A high depth leads to a complex decision function while a low depth leads to a simple function but probably to biased predictions. The basic version of decision tree algorithm used in our experiments was CART algorithm since it was identified to exhibit superior performance comparing to other decision tree algorithms [24]. On Naive Bayes (NB) [20] classifier, no parameters were specified.

All Neural Networks (NNs) are fully connected networks composed by two hidden layers each and N.L.x refers to the number of Neurons in Layer x. The basic tuning parameter of a Logistic Regression (LR) constitutes the regularization parameter C, just like in Support Vector Machine (SVM) [25], where small values specify stronger regularization. All SVM models were composed by a radial basis function kernel. We have to mention that all these models' parameters were identified via exhaustive and thorough experiments in order to incur the best performance results. Finally, the k-NN [26] was implemented based on the Euclidean distance metric, while the basic tuning parameter is the number of neighbors k.

3.1. Experimental Results

Table 6 presents the performance comparison of WB models regarding the predefined performance metrics. LR_1 exhibited the best classification score (94%) while NB exhibited the worst (77%). Table 7 presents the performance comparison of the best identified WB model (LR_1) comparing to the BB models. LR_1 managed to be as accurate as the best identified BB models (NN_3 and SVM_2). This probably means that our feature extraction framework managed to filter out the noise and the complexity of the initial image representation. As a result, this framework creates a robust and simpler data representation that simple linear models can efficiently be applied on, while powerful BB models like NN are becoming unnecessary.

Table 6. Performance comparison of white box (WB) models.

WB Model	*Acc*	F_1	*sen*	*spe*	*PPV*	*NPV*	*AUC*
DT_1	0.87	0.86	0.83	0.92	0.9	0.86	0.87
DT_2	0.89	0.87	0.86	0.91	0.89	0.88	0.88
DT_3	0.87	0.86	0.86	0.88	0.87	0.88	0.87
NB	0.77	0.74	0.69	0.84	0.79	0.76	0.77
LR_1	**0.94**	**0.93**	**0.94**	**0.94**	**0.93**	**0.95**	**0.94**
LR_2	0.93	**0.93**	0.93	0.93	0.92	0.94	0.93
LR_3	0.93	**0.93**	0.93	0.93	0.92	0.94	0.93

Table 7. Performance comparison of black box (BB)–WB models.

Model	*Acc*	F_1	*sen*	*spe*	*PPV*	*NPV*	*AUC*
NN_1	0.93	0.92	0.92	0.94	0.93	0.93	0.93
NN_2	0.94	0.93	0.92	0.94	0.93	0.94	0.93
NN_3	0.94	0.93	0.92	**0.95**	**0.94**	0.93	0.94
SVM_1	0.92	0.91	0.9	0.93	0.92	0.92	0.92
SVM_2	0.93	0.93	0.92	**0.95**	**0.94**	0.93	0.93
SVM_3	0.93	0.93	0.92	0.94	0.93	0.93	0.93
k-NN	0.89	0.87	0.83	0.94	0.92	0.86	0.88
LR_1	0.94	0.93	**0.94**	0.94	0.93	**0.95**	0.94

3.2. Predictions Explanations

In the sequel, our framework's explanation output is presented for some case study predictions. The final prediction model is the LR_1. Let assume two new instances as presented in Figure 6.

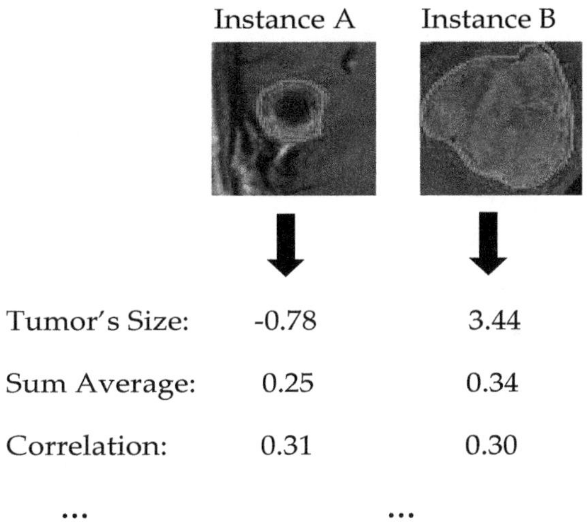

Figure 6. Two case study instances. Instance A is GLIOMA while Instance B is NON GLIOMA.

Two basic language forms are proposed for our model's explanation output, graph diagrams and questions–answers forms as presented in Figures 7 and 8, which were extracted via the formulas described in Section 2.3.4 regarding the predefined conditions A, B and C. The graph diagram provides in a compact, comprehensive and visual form, information which can easily fast extracted by just investigating every node. Each node represents one feature followed by an explanation rule in which a specific prediction output is qualified. The three displayed nodes represent the three most important identified features while the size of each node represents the importance factor of the corresponding feature.

A questions–answers form is probably one of the best ways to provide explanations since this is the main fundamental way that humans make explanations (more details in Section 2.3.2). As already mentioned before, the proper choice of the language is highly depended by the audience. Therefore, we also propose two types of questions–answers forms, Specific and Humanistic form. In specific form, the answers are extracted directly by the graph diagram without any information loss providing all details of graph's information. In humanistic form the answers are extracted via a preprocessing step aiming to simplify the explanation and convert it to a more human like explanation, by approximating the initial model's features to easier understandable abstract features (meta-features) specified by the application domain. For example, in our case the Object size can be converted to Tumor Size, the Sum Average to Tumor's Color (more details for Sum Average feature are presented in Section 2.4). Additionally, every quantitative value has to be converted to qualitative such as Small, Average, Large. For this step is essential the knowledge of a High and Low value of each feature in order to create such qualitative terms.

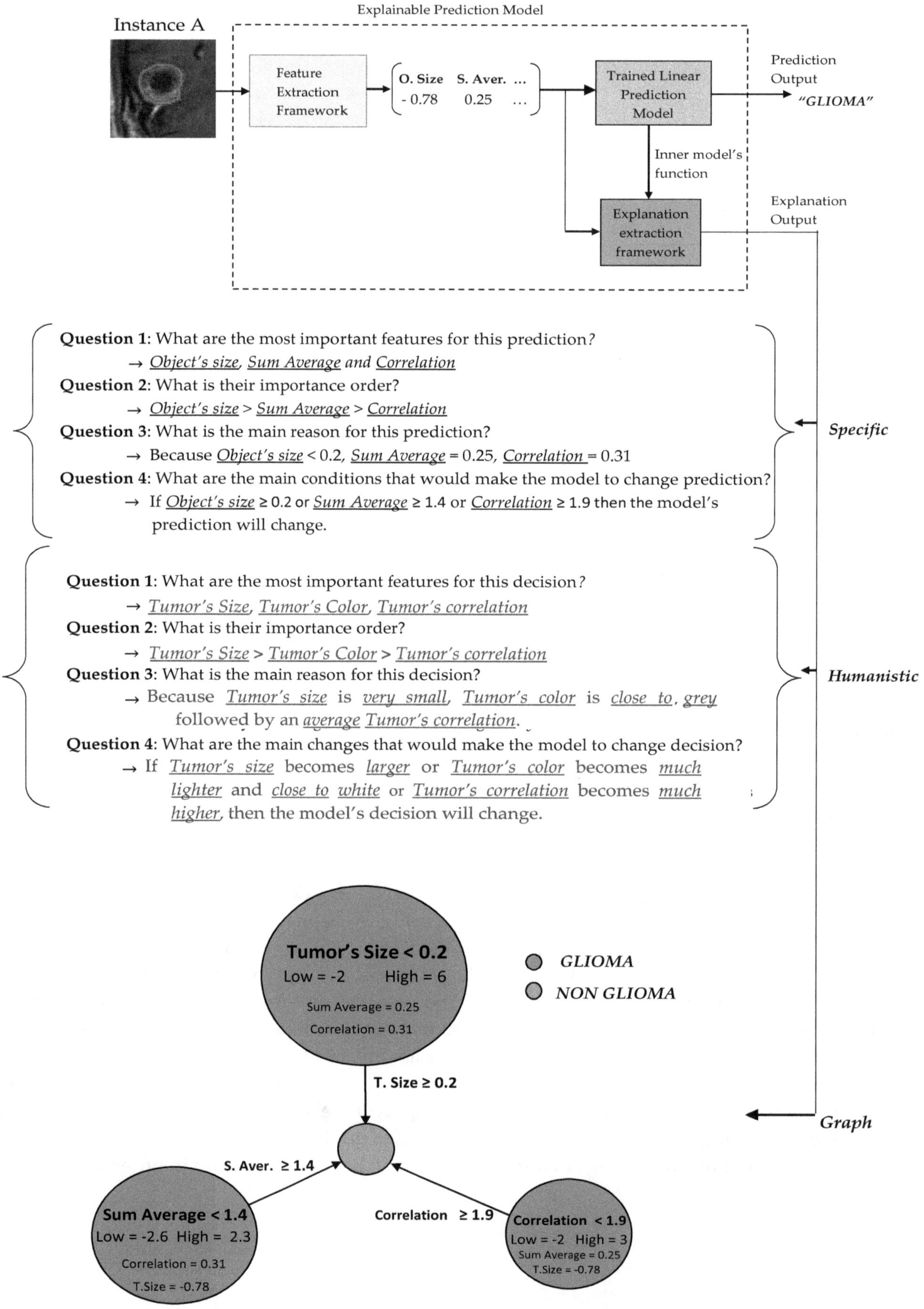

Figure 7. Explanation output for Instance A.

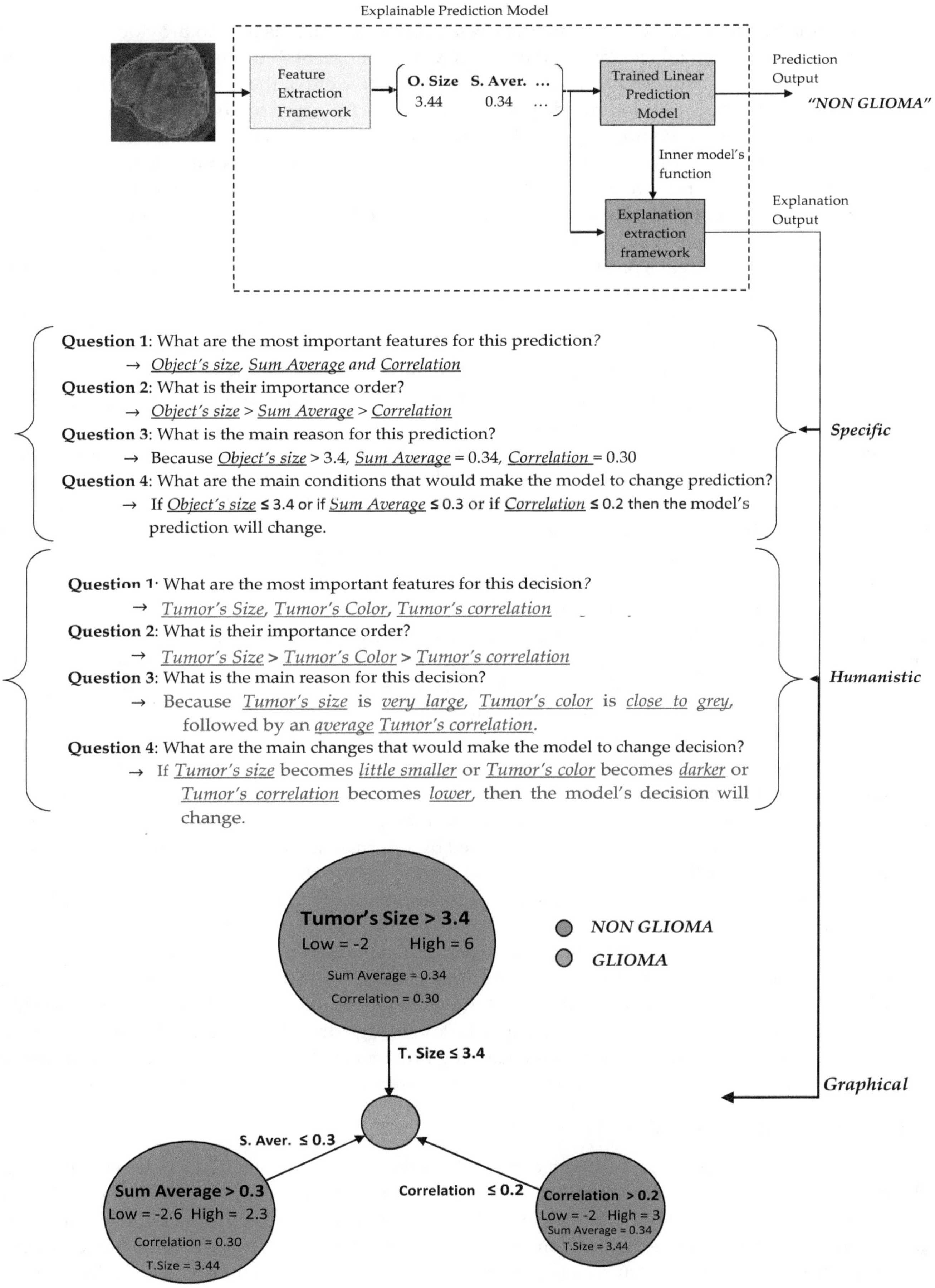

Figure 8. Explanation output for Instance A.

4. Discussion

In this study, a new prediction framework was proposed, which is able to provide accurate and explainable predictions on image classification tasks. Our experimental results indicate that our model is able to achieve a sufficient classification score comparing to state of the art CNN approaches being also intrinsic interpretable able to provide good explanations for every prediction/decision result.

One major difference comparing to other state of the art explanation frameworks for image classification tasks, is that our approach is not performing pixels based explanations. By the term pixels based (or pixel returns) we mean that the explanations are based on the visual interpretation of the most important identified pixels that determined a specific prediction. For example, if a model classified as a cat, an image which presents a cat and a dog, then meaningful pixel base explanation would probably return the cat's pixels revealing that the model classified the image utilizing the proper area of pixels. However, if the task was to recognize an owner's missing cat, then the identification of high level features which uniquely describe this cat would be essential. Such features could be cat's size, cat's color, cat's color irregularity level and cat's number of legs. In such cases, the model's prediction explanation would be useful to rely on such high level features instead of just specific pixels. If the main reason for this prediction was just that this cat has 3 legs and blue color then pixel returns probably could not reveal any useful explanation and reasoning.

As already mentioned our explanation approach is not pixel based but higher level feature based. By this term it is meant that the explanations are performed via a higher level feature representation input, in contrast to raw pixels which are the lowest level input (initial representation). Such high level features can describe the unique properties that groups of pixels possess in every image such as color of an image, color irregularity level, shape irregularity of objects lied in an image, number of objects lied in an image and so on. Obviously, these high-level feature inputs have to be understandable to humans since the model's predictions' explanations would be useless. For example, if a model classified an image as a dog because $x = 5$ without any knowledge about what the feature x means and how was calculated, then such explanation can be considered meaningless. Where instead if it was known that the feature x is the size of an object in an image or the color value of an image and so on, then we would be able to make reasoning about the model's decision and easily understand it.

Nevertheless, creating high level image features being also understandable to humans is a complex task. There is no guarantee that utilizing these features as an input for the machine model would lead to high prediction performance, as probably there are a lot of other hidden unutilized features lied in an image that are probably useful for the specific classification problem. It is hard to identify a priori such features since they are actually found out and crafted by a human sense based approach, while it could make more sense to seek the assistance of an expert with respect to the application domain. In contrast, automatic methods such as CNN models manage to automatically identify useful features in images avoiding this painful human based feature extraction process. However, these features that automatic methods manage to identify are not interpretable and explainable to humans, whereas features crafted by humans can be transparent, meaningful and understandable. This is the trade-off that we need to endure if the objective is the development of interpretable prediction models. Traditional feature extraction approaches, specialized expertise, specific knowledge domain regarding the application and the art of creating useful features for machine learning problems followed by new innovative strategies and techniques can constitute essential key elements in explainable artificial intelligent era.

5. Conclusions and Future Work

In this work, an accurate, robust and explainable prediction framework was proposed for image classification tasks proposing three types of explanations outputs with respect to the audience domain. Comparing to most approaches, our method is intrinsic interpretable providing good explanations relying on high-level feature representation inputs, extracted by images. These features aim to describe the properties that the pixels of an image possess such as its texture irregularity level, object's shape, size, etc. One basic limitation of our approach is that some of these features are probably only understandable by image analysts and specific human experts. However, we made an attempt to qualitatively explain what such features describe in simple human terms in order to make our model's explanation output more attractive and viable to a much wider audience.

Last but not least, in our experiments we utilized all features, even the least significant. We attempted to reduce the number of features in this dataset by analyzing the correlation between the features as well as their significance and by applying some feature selection techniques [27–29]. However, any attempt of removing any features was leading to decrease the overall performance of the prediction model; hence, no feature was removed. We point out the feature selection processing was not in the scope of our work since our main objective was the development and the presentation of an explainable machine learning framework for image classification tasks. Clearly, an interpretable prediction model, exhibiting even better forecasting ability, could be developed through the imposition of sophisticated feature selection techniques as a pre-processing step.

In future work, we aim to incorporate and identify features more understandable to human, being also very informative for the machine learning prediction models. In addition, it is worth investigating whether an interpretable prediction model exhibiting even better forecasting ability could be developed through the imposition of penalty functions together with the application of feature selection techniques or through additional optimized configuration of the proposed model. Finally, we also aim to develop more sophisticated algorithmic methods in order to improve the prediction performance accuracy of intrinsic white box models. Such algorithms could simplify the initial structure complexity and nonlinearity level of the initial dataset, in order to efficiently train simple white box models.

Author Contributions: Conceptualization, E.P.; methodology, E.P., M.L., I.E.L., S.K. and P.P.; validation, E.P., M.L., I.E.L., S.K. and P.P.; formal analysis, E.P., M.L., I.E.L., S.K. and P.P.; investigation, E.P., M.L., I.E.L., S.K. and P.P.; resources, E.P., M.L., I.E.L., S.K. and P.P.; data curation, E.P., M.L., I.E.L., S.K. and P.P.; writing—original draft preparation, E.P., M.L., I.E.L., S.K. and P.P.; writing—review and editing, E.P., M.L., I.E.L., S.K. and P.P.; visualization, E.P., M.L., I.E.L., S.K. and P.P.; supervision, S.K. All authors have read and agreed to the published version of the manuscript.

References

1. Rawat, W.; Wang, Z. Deep convolutional neural networks for image classification: A comprehensive review. *Neural Comput.* **2017**, *29*, 2352–2449. [CrossRef] [PubMed]
2. Arrieta, A.B.; Díaz-Rodríguez, N.; Del Ser, J.; Bennetot, A.; Tabik, S.; Barbado, A.; García, S.; López, S.G.; Molina, D.; Benjamins, R.; et al. Explainable Artificial Intelligence (XAI): Concepts, taxonomies, opportunities and challenges toward responsible AI. *Inf. Fusion* **2020**, *58*, 82–115. [CrossRef]
3. Robnik-Šikonja, M.; Kononenko, I. Explaining classifications for individual instances. *IEEE Trans. Knowl. Data Eng.* **2008**, *20*, 589–600. [CrossRef]
4. Kuhn, M.; Johnson, K. *Applied Predictive Modeling*; Springer: New York, NY, USA, 2013; Volume 26.
5. Edwards, L.; Veale, M. Slave to the Algorithm? Why a 'Right to an Explanation' Is Probably Not the Remedy You Are Looking For. *Duke Law Technol. Rev.* **2017**, *16*, 18.
6. Molnar, C. Interpretable Machine Learning: A Guide for Making Black Box Models Explainable. Available online: https://christophm.github.io/interpretable-ml-book (accessed on 6 June 2018).
7. Pintelas, E.; Livieris, I.E.; Pintelas, P. A Grey-Box Ensemble Model Exploiting Black-Box Accuracy and White-Box Intrinsic Interpretability. *Algorithms* **2020**, *13*, 17. [CrossRef]
8. Ribeiro, M.T.; Singh, S.; Guestrin, C. "Why should I trust you?" Explaining the predictions of any classifier. In Proceedings of the 22nd ACM SIGKDD International Conference on Knowledge Discovery and Data Mining August 2016, San Francisco, CA, USA, 13–17 August 2016; pp. 1135–1144.
9. Robnik-Šikonja, M.; Bohanec, M. Perturbation-based explanations of prediction models. In *Human and Machine Learning*; Springer: Cham, Switzerland, 2018; pp. 159–175.
10. Wachter, S.; Mittelstadt, B.; Russell, C. Counterfactual Explanations without Opening the Black Box: Automated Decisions and the GPDR. *Harv. JL Tech.* **2017**, *31*, 841. [CrossRef]
11. Selvaraju, R.R.; Cogswell, M.; Das, A.; Vedantam, R.; Parikh, D.; Batra, D. Grad-cam: Visual explanations

from deep networks via gradient-based localization. In Proceedings of the IEEE International Conference on Computer Vision 2017, Venice, Italy, 22–29 October 2017; pp. 618–626.

12. Goodenberger, M.L.; Jenkins, R.B. Genetics of adult glioma. *Cancer Genet.* **2012**, *205*, 613–621. [CrossRef] [PubMed]
13. Cheng, J. Brain tumor dataset. Available online: https://figshare.com/articles/brain_tumor_dataset/1512427 (accessed on 2 April 2018).
14. Haralick, R.M.; Shanmugam, K.; Dinstein, H. Texture features for Image Classification. *IEEE Trans. Syst.* **1973**, *SMC-3*, 610–621.
15. Vyas, A.; Yu, S.; Paik, J. Wavelets and Wavelet Transform. In *Multiscale Transforms with Application to Image Processing*; Springer: Singapore City, Singapore, 2018; pp. 45–92.
16. Galloway, M.M. Texture analysis using gray level run lengths. *Comput. Graph. Image Process.* **1975**, *4*, 172–179. [CrossRef]
17. Tang, X. Texture information in Run-Length Matrices. *IEEE Trans. Image Process.* **1998**, *7*, 1602–1609. [CrossRef] [PubMed]
18. Daniel, G. *Principles of Artificial Neural Networks*; World Scientific: Singapore City, Singapore, 2013; Volume 7.
19. Su, J.; Vargas, D.V.; Sakurai, K. One pixel attack for fooling deep neural networks. *IEEE Trans. Evol. Comput.* **2019**, *23*, 828–841. [CrossRef]
20. Ng, A.Y.; Jordan, M.I. On discriminative vs. generative classifiers: A comparison of logistic regression and naive bayes. In *Advances in Neural Information Processing Systems*; MIT Press: Cambridge, MA, USA, 2002; pp. 841–848.
21. Raschka, S. An overview of general performance metrics of binary classifier systems. *arXiv* **2014**, arXiv:1410.5330.
22. Deepak, S.; Ameer, P.M. Brain tumor classification using deep CNN features via transfer learning. *Comput. Biol. Med.* **2019**, *111*, 103345. [CrossRef] [PubMed]
23. Rehman, A.; Naz, S.; Razzak, M.I.; Akram, F.; Imran, M. A deep learning-based framework for automatic brain tumors classification using transfer learning. *Circuits Syst. Signal Process.* **2020**, *39*, 757–775. [CrossRef]
24. Priyam, A.; Abhijeeta, G.R.; Rathee, A.; Srivastava, S. Comparative analysis of decision tree classification algorithms. *Int. J. Curr. Eng. Technol.* **2013**, *3*, 334–337.
25. Deng, N.; Tian, Y.; Zhang, C. *Support Vector Machines: Optimization Based Theory, Algorithms, and Extensions*; Chapman and Hall/CRC: Boca Raton, FL, USA, 2012.
26. Aha, D.W. (Ed.) *Lazy Learning*; Springer Science & Business Media: Berlin, Germany, 2013.
27. Benesty, J.; Chen, J.; Huang, Y.; Cohen, I. Pearson correlation coefficient. In *Noise Reduction in Speech Processing*; Springer: Berlin/Heidelberg, Germany, 2009; pp. 1–4.
28. Hall, M.A. Correlation-based Feature Subset Selection for Machine Learning. Ph.D. Thesis, University of Waikato, Hamilton, New Zealand, 1998.
29. Kira, K.; Larry, A. Rendell: A Practical Approach to Feature Selection. In *Ninth International Workshop on Machine Learning*; Morgan Kaufmann: Burlington, MA, USA, 1992; pp. 249–256.

Permissions

All chapters in this book were first published by MDPI; hereby published with permission under the Creative Commons Attribution License or equivalent. Every chapter published in this book has been scrutinized by our experts. Their significance has been extensively debated. The topics covered herein carry significant findings which will fuel the growth of the discipline. They may even be implemented as practical applications or may be referred to as a beginning point for another development.

The contributors of this book come from diverse backgrounds, making this book a truly international effort. This book will bring forth new frontiers with its revolutionizing research information and detailed analysis of the nascent developments around the world.

We would like to thank all the contributing authors for lending their expertise to make the book truly unique. They have played a crucial role in the development of this book. Without their invaluable contributions this book wouldn't have been possible. They have made vital efforts to compile up to date information on the varied aspects of this subject to make this book a valuable addition to the collection of many professionals and students.

This book was conceptualized with the vision of imparting up-to-date information and advanced data in this field. To ensure the same, a matchless editorial board was set up. Every individual on the board went through rigorous rounds of assessment to prove their worth. After which they invested a large part of their time researching and compiling the most relevant data for our readers.

The editorial board has been involved in producing this book since its inception. They have spent rigorous hours researching and exploring the diverse topics which have resulted in the successful publishing of this book. They have passed on their knowledge of decades through this book. To expedite this challenging task, the publisher supported the team at every step. A small team of assistant editors was also appointed to further simplify the editing procedure and attain best results for the readers.

Apart from the editorial board, the designing team has also invested a significant amount of their time in understanding the subject and creating the most relevant covers. They scrutinized every image to scout for the most suitable representation of the subject and create an appropriate cover for the book.

The publishing team has been an ardent support to the editorial, designing and production team. Their endless efforts to recruit the best for this project, has resulted in the accomplishment of this book. They are a veteran in the field of academics and their pool of knowledge is as vast as their experience in printing. Their expertise and guidance has proved useful at every step. Their uncompromising quality standards have made this book an exceptional effort. Their encouragement from time to time has been an inspiration for everyone.

The publisher and the editorial board hope that this book will prove to be a valuable piece of knowledge for researchers, students, practitioners and scholars across the globe.

List of Contributors

Yi Guan, Chia-Hsin Cheng, Weifan Chen, Yingqi Zhang, Sophia Koo, Maxine Krengel, Rosemary Toomey and Bang-Bon Koo
School of Medicine, Boston University, Boston, MA 02118, USA

Patricia Janulewicz and Kimberly Sullivan
School of Public Health, Boston University, Boston, MA 02118, USA

Ehwa Yang and Jae-Hun Kim
Department of Radiology, Samsung Medical Center, Sungkyunkwan University School of Medicine, Seoul 06351, Korea

Rafeeque Bhadelia
Department of Radiology, Beth Israel Deaconess Medical Center, Harvard Medical School, Boston, MA 02115, USA

Lea Steele
Neuropsychiatry Division, Department of Psychiatry and Behavioral Sciences, Baylor College of Medicine, Houston, TX 77030, USA

Naira Elazab, Hassan Soliman and Mohammed Elmogy
Information Technology Department, Faculty of Computers and Information, Mansoura University, Mansoura 35516, Egypt

Shaker El-Sappagh
Centro Singular de Investigación en Tecnoloxías Intelixentes (CiTIUS), Universidade de Santiago de Compostela, 15705 Santiago de Compostela, Spain
Information Systems Department, Faculty of Computers and Artificial Intelligence, Benha University, Benha 13512, Egypt

S. M. Riazul Islam
Department of Computer Science and Engineering, Sejong University, Seoul 05006, Korea

Lucia Billeci, Lorenzo Bachi and Alessandro Tonacci
Institute of Clinical Physiology-National Research Council of Italy (IFC-CNR), Via Moruzzi, 1, 56124 Pisa, Italy

Asia Badolato
School of Engineering, University of Pisa, Largo Lucio Lazzarino, 1, 56122 Pisa, Italy

Guillaume Dupont, Ekaterina Kalinicheva and Florence Rossant
ISEP, DaSSIP Team, 92130 Issy-Les-Moulineaux, France

Jérémie Sublime
ISEP, DaSSIP Team, 92130 Issy-Les-Moulineaux, France
Université Paris 13, LIPN - CNRS UMR 7030, 93430 Villetaneuse, France

Michel Pâques
Clinical Imaging Center 1423, Quinze-Vingts Hospital, INSERM-DGOS Clinical Investigation Center, 75012 Paris, France

Amitojdeep Singh, Sourya Sengupta and Vasudevan Lakshminarayanan
Theoretical and Experimental Epistemology Laboratory, School of Optometry and Vision Science, University of Waterloo, Waterloo, ON N2L 3G1, Canada
Department of Systems Design Engineering, University of Waterloo, Waterloo, ON N2L 3G1, Canada

Subrata Bhattacharjee, Deekshitha Prakash, Hyeon-Gyun Park and Heung-Kook Choi
Department of Computer Engineering, u-AHRC, Inje University, Gimhae 50834, Korea

Cho-Hee Kim
Department of Digital Anti-Aging Healthcare, Inje University, Gimhae 50834, Korea

Nam-Hoon Cho
Department of Pathology, Yonsei University Hospital, Seoul 03722, Korea

Mauricio Alberto Ortega-Ruiz
Universidad del Valle de México, Departamento de Ingeniería, Campus Coyoacán, Ciudad de México 04910, Mexico
Department of Electrical & Electronic Engineering, School of Mathematics, Computer Science and Engineering, City, University of London, London EC1V 0HB, UK

Cefa Karabağ
Department of Electrical & Electronic Engineering, School of Mathematics, Computer Science and Engineering, City, University of London, London EC1V 0HB, UK

Victor García Garduño
Departamento de Ingeniería en Telecomunicaciones, Facultad de Ingeniería, Universidad Nacional Autónoma de México, Av. Universidad 3000, Ciudad Universitaria, Coyoacán, Ciudad de México 04510, Mexico

Constantino Carlos Reyes-Aldasoro
giCentre, Department of Computer Science, School of Mathematics, Computer Science and Engineering, City, University of London, London EC1V 0HB, UK

Stefanus Tao Hwa Kieu and Abdullah Bade
Faculty of Science and Natural Resources, Universiti Malaysia Sabah, Kota Kinabalu 88400, Sabah, Malaysia

Mohd Hanafi Ahmad Hijazi
Faculty of Computing and Informatics, Universiti Malaysia Sabah, Kota Kinabalu 88400, Sabah, Malaysia

Hoshang Kolivand
School of Computer Science and Mathematics, Liverpool John Moores University, Liverpool L3 3AF, UK

Mizuho Nishio and Shunjiro Noguchi
Department of Diagnostic Imaging and Nuclear Medicine, Kyoto University Graduate School of Medicine, 54 Kawahara-cho, Shogoin, Sakyo-ku, Kyoto 606-8507, Japan

Koji Fujimoto
Human Brain Research Center, Kyoto University Graduate School of Medicine, 54 Kawahara-cho, Shogoin, Sakyo-ku, Kyoto 606-8507, Japan
Vahab Khoshdel, Mohammad Asefi, Ahmed Ashraf and Joe LoVetri
Department of Electrical and Computer Engineering, University of Manitoba, Winnipeg, MB R3T 5V6, Canada

Emmanuel Pintelas, Ioannis E. Livieris, Sotiris Kotsiantis and Panagiotis Pintelas
Department of Mathematics, University of Patras, GR 265-00 Patras, Greece

Meletis Liaskos
Department of Biomedical Engineering, University ofWest Attica, GR 122-43 Egaleo Athens, Greece

Index